The Impossible Return – Psychoanalytic Reflections on Breast Cancer, Loss, and Mourning

Anna Fishzon

Routledge
Taylor & Francis Group

LONDON AND NEW YORK

Designed cover image: "Cataclysm: Falling Figure" 18 × 60 oil on canvas 2021 @ Patrick Webb

First published 2026
by Routledge
4 Park Square, Milton Park, Abingdon, Oxon OX14 4RN

and by Routledge
605 Third Avenue, New York, NY 10158

Routledge is an imprint of the Taylor & Francis Group, an informa business

British Library Cataloguing-in-Publication Data
A catalogue record for this book is available from the British Library

ISBN: 978-1-032-81194-9 (hbk)
ISBN: 978-1-032-81195-6 (pbk)
ISBN: 978-1-003-49858-2 (ebk)

DOI: 10.4324/9781003498582

Typeset in Times New Roman
by codeMantra

"In this remarkable and vibrant book, Anna Fishzon has created a unique tapestry of cultural history, psychoanalysis, and her own journey through illness. Beautifully written, it is disturbing, funny, painful, and enlightening, offering important insights into not just the practice and theory of psychoanalysis but the intimate experience of illness and the body. This is a work of real generosity that deserves a wide readership."

Darian Leader, *psychoanalyst, Centre for Freudian Analysis and Research, UK*

"Does the psychoanalyst have a body? With courage and exquisite flair Anna Fishzon takes this question head-on through her lived experience of cancer, showing how the navigation of sickness, loss, and the reality of dying gives us the knot of *all* psychic transformations. Yes, the analyst has a body, one that is called upon to be irrepressibly alive until lost. I learned that there is no other way to understand psychoanalysis than in the experience of a body's breakdown and survival."

Jamieson Webster, *author of* On Breathing

"In *The Impossible Return*, Fishzon takes her personal experience as a breast cancer survivor and powerfully weaves and connects threads as diverse as psychoanalytic theory and clinic, opera, queer temporality, Chernobyl, philosophy, childhood in the Soviet Union/Ukraine, literature, and film, to name just a few. Crafting a book that not only works so stunningly well across such varied registers but also makes a truly remarkable contribution to all of these fields amounts to nothing short of achieving the impossible."

Alenka Zupančič, *author of* What Is Sex?

"By rights, *The Impossible Return* should be an impossible book: a cancer memoir unlike any other, it deftly combines the author's thoughts on the female body, Soviet animation, the Chernobyl disaster, and queer culture, not to mention Lacanian psychoanalysis. Her beautiful prose makes it all look effortless, weaving together all these topics in a thoroughly engaging manner. Fishzon eschews self-help in favor of self-analysis, but it is her readers who will reap the benefits."

Eliot Borenstein, *New York University, USA*

"Psychoanalyst and historian Anna Fishzon has produced a beautifully written, courageous, and utterly compelling book. Using psychoanalysis to reflect on opera, Soviet children's cartoons, the Chernobyl nuclear disaster, and much, much more, Fishzon moves gracefully between the theoretical and the concrete. Lending the book intensity and urgency is the fact that it is animated by the author's experience of breast cancer surgery. The book can be described as a literary free association engaging the cultural and the clinical, the historical and the psychoanalytic, all lent vital coherence through their relation to the body of the analyst-author."

Thomas Kohut, *Professor of History, Emeritus, Williams College, and President of the Freud Foundation U.S., USA*

The Impossible Return – Psychoanalytic Reflections on Breast Cancer, Loss, and Mourning

The Impossible Return – Psychoanalytic Reflections on Breast Cancer, Loss, and Mourning is a work of creative nonfiction and autotheory. It is part cancer memoir, part psychoanalytic theorizing, and part history of late Soviet Ukraine.

Anna Fishzon's personal narrative is interspersed with interludes exploring other "reconstructions" (Chernobyl's sarcophagus, the perestroika years) as well as psychoanalytic reflections on anxiety, prosthesis, hypochondria, and tattooing. The authorial voice is intentionally polyphonic: elegiac, humorous, at times academic and philosophical. Each chapter is set in the context of the writing process, with discussion of the COVID-19 pandemic and war in Ukraine. The prologue examines the psychoanalyst's bodily presence in treatment and includes clinical vignettes that discuss the impact of remote therapy sessions during lockdown, and an epilogue provides a meditation on repetition compulsion and the impossibility of mourning fully.

Through theoretical and personal reflections on mourning and recovery after catastrophic collapses of psyche, body, and place, this book makes original contributions to psychoanalysis, Slavic and cultural studies, trauma studies, film criticism, and history. This unique work will be relevant to readers interested in psychoanalytic studies, cancer and disability studies and critical theory, and academics of autotheory and memoir.

Anna Fishzon is a psychoanalyst in private practice in New York City. She is the author and coeditor of two previous books.

For Dorian

Contents

Preface

I first conceived this book as a love letter to women living with the ravages of breast cancer: mastectomy, reconstruction, unfulfilled promises, pink-tinted shame, disappointments, and hard-won celebrations. I wished to help myself and others grapple with embodiment, to make nonsense of the too-coherent and medicalized, to ponder how one might do the impossible, to mourn a body, and to come to terms with the mirror: aesthetic concerns, imperatives to beautify, certainly, as well as the longing for self-recognition after corporeal loss. I sought to understand how one might transform traumatic rupture into *prosthesis* as both appendage and subtraction, the traversal of animate and inanimate.

Soon after I began writing, I noticed I was prone to narrative digressions. An analysand and analyst, I heed the call to say whatever comes to mind, postponing sense-making until the end of the analytic hour, or the analytic week, or years after the termination of an analysis. And because I am also a former academic historian and Soviet refugee, I am preoccupied with time and its collapse. The loss of my breast and the telling of that story sparked meditations on other losses, recapitulations of other impossible mournings, failures in making things right. Accommodating a silicone implant, a numb extension of the flesh, evoked mute and generative aspects of various unfinished projects: Letting go of my breast became a goodbye to the Soviet Union—a no-longer extant place—and an elegy for my academic career. The subject of psychoanalysis is defined by creativity that springs from overwhelming grief. And, so, a study of the cuts surgery makes in memory led to an exploration of the ways the body archives other sorts of cuts—violence to one's childhood, to one's mind, to one's entire life.

In weaving together several leitmotifs, in allowing them to join, separate, and produce echoes and variations, *The Impossible Return* declares its loyalty to my two great loves: opera and psychoanalysis. In the psychoanalytic hour and in the many years that often constitute an analysis, themes that emerge at the start repeat and develop over time, intertwining and diverging as they are worked through. In opera, too, motifs might be introduced, abandoned, and reach full-throated effect only in the final act. There is a recursive movement by which early notes, words, passages, and half-sayings acquire sense. If my readers can sustain patience and attention, they will recognize that this book finally arrives at deferred meanings.

And yet, inevitably, as in both analysis and opera, some scenes and musical strands escape the recapitulating impulse, remaining enigmatic, solitary, or stubbornly insistent.

The Impossible Return is an experiment that aims to bridge critical writing, academic discourse, and the deeply personal. While it is informed by the conventions of autotheory and other types of autobiography, the present book draws inspiration from Jean-Luc Nancy's *Corpus*, its equal commitments to lyricism and philosophical rigor; from the passionate statements of the Soviet bard Vladimir Vysotsky; and from the philosophical flourishes of David Wills's *Prosthesis*, a work that explodes many literary sensibilities, every generic expectation, and makes no compromises in its theoretical aims. Intentionally out of tune, broken, and possessed, Nancy, Vysotsky, and Wills convey their devotion to language and characterization.

The Impossible Return owes much to the pioneering work of poet Wayne Koestenbaum, intersecting with its pathologies and concerns, its willingness to wax operatic, extravagant, and slightly embarrassing. My book ultimately seeks its own trespass, its own particular emancipation from convention, its own psychoanalytic reflections on survival, prosthesis, and mourning. The detours it takes through Brezhnev-era animation, the Chernobyl nuclear disaster, and opera may seem indulgent—and they probably are. But these sections, independently and in concert, offer arguments about the very concepts of reconstruction, repetition, haunting, and cure. They feature perestroika and the phenomenology of "late socialism," the object-voice as silence, the circular drive accompanying change.

It is my hope that the turbulences and provocations of *The Impossible Return*—the manner in which it intervenes in and disturbs genres and disciplinary knowledges—will contribute to the recovery of feeling and self in the breach of illness and to new ways of thinking impasse itself.

Acknowledgments

This book began as an unconventional cancer memoir and a work of autotheory. My previous writings had been narrowly academic, and I doubted whether I was capable of blending intensely private experiences with scholarly work. In those tentative, early stages of the manuscript, I relied on the spirited encouragement and critical acumen of my first-ever psychoanalytic writing group, led by Jill Gentile: Barbara Kane, Ryan Kull, Paul Sireci, Fredrika Stjarne, Francia White, and Kirsten Wittenborn. Later I was helped tremendously by other writing groups, which included Azeen Khan, Victoria Malkin, Sam Semper, Orna Shachar, Tracey Simon, and Fredrika Stjarne. Each of these talented analyst-writers in her own way stoked enthusiasm for the project, keeping it alive when the pandemic and a growing private practice competed for time and attention.

Sam Semper has been a stimulating interlocutor and guide from the earliest days of analytic training. Fredrika Stjarne, present in all manner of writing, reading, and study groups, has seen me through several crises of belief and will, and remains an unflagging friend, gracious colleague, and motivating force.

My deepest gratitude to Ian Beilin for reading every word and for suffering the seemingly eternal, coffee-fueled morning writing marathons that brought this book to completion. And to Yarden Avital for poring over the manuscript and for her invaluable friendship. It was only when Ian and Yarden finished reading a chapter that I felt I could move on to the next.

Big thanks to Carla Levy and Kabir Dandona for commenting on chapters and keeping faith in my writing. To Igal Halfin for reading all of it and for decades of stalwart friendship and intellectual exchange. Juliane Fürst and Anna Paretskaya read, edited, and advised, holding me during critical moments of the book's development. Kathryn Kuitenbrouwer carefully edited the manuscript and provided constructive feedback. My editor at Routledge, Susannah Frearson, exhibited consummate patience and clarity during the manuscript submission process.

I extend much gratitude to dear friends and colleagues, family, chosen family, and all those who fortified me through cancer, and through the final round of editing: Eric Barry, Nick Boston, Jon Carnero, Georgia Ede, Kate Glazer, Gayle Goren, Ranjana Khanna, Tom Kohut, Natasha Kurchanova, Emma Lieber, Tracy Morgan,

Chris Nelson, Olga Poznansky, Richard Rhorer, Monroe Street, Aleksandra Wagner, Mary Yordy, and the ever-brilliant Julia Zarankin.

My comrades at the Institute for Psychoanalytic Training and Research were a vital part of my analytic formation. This book has benefited from their wisdom and clinical insights, offered over many years: Masha Mimran, Eric Shorey, Raluca Modica, Nadia Bassino, Aneta Stojnić, Lee Share, Alex Cyr, Polina Mariani, Ludovica Lumer, Gila Ashtor, Alexandra Petrou, and Diana Wolkind.

Thanks to supervisor-teachers, erstwhile supervisors-now-friends, fellow participants of reading groups, and members of the Après-Coup Psychoanalytic Association, all of whom taught me much about psychoanalysis and shaped this book: first and most, Alan Bass, Eliana Betancourt, Lillian Ferrari, Bruce Fink, Paul Geltner, Patricia Gherovici, Brian Kloppenberg, David Lichtenstein, Ellen Marakowitz, Paola Mieli, Donald Moss, Jamieson Webster, and Yukari Yanagino. And to those no longer here to accept my acknowledgments: Sheldon Bach, Elliot Kronish, and Jared Russell.

I am grateful to the spouses and partners of close friends who also became friends and endured many conversations about the book and its difficulties: Assi Dadon, Suzi Smith, Ron Weinstock, and Boris Ingberg. Special thanks to Patrick Webb for opera companionship and for contributing the cover art.

I carry with me the voices of IPTAR teachers and advisors who shepherded my full immersion in psychoanalysis: Eva Atsalis, Nancy Einbinder, Carolyn Ellman, Steven Ellman, Susan Finkelstein, Joan Hoffenberg, Judy Ann Kaplan, Laura Kleinerman, Naama Kushner-Barash, Janice Lieberman, Bruce Reis, Carla Rentrop, Aaron Thaler, and Neal Vorus.

My supervisor and mentor Richard Lasky died before I finished this book. I wish he could have read it; perhaps he would have heard its music. Richie always approached my theoretical papers and case reports with heartfelt curiosity and openness. His warmth, generosity, and rigor helped me become an analyst who writes.

I am grateful for the good humor and tolerance of my son Dorian, to whom this book is dedicated. His love of writing and research inspires me every day. And to the Fishzon, Beilin, Nastashkin, Vizelberg, and Zarankin families, especially my parents, Polina and Sam, for emotional sustenance.

I continually learn from my analysands, supervisees, student-colleagues, and colleagues affected by breast cancer. Their courage and devotion to analytic work are in my reverie as I elaborate the themes of this book.

This project would not have been conceived without Arnold Wilson. I thank him for reading the manuscript, for enabling me to question why it is I write, for the gift of his silence—and for analysis, which permeates every page.

Short sections from Chapters 1, 4, and 12 appeared in my first book, *Fandom, Authenticity, and Opera: Mad Acts and Letter Scenes in Fin-de-Siècle Russia* (Palgrave Macmillan, 2013). Sections of Chapter 8 appeared in "The Place Where We [Want to] Live: East–West and Other Transitional Phenomena in Vladimir Vysotskii's *Alisa v strane chudes*," in *Russian Literature* (2018), *96–98*, 167–193;

reprinted with permission of Elsevier. Earlier versions of sections in Chapters 8, 10, and 13 were included in "The Fog of Stagnation: Explorations of Time and Affect in Late Soviet Animation," in *Cahiers du monde russe* (2015), *56*(2–3), 571–598, and are reprinted with permission of the publisher. Sections of Chapter 8 were included in "Introduction: The Queer Child and the Childish Queer," in A. Fishzon & E. Lieber (Eds.), *The Queerness of Childhood: Essays From the Other Side of the Looking Glass* (Palgrave Macmillan, 2022), pp. 1–13, and are reprinted with the kind permission of my coauthor Emma Lieber. Earlier versions of sections in Chapters 1, 4, 9, and 12 appeared in my chapter, "Queue Time, Animation, and the Queer Childhood of Late Socialism," in *The Queerness of Childhood*, pp. 239–266, and are reproduced with the kind permission of the volume's coeditor, Emma Lieber. Sections of the Epilogue appeared in my review of the book *Sound, Speech, Music in Soviet and Post-Soviet Cinema*, by L. Kaganovsky & M. Salazkina (Eds.), in *Laboratorium: Russian Review of Social Research* (2017), *8*(3), 146–150, reprinted with the journal's permission. Revised portions of Chapters 5, 9, and 13 appeared in "The Queer Legacies of Late Socialism, or What Cheburashka and Gary Shteyngart Have in Common," in Olga Voronina (Ed.), *A Companion to Soviet Children's Literature and Film* (Brill, 2019), pp. 440–473, and reprinted here with permission of the publisher. Extensive quotations from the film *Chernobyl's Heritage: The Zone* (2011) appear in Chapter 6 with the kind permission of directors Anton Bendarjevskiy and Márk Maczelka. Quotations from Audre Lorde's *The Cancer Journals* are reprinted in Chapter 7 with the permission of Abner Stein. Finally, I thank Margarit Ordukhanyan for permission to use her translations of Azazello's poetry and manifesto and the Wende Museum for permission to cite from the Azazello (Anatolyi Kalabin) Collection.

Most transliterations in this book conform to the Library of Congress style. Exceptions are made in the cases of a few names with well-known English variants: for example, Modest Mussorgsky, Petr Tchaikovsky, and Vladimir Vysotsky. I also retain the original spelling in quoted material and when referring to works in lists of references. Most transliterated Russian titles at their first appearance are followed by common English translations in parentheses. Unless otherwise indicated, all translations from Russian are mine.

Prologue

The Body of the Analyst

For over a decade I attended conferences and panels on the psychoanalyst's body only to hear instead papers about the bodies of patients, bodies generally, body odors, eating disorders, feminine sexuality, and terminal illness. Anything is more palatable—more discussable—it seems, than the body of the analyst. This is not entirely surprising. The analyst's body is both a scandal and a silent agency, crucial to the psychoanalytic setting. It is the incarnation of the drive, an expression of libidinal tension; and it is also unspeakable, evacuated of meaning, a vehicle of transference.

I was diagnosed with breast cancer in September 2017. In February 2019, after I'd been declared cured and had begun this book, I knew that if I was going to risk writing, and having my patients read, about my broken body, I would have to address the role of the analyst's Real body in the consulting room; not the frequently discussed analyst's reality or "real presence" (Kirshner, 2018) but, rather, my body as a repository of the drives, a placeholder for my analysands' unconscious wishes and not-yet-imagined causalities. In writing about cancer and mastectomy, would I irrevocably damage my analytic function, inhibit my ability to act as a container of projected fantasies? And then, implausible events took discussions of the analyst's body in startling directions.

In March 2020, when New York, my home city, emerged as COVID ground zero of the United States, many analysts took flight, abandoning their offices. Their bodies went to Shelter Island, Upstate New York, Florida, and other bucolic oases. Those less established retreated to their Brooklyn studio apartments, holding phone sessions from bathrooms. What choice did they have? After the initial shock, a flood of online professional meetings provided platforms to discuss the absence of bodies, our own and those of our patients. Analysts spoke of hitherto unknown exhaustion after days of phone, Zoom, and Skype sessions. Some wondered about the effects of remote treatment on "the transference": Was the virtual consulting room a space hospitable to the recrudescence of infantile desires? Others shared confusion and irritation about the near dissolution of the classical psychoanalytic frame. I will offer a few examples from my practice. Sessions punctuated by the slurping of cereal, coffee, and Red Bull; the filing of fingernails and an occasional full manicure masterfully executed while free associating; distracted scanning of

DOI: 10.4324/9781003498582-1

news headlines during interpretations, and, inevitably, bodies in various states of half-dress, in pajamas and under bed sheets. In analysts' early online exchanges, frank concern about patients' free-fall regression and unkempt appearance followed confessions of conducting Zoom sessions without pants.

A few months into the pandemic, another shift in the discourse took place—a more self-affirming position arose—an attempt to recuperate or redeem, if not deny, the loss. Perhaps we, creative analyst-heroes on the front lines, had not lost as much as we'd initially believed. Swift adaptations had been made. Online there was still transference, and there was still a frame, different but undeniable. We retained important analytic instruments: our voices and ears, and on Zoom, our eyes. Indeed, the lack of physical presence was deeply paradoxical, introducing a troubling *over*proximity. Analyst and analysand now peered into each other's homes, and some Zoomed from childhood bedrooms; intrusive disembodied voices and new sounds echoed in our headsets. Patients listened to my child throw a tantrum in an adjacent room. My analyst's dog could not be muted (though the phone sometimes was). We heard and saw too much: a too-stimulating maternal symbiosis posed novel dangers to the analytic frame (Perelberg, 2021).

When psychoanalysis confronted the pandemic, it yielded instantly its core principles and doxa: two bodies in a room as constitutive of treatment, the privileging of suspense and risk over neurotic safety and the urge to cure. Many analysts focused on "staying safe," choosing to plug up or turn away from the hole the virus had torn in our reality. But Sigmund Freud's oft-repeated (likely apocryphal) declaration on his way to America, "they don't realize we are bringing them the plague," yoked psychoanalysis to viral illness (Rousselle, 2020). The gradual return to offices and in-person work prompted more reflection on what we had lost in the intervening remote sessions. As many continue to work remotely, questions of "presence" acquire new relevance. What is the function of the analyst's Real body in the transference and in the frame, and what, precisely, is the risk involved in having two bodies in a room?

In calling attention to the Real of the analyst's body, I am referencing Jacques Lacan's notion of the Real, the inassimilable, inarticulable aspect of being, the sheer thingness of the material and biological that cannot fully be grasped by the speaking subject. I am also alluding to Lacan's understanding of the analyst as the *objet petit a* for the analysand: the beyond of the pleasure principle, the aphonic remainder of speech that elicits the subject's desire and evokes the drive, the libidinal excess or painful satisfaction (jouissance) the subject derives from her symptoms.

The analyst's body, as object *a*, ought to be a corporeal representation of primal repression, the lost object that resists symbolization. Psychoanalysts Dries Dulsster and Stijn Vanheule (2019) instruct, citing fellow Lacanian Eric Laurent:

> The analyst must "mount the stage." … The analyst should be able to incarnate a presence, sometimes very active, sometimes absent, sometimes discrete, depending on the case. According to Laurent (1992) this is the dimension of "knowing-how-to-act" … in clinical work. One should explore what kind of drive-related object one is for the analysand, and actively work with this

dimension. The analyst should be present in the analytic work, but his actions should be emptied of private *jouissance*.

(p. 64)

I would augment Laurent's formulation: The analyst's Real body always has the potential to become obscene, evidencing something of her personal jouissance. The sneeze behind the couch, a scratch of the head, the rustle of trousers, a deep sigh or suppressed yawn could arrest or enrage the analysand, inhibiting or inciting speech. Even such incidental manifestations of jouissance invite transference and propel the analysis.

She enters, double-masked, with a full cup of coffee she could not drink anyway. It is her first session in the office since lockdown—not "our" old office, but a new space I'd leased only weeks before. With her back to me, she drapes her coat on an armchair at the other end of the room, poised to place her coffee on a side table, within reach. Then it happens. The cup flies out of her hand and through the air in slow motion, coffee splattering promiscuously on the desk, the couch, my laptop, and the bookcase, before finally making its descent and alighting as a huge Rorschach stain on my recently purchased beige rug. We both stand frozen for a few seconds. Alarmed, she raises her arms and clasps her head, emitting a choked cry. Tears streaming down her cheeks, she offers to clean up and runs to the bathroom for some paper towels. Devastated but composed, I reassure her: "I have a good spot remover."

"It's like a fairy tale in here," she later declares as she stretches out on the couch, peering at the big window facing a garden. I am behind her, sharing the view. She talks without pause for over 30 minutes. At the conclusion of the session, she is eager to tear off the mask: "I cannot stand this anymore! I cry and it sticks to my face! I feel better at home, without it! Here I'm muzzled and then asked to talk. I am so anxious! Maybe we should go back to remote sessions where I am comfortable and safe in my bed. The mask feels like a barrier ..."

Lacanian psychoanalysis asserts that one's sense of self (and specular unity as such) is created through an internalized understanding of oneself as an object (*I have*, rather than *I am*, a body), a framing or delimitation of one's perspective. The subject of the unconscious depends, in other words, on exclusion, difference, and self-distanciation. Fundamentally split, subjects view themselves from a gaze located elsewhere, a gaze supported by the social world and by language, which in turn lend validation and coherence to identity and self-possession. And since human beings are also subjected to the demands of culturally informed bodily urges called drives—repetitive, dumb, and insistent on satisfaction—their self-images and symbolic identifications are marked by uneasiness, continually threatened by irruptions of scandalous enjoyment, or jouissance. I repress my own gaze, the inside of my body; I cede the Real in order to acquire surface, a reality. The lost object and its drive elements, objects *a*, can be encountered by the subject in ephemeral traces, returned in the Other's gaze (as opposed to the eye) and the voice (as opposed to speech). In taking myself as the subject I become an object in fantasy, that is, in *my* frame of reality. This procedure is primary repression, a fissure in myself that I do not wish to know.

Just as the analyst's embodiment of the drive—the use of her gaze, her voice, her silence—has repressive effects that enables analysis, it also jeopardizes framed reality. The analysand might for an instant identify with object *a* (that is, merge with the picture, be inside), and this prospect provokes acute anxiety. Self-distance momentarily shrinks, and the subjective viewpoint collapses. Such a situation cannot be realized on Zoom because the analysand sees his two-dimensional analyst within the frame, in the picture, while he remains safely outside and in control. He feels secure, perhaps very close to the analyst, entombed in a portable device. There are many therapeutic effects and formations of the unconscious; but is there analysis?

The analytic encounter is analytic due to the risk of two bodies in shared space. This risk, to be sure, is generated by the possibility of a body jumping out of the chair and striking the other, and by tension arising from the physical proximity of two people who could have sex but choose not to. But the biggest, most essential risk is in becoming object *a*, incarnated by the analyst: in merging with one's own scene, with potentiality as such. This is the risk that allows the analysand fleetingly to experience his unconscious and to identify with his once-repressed cause of desire.

"I really miss being with you in the office. There is something different about remote analysis—I can't quite articulate it. I mean, I still get something out of it, it's productive I guess, but I never get to a totally associative point. I feel more defended. Like, when I used to come in person, sometimes, once in a while, I'd get into a kind of zone ... like I was dissolving, lost, dizzy. My words, your words, would float above me like material objects. The light in the room would change, and my vision would get blurry. I felt very vulnerable, and sometimes there was even a palpable internal shift after a session ... I mean, I feel vulnerable even now, but not like that."

Early in the pandemic he described what he called "an incestuous feeling," severe, inhibiting anxiety just before, and sometimes during, sessions. After several weeks he acclimated to Skype. He had decided to move to the West Coast. Skype would be our medium for the foreseeable future. But in another 6 months he voiced disappointment and sadness. An entire realm of experience had become inaccessible.

The body both instantiates risk and performs a repressive function in the transference. As embodiments of objects *a*, the analyst's spatiotemporally situated enunciations can highlight the split between the intended meaning of the analysand's speech and its asemantic, tonal aspect: the equivocality of sounds (rather than conceptual connections among words) that cleave to drive derivatives, the uncanny materiality that exceeds grammatical language and mediates utterance. The analyst's physicality as gaze, voice, and silence allows for the emergence of such destabilizing libido-conveying effects while simultaneously binding them to the symbolic and visual dimensions of being. In anchoring the frame, the living presence of the analyst also provides a temporal elasticity, a suspension that nonetheless moves and transforms. Holding drive elements and regulating jouissance, the analyst's body permits the analysand to hear herself anew, to oscillate between past and present in the service of a suppler and more open-ended future.

"'Tell me what I should do,'" writes analyst Anne Dufourmantelle (2011/2019), "'I just don't know anymore. I don't understand anything anymore. I obsess. I haven't been able to sleep. What should I do? Give me an answer ...' The silence of the analyst opens a suspense. It is not a non-response or a non-reception; it is an engagement with the non-resolution of an act, an invitation to take further risks, to hold the unbearable contradictions within oneself and bring them alive" (p. 15).

What can one ultimately say about the living presence of two bodies, the ephemeral residue of the analytic session? One would have to speculate about the medium of speech divorced from sonority, an interpsychic reverberation, a silence left hanging in the air after an interpretation. There is an empty space in which the voice resonates, the void in the Other: drives that come back to us in the form of alterity—and disturb our poetry—when we speak.

But can one really hear or isolate this silence? And whose voice is one even talking about? Sound theorist Mladen Dolar (2006) proposes a simple synthesis: "The analyst's stance consists in turning herself into the agent of the voice, which coincides with the silence of the drives, by assuming this silence as the lever of her position, thus turning the silence into an act" (p. 157). Dolar here refers to the Lacanian psychoanalytic act: the identification with object *a*, a fragment of the drive—the cause of the subject's repetitions. Counterintuitively, then, it is not the analysand's speech that produces the sonic residue, but the analyst's silence, which functions as the embodiment of the voice as object, the mute voice that alternately halts and fuels the temporally situated chain of the analysand's associations.

She speaks to me on Facetime while lying on her own couch. "We're almost out of time, and do you realize you've said nary a word this entire session?! You tell me nothing! ... What are you doing, anyway? You're probably bored after long days of remote sessions. Are you texting your friends? Shopping online? I think I heard you typing earlier. Sometimes I think you mute yourself because I don't hear you breathing anymore ... all I hear is a kind of soft static, maybe a computer fan. I am searching for evidence of your presence, and instead I get this stupid crackle! It's much more difficult to tolerate your silence like this!"

The analyst's silence figures the subject's constitutive gap, the primordial loss: It is the broken cry, the blind spot in the visual field. A solicitation of transference, and an appeal to assume one's position as a subject, it prompts the need to speak so as to fill the void, to quash the silence. Can silence as object-voice be rendered present via computers and phones? Subjectivity is an edge-condition traced by the rims of the eyes, the mouth, the nostrils. Corporeal borders mark the drive's circular route, where outside meets inside through voice, gaze, and smell. The mediation and flatness of screens disturb the overlapping circuits of the invocatory and scopic drives, such that bodily emissions and residues—the ungraspable byproducts of sexuation—cannot "appear" to, and be used by, the analysand.

What is lost, then, in remote sessions? Contact is lost with the Real of the analyst's body, breath, the uncanny remainder; the body as a signified that brushes against sexuality and death; the difference between speech and voice, between the eye and the gaze. The image of the body is not an object. On Zoom, analysts sit in two dimensions, exhausted by an excess of seeing and sense, having forfeited the materiality of their silences, the very medium of therapeutic action.

Given the importance of the Real presence of the analyst's body—a material substance emptied of the analyst's private suffering—am I putting too much flesh on the bone by writing this book, putting my body, in other words, in the frame of my own imaginary, depriving my analysands of coating it with their unconscious fantasies? After this, will I continue to function as the cause of their desire, as outline and mediator of new thoughts and self-assemblages, a sort of husk to be discarded eventually? What will be the fate of my analytic body when it is elaborated through personal narrative, shot through with illness? I do not know, and I worry about it. But I must hazard the endeavor, for in the interstice of shame and embarrassment there are lessons in mourning: mourning a body, a homeland, and an object of study. This book is not a confession. It is an effort at representing corporeal loss in the shadow of other improbable losses, a restitution of the self within the void of subjectivity.

References

Dolar, M. (2006). *A voice and nothing more*. MIT Press.

Dufourmantelle, A. (2019). *In praise of risk* (S. Miller, Trans.). Fordham University Press. (Original work published 2011)

Dulsster, D., & Vanheule, S. (2019). On Lacan and supervision: A matter of super-audition. *British Journal of Psychotherapy*, *35*(1), 54–70.

Kirshner, L. (2018). The presence of the analyst. English version. Retrieved August 20, 2024, from https://www.academia.edu/38092225/The_Presence_of_the_Analyst_docx. (Original work published 2018 in German)

Laurent, E. (1992). Quatre remarques sur le souci scientifique de Jacques Lacan [Four remarks on Jacques Lacan's scientific concerns]. In M.-P. de Cossé Brissac, F. Giroud, R. Dumas, et al. (Eds.), *Connaissez-vous Lacan?* [Do you know Lacan?] (pp. 41–43). Seuil.

Perelberg, R. J. (2021). The empty couch: Love and mourning in times of confinement. *International Journal of Psychoanalysis*, *102*(1), 16–30.

Rousselle, D. (2020). *The truth about coronavirus*. Ebrary. Retrieved August 28, 2024, from https://ebrary.net/141868/psychology/truth_coronavirus

1

Technology

"Here, let me show you," she exclaimed, rotating the computer screen. "You see those white dots?"

I strained to make them out, putting on my glasses. "Yes, uh-huh, now I do." They looked so tiny, innocuous, diffuse.

"All that is cancer. They're clustered in two areas, mainly. The mammogram picks up the calcifications."

I stared silently at the side-view X-ray image of my breast. Was it really mine?

The oncologist shifted the screen further toward me.

"Here, you see how they form a radial pattern—like the spokes of a bicycle wheel? That's why you're not a candidate for a lumpectomy."

I wasn't immediately sure about the wheel analogy, but I noticed my husband vigorously nodding and taking notes.

"We'll do an MRI to check, but I'm pretty certain we will not be able to spare the nipple."

It was all moving too fast for me. I hadn't known nipple-sparing mastectomies were even an option.

"Are you sure? Is sparing the nipple a possibility?"

She pointed at the screen emphatically: "You see how the dots radiate from the nipple? Probably too close. You wouldn't have any feeling in it anyway. It wouldn't be a functional nipple, purely aesthetic."

The oncologist shrugged as her phone pinged, competing for attention with the larger screen.

"Hold on," she muttered, perusing a long string of texts. "The basement of my house flooded this morning, and the nanny is having an issue. I'm trying to deal with it. I'll be right back."

She sprang from the chair and darted out of the consulting room, her petite frame tenuously supported by a white coat and 4-inch stilettos.

And so the fate of my right breast was decided.

~

The appointment was at Famous Cancer Hospital, one of the best in the world. Yet I had difficulty convincing myself the whole thing wasn't a sham, a ruse, a mistake. I stood naked in my bedroom and looked down at my innocent breast, destined for

DOI: 10.4324/9781003498582-2

imminent execution: my beautiful and good breast that gave me sexual pleasure and nursed my son. What relationship could its warm alabaster surface possibly have to the speckled, grainy image now deemed the consummate evidence of my fragile corporeality? How could I have faith that those little dots—quiet, invisible, and unfelt—threatened my life? Milk ducts that once provided nurturance and fattened my baby were jammed with carcinoma. The proof? White flecks on a computer screen.

~

I am decidedly lo-fi, deeply suspicious of new audiovisual technologies. For 10 years I researched and wrote about early sound recording—gramophones and records of the acoustic era—before high fidelity, before stereo, before mono and electrical recording. Gripped by nostalgia for the present—a yearning to belong that will not be soothed by Instagram—I cling to belongings from bygone eras: over 10,000 recordings on CD and vinyl. I love art forms that are perpetually dying or routinely declared to be dead: opera and psychoanalysis. Because I'm a Soviet refugee, the embodiment of kitsch, I feel at home with the untimely and outmoded. In my solitude and in listening, I am finally *inside*: inside opera, inside the Soviet past, inside the Other. Paradoxically, I am also separate, comfortably removed, producing narrative.

The last Soviet generation experiences its childhood as a lost object. Not just lost in the common way—to memory, repression, or cynicism—but as a repository of potentialities, medium of temporality, and culturally situated iterative process of subjectivization. The sad contemplation evoked by artifacts of that childhood cannot be reduced to nostalgia for a country one has left because the Soviet Union is dead. Its deadness and irretrievability produce a melancholic stance, as does the disillusionment with Soviet myths and their progenitors. What is more, radical discontinuity itself, a traumatic breach in one's relationship to time, becomes the object of melancholic identification, a constitutive component of the ego.

In my attempt to mourn the Soviet Union, I chose to study the vicissitudes of old technologies, precisely, the ways in which people developed (and lost) faith in machines. Early 20th-century consumers were trained in modalities of listening and perception, immersed in discourses that enabled them to believe that film and gramophones reproduced reality and captured human bodies and voices.

~

Throughout the 1910s and 1920s, the Edison Phonograph Company conducted so-called tone tests, a publicity campaign organized across the United States to show the superior fidelity of its machines. In darkened rooms, sometimes concert halls, audiences would listen to the singing of famous Edison recording artists and then try to determine whether the voices were "live" or recorded. Often they would guess wrong and gape in amazement when the lights came on to reveal a machine playing. Now, when listening to early vocal recordings, I cannot help but smile with incredulity and bemusement at this story. To the contemporary ear, the hissing, crackling, pitch distortion, and limited dynamic range of acoustic opera recordings make the distinction between them and "real" voices so stark that I'm tempted to ask: Did early 20th-century listeners hear differently than we do today?

Theodor Adorno's 1928 essay "The Curves of the Needle" offers an answer. In it he argues that gramophones do not act as vanishing mediators of voices and the intrusion of technology facilitates rather than hinders authenticity. The residue of incidental noises and other imperfections, paradoxically, make recordings sound human. What could he have meant? Despite the efforts of early gramophone companies to perfect records by removing evidence of reproduction, one needed to be made aware of the machine's presence to distinguish and name that which was human and "real." The pure voice, exactly reproduced, fully detached from a mediating corporeality, was uncanny and unnatural seeming. It was in the excess, as it were, that humanity was expressed (Adorno, 1928/1990).

I spent many pages arguing that the frequent invocations of "natural sound" or "authenticity" in the first record reviews referenced not an exact reproduction but this very excess.

~

Since the advent of the recording industry, inventors, manufacturers, retailers, and record reviewers have been obsessed with sound fidelity. Early recording mogul Fred Gaisberg was committed to producing records that did not sound mediated, that is, recordings free of surface noise and distortion. The advertisements and trademarks of the Gramophone and Victor companies claimed that their records were faithful to "living" voices and went still further to equate record and singer. Emile Berliner's famous HMV (His Master's Voice) trademark, based on Francis Barraud's painting of his terrier Nipper peering into the horn of a phonograph (originally an Edison machine), suggests that the dog is unable to distinguish between a record of his master's voice and his real master. Widely disseminated Victor ads from the 1910s featured tenor Enrico Caruso standing next to a disc roughly the size of his torso with the caption: "Both are Caruso." These ads went on to boast that "the record of Caruso's voice is just as truly Caruso as Caruso himself. It actually *is* Caruso—his own magnificent voice, with all the wonderful power and beauty of tone that make him the greatest of all tenors" (Symes, 2004, pp. 27–29).

The early discourse of sound fidelity or verisimilitude thus suggested that "perfect" fidelity was achieved when the technology enabling sound reproduction, acting as a mediator, vanquished itself and the relation between "living" and reproduced sound was rendered transparent. But while the Victor ads claimed to erase the distinction between the original and copy, they also alluded to an external reality or original that looked quite different from the disc beside it—the picture of Caruso. The assertion that both were Caruso, in other words, introduced the very idea of "originals" and "copies"—and the notion that there could be a difference between the two.

In *The Audible Past*, historian Jonathan Sterne (2003) argues that an idea of sound fidelity based on a "fundamental distinction between original and copy will most likely bracket the question of what constitutes originality itself," emphasizing the technology rather than the process of reproduction (p. 219). But both originals and copies actually are mediated:

> The efficacy of sound reproduction as a technology or as a cultural practice is not in its keeping the faith with a world totally external to itself. On the contrary, sound reproduction, from its beginnings ... implied social relations among people, machines, practices, and sounds. The very concept of sound fidelity is a result of this conceptual and practical labor.
>
> (Sterne, 2003, p. 219)

Sterne (2003) then turns to Walter Benjamin's classic essay "The Work of Art in the Age of Mechanical Reproduction" (1935/1968), in which aura is defined as "the unique presence in time and space of a particular representation, its location in a particular context and tradition" (p. 220). Sterne highlights not the part of Benjamin's essay that expresses regret over the "withering" of aura, freed from its time, space, and tradition in the age of mechanical reproduction, but a footnote that qualifies his definition of aura: "Precisely because authenticity is not reproducible, the intensive penetration of certain (mechanical) processes of reproduction was instrumental in differentiating and grading authenticity" (as cited in Sterne, 2003, p. 220).

Sterne (2003) elaborates on aspects of Benjamin's analysis of film to assert that the mediation resulting from sound reproducing technologies is a cultural rather than an ontological problem:

> The very construct of aura is, by and large, retroactive, something that is an artifact of reproducibility rather than a side effect or an inherent quality of self-presence. Aura is the object of a nostalgia that accompanies reproduction. In fact, reproduction does not really separate copies from originals but instead results in the creation of a distinctive form of originality: the possibility of reproduction transforms the practice of production. ... Authenticity and presence become issues only when there is something to which we can compare them.
>
> (p. 220)

Notions of sound fidelity changed fundamentally in the 1930s, as record producers and companies increasingly announced that their products were superior to live performances. In the era of electrical recording, fidelity could connote the correspondence between two different reproduced sounds, a measurement of recordings against other recordings. But even purists like Gaisberg, producers of the acoustic age whose modest aim was to make faithful recordings of the best "living" voices, referred to a living voice or reality already mediated by the idea and process of reproduction. When Gaisberg recorded the "Volga Boat Song" with the famous Russian bass Fedor Shaliapin, "together [they] produced two more stanzas and conceived the idea of beginning the number softly, rising to a forte and fading away to whisper, to picture the approach and gradual retreat of the haulers on the riverbanks" (Gaisberg, 1946, p. 68). Gramophone chose to record Caruso in part because the "overtones and strong vibrato in his voice etched a particularly 'brilliant' tone—it suited the technology well, and enhanced 'fidelity'" (Siefert, 1995, p. 439).

~

My noninvasive cancer, "high-grade" ductal carcinoma in situ, or DCIS, is perfectly suited to mammography. That's because abnormal cells grow and die too quickly for the body to clear them away. They pile up in ducts like dust on a New York City windowsill and then petrify, eventually forming tiny specks of calcium. Mammograms have received a lot of bad press for their imprecision and inaccuracy. They miss small tumors, especially in younger women with dense breasts. Some gynecologists even proclaim mammograms useless, advising their patients to wait until age 50 (rather than the typically recommended age 40) to screen for breast cancer. But mammograms are expert at detecting calcifications. You'll never feel or see DCIS in the form of a lump during a physical exam, but mammography will reveal its attendant microcalcifications in several common patterns: spokes of a wheel and tree branches are the preferred descriptions. When a radiologist sees those patterns and they are multifocal, she sends you for a needle biopsy straight away.

Approximately 25% of all breast cancer diagnosed in the United States is DCIS, and 20%–60% of DCIS progresses to invasive ductal carcinoma. Fast-growing, high-grade DCIS is more likely to become invasive than the low- and intermediate-grade varieties (Wang et al., 2024, para. 1). Several large areas of my breast were sprinkled with microcalcifications. But in order to assimilate the idea that I had cancer, I had to have faith in machines and their hermeneuts. I had to believe the uncanny cancerous dots were me and that mammography, stereotactic biopsies, and MRIs, offering visual evidence, do not lie.

References

Adorno, T. W. (1990). The curves of the needle (T. Y. Levin, Trans.). *October, 55*, 49–55. (Original work published 1928)

Benjamin, W. (1968). The work of art in the age of mechanical reproduction (H. Zohn, Trans.). In H. Arendt (Ed.), *Illuminations* (pp. 217–251). Harcourt Brace Jovanovich. (Original work published 1935)

Gaisberg, F. (1946). *Music on the record*. Robert Hale Ltd.

Siefert, M. (1995). Aesthetics, technology, and the capitalization of culture: How the talking machine became a musical instrument. *Science in Context, 8*(2), 417–449.

Sterne, J. (2003). *The audible past: Cultural origins of sound reproduction*. Duke University Press.

Symes, C. (2004). *Setting the record straight: A material history of classical recording*. Wesleyan University Press.

Wang, J., Li, B., Luo, M., Huang, J., Zhang, K., Zheng, S., Zhang, S., & Zhou, J. (2024). Progression from ductal carcinoma in situ to invasive breast cancer: Molecular features and clinical significance. *Signal Transduction and Targeted Therapy, 9*, Article 83. https://doi.org/10.1038/s41392-024-01779-3

2

Looking Inside

I scheduled my first mammogram for lunchtime, between my patients. There would be an hour to grab a coffee afterward, maybe even stop at the DACA rally nearby. My hard-nosed East European ob-gyn had been urging me to get a mammogram for the past 3 years, since I had weaned my son. I'd procrastinated, explaining that I had no lumps, no issues, and no family history of breast cancer. But she kept insisting. "You have a young child," she warned.

I am not sure why I hesitated. My mother complained that it hurt mightily. Friends related stories of breasts compressed like panini. A flurry of articles cast doubt on the value of mammography screening in women under 50. I was nervous, mostly about the pain.

After 15 minutes in the general waiting area, I was shown to a changing room and given a bubblegum-pink robe. The technologist was a model of kindness and reassurance. She peppered her What to Expect spiel with anecdotes of her own unwarranted scares and false positives. The rush of pink and anecdotes was oddly comforting: The appointment was proceeding according to expectation. The first set of pictures was a breeze; some mild discomfort—and the procedure was over. I waited half-naked while the tech took the images over to the radiologist to be read. It was an impossibly long 10-minute interval. She came back with a broad smile. "The doctor wants more views of the right breast. It happens a lot, as I told you. Just try to relax."

Waves of racking anxiety ushered the second round of imaging. Another angst-ridden wait. The radiologist entered the room. He was corpselike and dissociated, straining to make minimal eye contact. The sallow corpse spoke aridly about extensive areas of calcification, multifocal. The next several minutes were a blur.

"We would like you to schedule a biopsy of the right breast. Preferably before you leave today."

"Today? Is it really that urgent? Can't we wait 6 months and rescreen?"

The corpse showed hints of life: "Err … There's a lot of it …"

Several sentences later, I was alone again with the spunky technologist.

"About 80% of the time it's nothing," she chirped.

"Right," I said getting up, convinced that my knees would buckle.

DOI: 10.4324/9781003498582-3

I stopped at the reception desk on my way out. And then continued walking, through the automated doors and into the sun-drenched early September afternoon. After two laps around the block, I returned.

"I'd like to make an appointment, a biopsy of the right breast."

"Yes, Ms. Fishzon."

The receptionist knew my name. Surely a bad sign.

"When is your next available time?"

"Thursday at noon," she said with a tinge of pity.

It couldn't happen soon enough.

~

During the biopsy I was told to stay perfectly still for 20 minutes so that a good sample could be obtained. Afterward, I was complimented multiple times for being an exemplary patient. No other patient had ever managed such impeccable rigidity! Later, during the MRI, I was told again to remain still while lying face down for 30 minutes with a needle in my vein, injecting dye. Frozen and mute in the roaring MRI tube, I felt my world collapsing. I tried to cling to music, to my humanity. Schubert's last sonata? No, too dark. Bach's Preludes, maybe? Too strongly linked to my mother. I turned ineluctably to opera.

While waiting for the biopsy results, I dreamed that I ate my eyeglasses. I still recall the texture and crunch of the wire frames and the taste of plastic and metal in my mouth. The dream produced what for me was an unprecedented gustatory memory. I brought it to my analyst, who said, "You wanted to look inside." I had, indeed. But the experience was much more literal than I'd imagined.

~

The MRI and analysis revived my first operatic loves: Giuseppe Verdi's middle-period works, *Rigoletto* (1851) and *La Traviata* (1853). Both feature glorious duets for soprano and high baritone. Both treat one of the composer's great themes: the father–daughter bond. When I was 12, these musical and dramatic choices tempted, embarrassed, and sustained me. They filled me with a vertiginous disquiet I now call jouissance.

The hunchbacked Rigoletto loves Gilda madly. The problem is that he is her only parent and she is his only child. Verdi invests the father–daughter relationship and its music with the sort of propulsive passion and catastrophic consequences one normally finds in depictions of romantic love. Gilda's mother died in her daughter's infancy, leaving Rigoletto with no significant human attachment other than his child. The father's desire to protect his daughter is so ferocious and stifling that it ultimately kills her (Robinson, 2002, pp. 113–114).

Rigoletto is a jester in the court of the Duke of Mantua, a notorious seducer and cad. The hunchback keeps Gilda in seclusion knowing full well that because his job entails ridiculing courtiers, she is vulnerable to their vengeful pranks, humiliation, and rape. Gilda, in fact, is so naive and sheltered, she fails to recognize that the handsome young man wooing her en route to church is actually the Duke. Inevitably, she is abducted by courtiers and delivered to the Duke's bedroom. Rigoletto discovers his daughter's dishonor, vows revenge, and hires an assassin to murder the Duke. The tragic denouement is achieved through a sequence of melodramatic plot devices and a musically innovative quartet sung on a stormy night, with Gilda's sacrificing herself to save her lover's life. In the final scene, Rigoletto discovers that the sack he has been given by his hitman contains not the body of his daughter's seducer, but the wounded and dying Gilda.

Death is drawn out and attractive in opera, music slowing the pace of final laments, allowing time for soaring arias and exhilarating farewells. Expiring bodies of prima donnas and slain heroes, tranquil and sublime, are displayed for sympathy and adoration. The death scene duet commences with Gilda's "Lassù in cielo, vicina alla madre," through which she summons the fantasy of a heavenly reunion with her mother. In song she reconstitutes the nuclear family that eluded her for much of her short life. Gilda's lines, vocalized while supine, are aptly set to an ethereal "arc (rising a sixth) and supported by high violins" (Robinson, 2002, p. 120). Rigoletto then contributes his motif ("Non morir, mio tesoro, pietate ... Oh mia figlia! Oh mia Gilda!"):

Do not die, my treasure, have pity!
Oh, my dove, you must not leave me!
If you go, I will be all alone!
Do not die, or I shall die beside you!
Oh, my daughter, my Gilda!
(Verdi & Piave, 1851/1997)

I imagine Tito Gobbi and Maria Callas: his lachrymose timbre, her wobble above the staff. There is a surge of devastation in the words, "You must not leave me! ... I will be all alone," accompanied by a crescendo in the low strings. The two voices soon meet and entwine, producing a transcendental union. Gobbi's hulking chest hovers over the diminutive Callas. Then the half-whispered and chilling, "Gilda! Mia Gilda ... è morta!" followed by a bloodcurdling cry (Verdi & Piave, 1851/1997).

La Traviata also ends with the death of a self-sacrificing daughter figure. The rapport between Violetta Valéry and the patriarch Giorgio Germont bears the characteristics of a father–daughter relationship. Their sweeping duet in act 2 is the opera's emotional center and includes its most exquisite music. The consumptive Violetta sings, "Embrace me as a daughter," and when Germont shows up at her deathbed in the final act, he rejoins, "I come to keep my promise and embrace you as a daughter."

Violetta wants to leave the demimonde to marry Alfredo Germont, a dashing young nobleman from Provence. But the elder Germont sternly urges the erstwhile courtesan to choose a different path. Her liaison with his son has brought disgrace upon the family and ruined his daughter's marriage prospects. Violetta agrees to give up Alfredo for the sake of his sister, though she knows the decision will hasten her own end. Catherine Clément (1988) would have us believe that the patriarch is dryly conducting "business" (p. 63), but the pair's mezza voce eloquence suggests a libidinal valence.

Strangely, almost counterintuitively, the opera's tenor fades into the background. Armed with a serenade, two cabalettas, and a dramatic party scene, Alfredo is nonetheless musically flimsy, gullible, and pusillanimous. He lives off Violetta's savings, runs to daddy for financial help, and is quick to believe her recidivism. Convinced that Violetta abandoned him impulsively to resume her former life, he publicly insults her by flinging money at her feet. Even his presence at her bedside in act 3 has little impact. He has learned the truth and begs her forgiveness, but it is too late.

When I think of *Traviata*, it is clear what matters: not the flaccid and forgettable tenor, strained and unconvincing in his high-C passion, but the gentle, lower-toned Germont and his enduring connection to the principled and daring heroine.

~

"I'm going to sit up today; I'm too anxious," I announced as I made my way to the leather armchair.

He ambled across the consulting room and sat in the identical chair, facing me.

I'd moved to the couch a few weeks into the treatment and had been lying down for over a year. The room looked eerily unfamiliar from the upright, seated perspective. It was bigger and colder than I'd remembered. I noticed my analyst's fingers wrapped around the armrests, gripping them tightly, as if braced for a plane crash. Behind him loomed a Georgia O'Keeffe print, trite and hideous; like my analyst, it was positioned beside the couch, usually out of my sight. What would he and the analysis mean to me now, in this catastrophic moment? Our work together seemed ill-timed, irrelevant. A paraphrase of Slavoj Žižek's quip about philosophy resounded in my mind: Psychoanalysis "does not solve problems" … its "duty is to redefine problems, to show that what we experience as a problem is a false problem." When faced with a true problem, let's say, a natural disaster or a deadly virus—a real threat—you don't need psychoanalysis! You need "good science to find a solution" (Taylor, 2005, 30:18). Xanax, oncologists, imaging, and surgery were required at present. I dreaded and hoped for hollow reassurance and the promise of phone sessions.

Desperate, I searched his face for evidence of panic. He appeared serious and thoughtful, but calm. His hands remained glued to the armrests. "I have cancer," I heard myself say.

~

Anticipating Sigmund Freud, Verdi demonstrated the importance of the family romance for the Victorian imagination, and for the 21st century. The composer well understood the overinvestment in the emotional bond between parent and child. At age 12, long before I read the father of psychoanalysis, I learned from Verdi something of the Oedipus complex, as well as the pleasures and perils of being an oedipal winner. I adore Verdi's baritone-fathers. My attitude toward my own father is more ambivalent. Not that Rigoletto and the elder Germont are unfailingly dignified. They are weak men, flawed and destructive. Yet they respect sopranos and aim to protect their children.

When I came home after learning I had cancer, my parents, who had been minding my 4-year-old, greeted me at the door. My father embraced me, probably for the first time in many years, and cried, "My daughter! My daughter!"

After the mastectomy, I listened again and again to the Callas–Gobbi 1955 recording of Gilda's death scene, Verdi's testament to the searing love between fathers and daughters and to the tectonic shifts in 19th-century Europe that transformed the family from a primarily economic to an affective unit, the seedbed of care and passion. Never had I longed for a father so much and never had my need felt so devouring. For 3 weeks my analyst and I were separated. During that period, I grasped my profound void and the analytic work that lay ahead.

References

Clément, C. (1988). *Opera, or The undoing of women*. University of Minnesota Press.

Robinson, P. A. (2002). *Opera, sex, and other vital matters*. University of Chicago Press.

Taylor, A. (Director). (2005). *Žižek!* [Film]. Zeitgeist Films. YouTube. Retrieved August 13, 2024, from https://www.youtube.com/watch?v=7FItgC3H9xw

Verdi, G., & Piave, F. M. (1997). *Rigoletto* [Album recorded with the Orchestra and Chorus of Teatro alla Scala, Tullio Serafin conductor]. EMI. (Originally recorded in 1955, original work published 1851)

3

The Zone

I have a very clear memory of the day I became a cancer patient. I called surgical oncologist Dr. G's office at Famous Cancer Hospital (FCH) less than an hour after I had received the diagnosis from my stoically cheerful ob-gyn. "If I were you, I would not attempt to spare the breast," she'd advised upon delivering the news over the phone. "Look, they have all kinds of options now, but the way I see it, well, it's simple: no breast, no cancer!"

I sat on the hallway floor near one of the reading rooms in Columbia University's Butler Library, the place where I still did much of my writing; the place where I had studied for an embarrassingly long time and finished my PhD dissertation. My hands shook as I unfolded the scrap of paper bearing the referral information and the words "intraductal carcinoma." On the phone with FCH, affectionately called "Famous" by the staff, I immediately realized I was in the Big Leagues. The receptionist went out of her way to elicit a positive transference both to the hospital and to my prospective surgical oncologist. She told me the doctor would see me next week after reviewing the mammogram images, biopsy slides, and pathology report faxed over by the radiologist's office. "Here at Famous we prefer to redo the slides at our lab and generate our own pathology report," she explained in response to a medley of nerve-racked questions. "You're in good hands! Breasts are Dr. G's passion!"

~

When one becomes a patient at FCH, one enters a world unto itself, a cancer-treatment zone with its own geography, language, rhythms, and ethics. Suddenly you recognize Manhattan Island as an archipelago of FCH buildings that you are destined to shuttle between for many months. You are assigned a "peer" and a social worker, a medical care team, and a patient portal. You are encouraged to visit the library and the shop at the Breast Center. You are made to feel special. Except, in the world of FCH, I soon discovered I wasn't very special. Much to my chagrin and breathtaking relief, I quickly became rather ordinary, routine, even boring.

~

Perhaps the sole attribute saving me from FCH mediocrity was my reacquired youth. I had two consecutive miscarriages within a year before becoming pregnant with my son at age 40. Throughout my relatively uneventful third pregnancy,

DOI: 10.4324/9781003498582-4

I was reminded repeatedly of my "advanced age" and "high risk." At every appointment—every ultrasound, blood test, and consultation—I was told my eggs were decrepit and potentially defective. GERIATRIC PREGNANCY was scrawled in horrifyingly bold, red letters across the top of my chart. The pregnancy ended with a placental abruption and an emergency cesarean section in its 38th week. My son was born healthy. Placental abruptions happen in 1% of pregnancies, usually from a blow to the abdomen. In my case it was "probably due to being older."

Shortly after my 45th birthday celebration and 3 weeks prior to my first and fateful mammogram, I learned that I was menopausal. I hadn't menstruated in 6 months and my ob-gyn decided to do some bloodwork during the annual visit, "just in case." A few weeks later I received a voicemail that the pap smear was normal, the estrogen and prolactin were fine, and the follicle-stimulating hormone (FSH) levels were "postmenopausal." It was "on the early side" but technically not "early menopause." My "ovaries were failing."

I replayed the message several times, agape. I was certain she'd said, "Your organs are failing." My fertility, my femininity—a self-image informed by youthfulness and sexual power—were abruptly and seriously compromised. I dreamed of decay, mortality, and death. The words "middle-aged" and "geriatric" haunted each address of "ma'am" and "Madame."

But the cancer diagnosis instantly made me young again. The kind doctors and nurses at FCH never ceased telling me that I was "only 45." Because I am Ashkenazi Jewish and "developed breast cancer so young," I was tested for the BRCA1/2 and other gene mutations. BRCA genes protect people from breast and ovarian cancers. Between 8% and 10% of Ashkenazi Jewish women who develop breast cancer carry a BRCA1 mutation (only 2%–3% of non-Jewish White women diagnosed with breast cancer are carriers). Recent studies estimate that about 72% of women who inherit a BRCA1 mutation and about 69% of women who inherit a BRCA2 mutation will develop breast cancer by age 80. The lifetime risk of ovarian cancer for women with a BRCA1 mutation is 35%–70% and 10%–30% for women with a BRCA2 mutation (Susan G. Komen, n.d.).

I tested negative for the BRCA1/2 mutations, averting a double mastectomy and oophorectomy. I sweated the results. A TP53 gene anomaly was found, but neither the lab nor the genetic counselors knew what to make of it. The enigmatic signifier tortured me for weeks. Genetic testing and research often yield results for which there is no epistemological foundation: Without a frame, interpretation is impossible.

Soon I forgot about TP53. I got to keep my ovaries and one breast—and I got more opportunities to hear about my precocity.

~

When I wasn't in the world of FCH, I was surrounded by people who didn't have cancer. Scanning bodies and faces on subway platforms and on the street, I quietly brimmed with rage and envy. Pregnant women possessed breasts available for nursing; teenagers flaunted slender figures through diaphanous t-shirts; the old sagged and expanded, losing nothing. Menopausal runners, moms with strollers, backpacked students, octogenarians precariously draped on walkers. Carefree and untouched by cancer, these two-breasted women roamed the streets and led their lives unaware of the wounded among them. I couldn't have been the only breast cancer patient in the subway car, in the restaurant, in Washington Square Park. One of every eight women develops breast cancer in her lifetime. Yet I felt abject and isolated. The social link had been severed.

I tried to fill my days with people who'd had cancer, constructing my own cancer zone, a holding environment for my unformulated thoughts and overflowing anxiety. I called my breast cancer twin, a survivor paired with me through the FCH "peer-to-peer" program. I messaged everyone I knew who had been diagnosed: teachers, cousins, estranged friends, distant relatives, a colleague's sister in Mexico City. I called my former, Relational analyst and spoke with him for 50 minutes, out of habit. He had disclosed to me his own brush with early-stage cancer a year into my treatment.

Despite the nonstop talk, my anger and aloneness were largely incoherent and unsymbolized, failing to coalesce into *Why me?* or *Fuck cancer!* It was and remains difficult for me to claim an identity related to breast cancer. Can a person diagnosed with stage 0 ductal carcinoma in situ legitimately call herself a survivor? Inside FCH there are terminally ill 30-year-olds hooked up to chemo and bald children with rare leukemia. Concave-chested women meditate and read *Vogue*, awaiting PET scans. Wheelchair-bound men in hospital gowns feebly attempt gallows humor.

My blood pressure always spiked in the cancer zone. Its suffering was frank, pervasive, and difficult to bear. But over time, I noticed that I looked forward to each return. *Out there* I was a mastectomy freak and cancer victim. In the waiting rooms of FCH, I was lucky.

~

The Zone of Andrei Tarkovsky's film *Stalker* (1979) is Chernobyl's Exclusion Zone avant la lettre. In the film, the eponymous protagonist smuggles visitors into the Zone, guiding them through a mysterious and sealed-off industrial wasteland once inhabited by extraterrestrials. The Zone contains magical debris and uncanny abandoned places, most notably a Room where one's deepest wishes are realized. *Stalker* depicts a fundamental lesson of psychoanalysis: the impossibility of articulating unconscious desires and the absolute horror of their realization. Travelers to the Zone risk imprisonment and death only to balk at the room's threshold, arrested by the destructiveness of their drives and the fear and ignorance of their true intentions. The Stalker tells of his predecessor Porcupine, who entered the Room with the hope of resurrecting his dead brother. Instead of fulfilling Porcupine's conscious wishes, the Room brought him great wealth and drove him to suicide.

This explicit message of the film—that we do not want what we desire— reverberates in the fates of its director and actors. *Stalker* was shot near an abandoned hydroelectric power station in Estonia. Tarkovsky obsessed over the cinematography, deciding to shoot the entire script twice in the same location. His compulsive repetition proved lethal. Sound recordist Vladimir Sharun believes that the premature deaths of Tarkovsky, his wife Larisa, and actor Anatoly Solonitsyn from the same form of bronchial cancer were caused by exposure to toxic contaminants emitted by a chemical plant upstream from the set.

~

The letter arrived at its destination on April 26, 1986. In the early morning, at 1:23 a.m., the fourth reactor of the Chernobyl Nuclear Power Plant erupted in two massive explosions. But the meltdown was not the most historically ill-fated aspect of that day. Of rivaling importance was General Secretary Mikhail Gorbachev's decision to cover up the catastrophe. The Soviet government ordered a complete media blackout about the accident and blocked all communication channels of the power plant. In the neighboring city of Pryp'yat, just 3 kilometers away, phones fell silent, no mail was delivered, and no telegrams sent. The TASS news agency published terse reports some 2 days later, after word of the disaster spread around the world due to elevated radioactivity in European capitals (Bendarjevskiy & Maczelka, 2011).

By the evening of April 26, Pryp'yat's radiation levels climbed to 600,000 times the normal rate. Children rode bicycles, played in sandboxes, and sipped water from fountains; families picnicked and labored outdoors, unaware of what was happening. The following day, the 50,000 residents of Pryp'yat were evacuated in a 3-hour clandestine operation. They were instructed to pack only essential belongings since they would be home in less than a week. They never returned (Bendarjevskiy & Maczelka, 2011).

Leaked foreign broadcasts and rumors circulated, but the Ukrainian capital, my birthplace Kyiv—a city of over 2 million people about 130 kilometers from Chernobyl—received no official word about the magnitude of the situation. May Day parades proceeded throughout Ukraine as scheduled. Finally, on May 14, Gorbachev made a public statement about the crisis on Soviet television, after considerable pressure from the Swedish government and extensive reporting by Western media. As effects of the Chernobyl catastrophe rippled across Europe and throughout the world, a chastened Gorbachev launched glasnost and perestroika. This was the beginning of the end of the Soviet Union.

The abandoned city of Pryp'yat, frozen in the 1980s, is currently part of the Exclusion Zone, uninhabitable for the next 20,000 years. Once a communist city of the future, it boasted a "high-quality infrastructure and an effective network of local institutions" (Bendarjevskiy & Maczelka, 2011, 1:12:25). Its stores were fully stocked when goods deficits plagued other Soviet metropolises. Now Pryp'yat is a ghost town and disaster tourism destination. Popular spots include decaying apartment blocks, a high-rise topped by a hammer and sickle, assorted public buildings, an indoor swimming pool, and a Ferris wheel. In its deserted residential buildings, one finds cribs, clothes, unmade beds, open drawers, and numerous other artifacts in various states of decomposition: tea kettles on stoves, overturned refrigerators, photographs, and crumbling walls; suspended doll limbs and forsaken teddy bears. Nature has reclaimed much of the urban landscape. Trees have sprouted on the city's roads, and wild fauna populate its squares and man-made parks. When time stopped in Pryp'yat on April 27, 1986, it grew thick with objects.

~

In his analysis of *Stalker*, Slavoj Žižek points out that the "material density of the film is that of time itself. ... We are made to feel the inertia and drabness of time." In Tarkovsky's cinematography, time is not an invisible, weightless "medium through which things happen." The visual vocabulary and haptics of the film make everything—objects, people—into markers of time, first and foremost. The Stalker looks as if he has been "exposed to too much radiation," like a person "who is falling apart alive." This "disintegration of the material texture of reality," Žižek suggests, acts as a kind of spiritual motivating force for Tarkovskian subjects; it propels their relationships to God and to desire (Fiennes, 2006, 2:19:11). Similarly, Chernobyl's Zone renders time visible: Time sticks to objects and acquires a density. The suspension of subjective temporality in the Exclusion Zone turns time itself into an object, transforming it from an unfelt structure through which lives pass into a viscous and trapping substance.

Like the adventurers of Tarkovsky's film, people are drawn to the Exclusion Zone, sometimes hiring guides and tourist agencies to facilitate entry. Chernobyl's Zone is not off limits, as is its counterpart in *Stalker*, but visitors do require a permit. There are checkpoints and bodily inspections. Tourists are provided with dosimeters that bring radiation (and time) into view and audibility. Indeed, it seems that people go to the Exclusion Zone to see, hear, and experience time. Chernobyl is a time museum.

Žižek notes that there need not be anything "specific about the zone. It is purely a place where a certain limit is set." When you create a frame, a boundary around an area, "things might remain exactly the way they were, but it's perceived as another place" (Fiennes, 2006, 2:21:01). The zone, in other words, enables transference: It is a screen onto which the subject projects her innermost beliefs and fears. The Exclusion Zone's atemporality mimics the unconscious. No time passes within its borders, and yet time is represented there as an empty signifier that lends structural support to perception. The petrified landscape of Chernobyl's Zone offers a privileged and jouissance-laden perspective on the constitution of reality. It makes the Soviet Union appear again, and with it, the contingency of time.

~

FCH is a zone that makes cancer—the great thief of time—visible, so as to halt its progress. Radiation operates there as an acephalic and circular drive, cancer's cause and cure. Like radiation, cancer often moves stealthily, without odor, sound, or taste. Its arrival on the scene is unexpected, uncanny. Cancer's image, more than cancer-in-itself, incites anxiety and disavowal.

In his seminar on anxiety, Jacques Lacan (1962–1963/2014) claims that the uncanny is produced by the appearance in the visual field of that which is normally excluded. In the aftermath of the mirror stage, the subject's perceptual coherence depends on an anchoring exclusion of what Lacan calls object *a*: The infant can feel herself whole and experience her body as a surface she possesses because she does not see her own gaze, the back of her head, her eye sockets (and does not have to worry about them). The frame of fantasy—one's very autonomy—is maintained by the impossibility of fully experiencing one's own birth and death.

MRIs, CT scans, and mammograms reveal too much, capturing objects *a*: They rupture the subject's corporeal integrity, confusing inside and outside. The uncanniness of the X-ray resides, then, in its recovery of lost libido (once given up and transferred onto objects) and the partial collapse of the ideal, fixed place of the gaze from which the subject perceives herself. Disturbances in this third, objective field—the unconscious source of the subject's gaze—convert the self-image into the double. Breast MRIs are especially proficient at showing it *all*, more than necessary, yielding many false positives. In the mind of the cancer patient, the fullness of MRI, its denial of limits and death, becomes death's harbinger.

The promise of MRI and other medical technologies introduced to me the anxiety-provoking and paradoxical term, "occult microinvasion": the possibility that some of my high-grade and extensive DCIS had undetectably escaped the milk ducts and invaded surrounding tissue or would do so imminently. Bereft, and increasingly identifying with poet Audre Lorde, I hastened to chop off the agent of my destruction like "a she-wolf chewing off a paw caught in a trap" (De Veaux, 2004, p. 89).

References

Bendarjevskiy, A., & Maczelka, M. (Directors). (2011). *Chernobyl's heritage: The zone* [Film]. Urania Cinema. YouTube. Retrieved June 14, 2019, from https://www.youtube.com/watch?v=l-nvfu9QA8k

De Veaux, A. (2004). *Warrior poet: A biography of Audre Lorde* (1st ed.). W. W. Norton & Company.

Fiennes, S. (Director). (2006). *The pervert's guide to cinema* [Film]. Mischief Films; Amoeba Film. Vimeo. Retrieved August 19, 2024

Lacan, J. (2014). *The seminar of Jacques Lacan: Book X. Anxiety* (J.-A. Miller, Ed.; A. R. Price, Trans.). Polity. (Original lectures presented 1962–1963)

Susan G. Komen. (n.d.). *Breast cancer risk factors: BRCA1 and BRCA2 inherited gene mutations in women*. Retrieved August 12, 2024, from https://www.komen.org/breast-cancer/risk-factor/gene-mutations-genetic-testing/brca-genes/

Tarkovsky, A. (Director). (1979). *Stalker* [Film]. Mosfil'm.

4

Cut!

I told an analyst friend about my impending mastectomy. I wondered how it would feel to look down and see a breast missing. The thought was horrifying, but I tried to grow accustomed to it. She said, "Life is a series of cuts."

"I will be taking 3 weeks off because of a medical issue. Dr. M will cover while I'm away. I will send you her contact information in case you will want to see someone during that time. I will return on Monday, October 30th."

"You're having surgery, aren't you?!"

Silence.

"You are! ... I've had surgery so many times. Have you had general anesthesia before?"

"No, I haven't."

"I've had it five times. I was scared the first time. It's because you fear the loss of control. It's like death. It will be fine, no big deal. Very few people die from it. The doctors and nurses put you at ease—they'll joke with you as they put you under."

He and I lapse into a tense silence.

"Let me ask in this way: Do you think you're going to be okay?"

"I think I will be okay."

"... Three weeks."

He sits up suddenly and stares at me.

"You're having surgery."

Silence.

"I'm concerned. I want to ask questions."

"You can ask me anything you want."

"Yeah, I know. But I don't want to pry. And you won't answer anyway. You'll just ask me about my fantasies, about why I imagine you'll be away or whatever."

"You seem so certain of what I'll say."

He lies down again, silent for several minutes.

"I've had a difficult weekend. Mixed, actually. Isaac and I fought a lot. It started out good, I felt close to him. We cuddled in bed, but then he wanted me to help clean the apartment, of course. He's so controlling ..."

DOI: 10.4324/9781003498582-5

"I'll be back on October 30th. Dr. M—"
"Wait, wait! I'll make a note of it, hold on a minute!"
She pulls out her phone and looks at her calendar.
"I'll be away, too, actually, for part of that time. Perfect. Can we have phone sessions?"
"I will not be available, but Dr. M will be covering for me. I will text you her phone number later today, if you have an emergency—"
"Oh, okay! So! My opening was a big success. It was everything I'd hoped for and more ..."

"I will be away for 3 weeks to take care of a medical issue. Dr. M will be available if you need to see someone during that time. I will return on Monday, October 30th—"
"Uh-huh, right! I bet you're really going on vacation! Spain? Madrid! Barcelona? You're going to sip cocktails all day on a beach! Have fun!"

~

Because I am a collector, I am fond of wholeness: the complete set, the unabridged catalogue, the archive, the hunt for the crowning piece. I am gratified when nothing is missing from its place, when the objects are lined up, when their utility is irrelevant and their thingness is revealed. Collecting is the denial of death, an avoidance of reproduction. It is an amoral endeavor, the queerest of activities. I alphabetize my CDs and records, arranging them according to composer and period.

I collected vinyl before it became Vinyl, before it was elevated to the level of *das Ding*: when I was a pigtailed Soviet kindergartener smothered in freckles. My prized items were children's musicals with lavishly illustrated jackets and liner notes. Records brought saturated colors to our drab stagnation-era apartment block and provided a soundtrack to my oedipal years.

Collecting assumed its recognizable form in the 1830s. It evolved with the development of art history and other disciplines devoted to attribution and canon creation. A growing European bourgeoisie exhibited taste and status through the acquisition and curation of art objects and luxury goods. For nearly a century, consuming had been equated with Woman. Now a masculine arena of consumption was established, one associated with authenticity, individuation, and knowledge production. Wives shopped in placid department stores and pampering specialty shops, while husbands braved exotic flea markets and competitive auction houses (Auslander, 1996, pp. 85–86). Collections were amassed with the help of experts, men who helped other men select, build, and classify.

Dandyism marked the edge of masculine consumption, threatening its productive, national, and family-oriented cast. Dandies were abject, aristocratic, and, by the late 19th century, homosexual. They engaged in elaborate self-adornment and decorated interiors for themselves alone. Dandies' impractical collections of jewels, embroideries, perfumes, and baubles functioned as narcissistic extensions.

With the advent of sound reproduction, record collecting emerged as a major subset of masculine consumption, protected, at least for a time, from sliding into more degraded and darker variants: frivolous spending and hoarding.

~

In elaborating a sphere of consumption dissociated from the feminine, audiophile discourse from its inception linked the purchase of sound-reproducing commodities to autonomous selfhood, productivity, and mastery. Early 20th-century gramophone advertising tended to focus on the family, especially the relationship between paternal figures and impressionable youngsters. It identified authoritative men, calling on them to distinguish themselves as consumers and mold others in their image. Strapping fathers and uncles presided over teenage boys' developing interest in gramophones and record collecting with diligence and moral clarity. The principal messages of acoustic-era ads dripped with bombastic overstatement that betrayed the fledgling industry's insecurity: No matter concerning the gramophone was trivial, and every element of its construction deserved careful attention. Record collectors were to devise systems of categories that privileged sound fidelity and the latest engineering methods over famous performers.

To this day, consumption deemed suitable for men is scientific and tradition-making. It is premised on an epistemology and constructs a legacy, expertise passed down from one generation to the next. Above all, masculine consumption is conquest. Fin de siècle gentlemen ventured into a chaotic marketplace armed with enough knowledge and poise to outwit oleaginous retailers and successfully provide musical enjoyment for their families. Today's male consumers are tech savvy eBay geniuses scouring the internet for products and expertise.

Jacques Lacan, a notorious collector and dandy extraordinaire who had something to say about the "psychology of collecting," compressed the immensity of the subject into an amusing anecdote in Seminar VII (1959–1960/1992, pp. 113–114). In the days of Vichy austerity, Lacan's friend Jacques Prévert had a collection of empty match boxes. The items, needless to say, were affordable, and they were all the same, laid out "in an extremely agreeable way that involved each one being so close to the one next to it that the little drawer was slightly displaced" (Lacan, 1959–1960/1992, p. 114). Prévert's modest collection was a revelation. Lacan at once understood that the match box drawer, due to its emptiness and multiplicity, was liberated: "No longer fixed in the rounded fullness of a chest … it revealed the Thing beyond the object" (1959–1960/1992, p. 114). In other words:

> The arrangement demonstrated that a match box isn't simply something that has a certain [functionality] … that it isn't even a type in the Platonic sense, an abstract match box, that the match box all by itself is a thing with all its coherence of being. The wholly gratuitous, proliferating, superfluous, and quasi-absurd character of this collection pointed to its thingness as match box. Thus, the collector found his motive in this form of apprehension that concerns less the match box than the Thing that subsists in the match box.
>
> (Lacan, 1959–1960/1992, p. 114)

Collections are meant to be shown off. Obsessional neurotics collect so as to play at being elsewhere, to produce meta-theatrical spectacles for the Other in which they act as audiences of themselves, their own self-birthing. Whether straight or gay, masculine or effeminate, obsessionals do not retreat to secluded corners to listen to their records but, on the contrary, conspicuously display their collections and erudition, exposing the ears and eyes even of unconcerned guests to their entire inventory. For this reason, Dorian Gray in his latticed, vermilion-and-gold–ceilinged rooms and the hi-fi nerd living in his parents' suburban basement have a common queerness: Both eschew fatherhood and disavow finitude, striving to take masculine-coded consumption to its logical, sublimating end. Both, in short, are fetishists, throwing light on things and the Thing.

~

My *Goluboi shchenok* record was certainly my queerest childhood possession. I look at it now, ample scratches disfiguring its once sleek black surface, jacket tattered, sleeve in a state of appalling decay, and reminisce about the record, and myself, in our younger years. In Soviet Kyiv I found comfort, even love, in the India ink–drawn blue puppy, the familiar Melodiia label, the grooves, the crackling sound accompanying the initial meeting of needle and vinyl. My childhood records held unhatched and exquisite meanings, partially formed answers to future longing.

Goluboi shchenok, or *Blue Puppy*, a musical version of a Hungarian tale, first appeared as an animated film in 1976 directed by Yefim Gamburg. The Soviet writer Yuri Entin loosely adapted his screenplay from the story of Gyula Urbán, changing the color of the puppy from black to the less conventional blue. *Goluboi* is Russian slang for "gay," but Entin, in an interview of over a decade ago, denied having been aware of such an association in the 1970s. At age 6, I knew nothing about the animated film of 3 years prior and even less about the connotations of *goluboi*, potential or actual. My attention was focused on the revolving disc, its spindled hole, and a kiddie turntable—objects emitting sounds, telling a story about a sky-blue puppy teased mercilessly by other dogs: "You are blue! You are blue! We don't want to play with you!"

According to the lugubrious female narrator, Goluboi shchenok lives on an island where he is tormented and excluded simply because of the blue color of his coat. The first vocal number, a rather grating, cacophonous chorus of bullying, "normal-coated" dogs ("Until now there haven't been / any sky-blue dogs / You embarrass the entire neighborhood / You're an indisputable defect") is followed by the reedy lament of Goluboi shchenok: "Can it be that because of my coat / I will never know happiness? / I am cursed with a terrible fate. / Ah, why am I blue?" He wishes for a companion but has yet to find one. Next, the narrator introduces the funk-inspired song of a gravelly voiced evil pirate who arrives with resounding cannon fire to "do bad deeds." The inhabitants of the island recognize him as an inveterate kidnapper known for preying on stray dogs and flee into houses and hideouts while shunning the puppy, "slamming doors in his sky-blue face." A black cat finally offers shelter to the exposed Goluboi shchenok only to betray him inexplicably by delivering him to the pirate's ship (Entin & Gladkov, 1976).

As a child, I worried for the fate of the blue puppy and the fates of all outcasts and misfits, including my own. My parents, and the parents of many other Jewish children waiting to leave the Soviet Union, had lost their jobs, friends, and the respect of family members. Gazing into the ink-spot eyes of the puppy on the record jacket and humming his melancholic tune, I nursed a dim awareness of our impending refugee status and consequent dissolution of social ties, loyalties, and material life. I was preoccupied, too, with a more mundane childish loneliness elaborated during evenings spent with grandparents while mom and dad eked out their Soviet living, doing the few jobs Brezhnev-era Jewish intelligentsia 20-somethings were permitted to do, according to gender prescriptions: electrical engineering and teaching piano.

In middle age I marvel at the queerness shared by the excluded, "defective" (read "gay") blue puppy and Jewish soon-to-be ex-Soviet citizens, especially if "queer" refers to subversive logics and communal arrangements, a "deviation of sense," acts and subjectivities that disturb dominant categories, assimilationist strategies, and ideological interpellation (Cleto, 1999, p. 14). The affinity between the outsider characters of late socialist stories and the Soviet generation that emigrated as children in the 1970s and 1980s led me to write articles about the queer aesthetics and temporality of *Goluboi shchenok* and other Brezhnev-era animation.

~

The film version of *Goluboi shchenok* employs multiple musical styles, ambiguous lyrics, and innovative animation to confound binaries (masculine/feminine, self/other, natural/artificial, and foreign/native) and, in camp fashion, portray the constructedness of personality (Cleto, 1999, pp. 15, 18). After the puppy is abducted, the Black Cat, sung by Andrei Mironov in an exaggerated and self-mocking cabaret style, performs a catchy number in which he declares: "One must live skillfully, brothers, one must know how to live!" (Gamburg, 1976, 4:15). Originally appearing as a black Harlequinesque figure, the India ink Cat, like the Pirate, demonstrates his impressive plasticity, changing shape, shrinking into nothingness and inflating in seconds. What is more, the Black Cat is the only character protean enough to assume the color of the character he is trying to seduce or lure, turning blue when in the presence of the puppy. His unctuous voice, slick manner, and formlessness bespeak inauthenticity. The Cat's musical genre reveals him as a Wildean aesthete, a decadent prerevolutionary type or interwar hedonist who flouts convention. He puts on airs, camps it up, proudly proclaims his artifice, and broadcasts his model of living.

We learn later that the Black Cat's duplicity toward the puppy was part of a plan to cozy up to the feared Pirate. The reason for the Cat's interest in the Pirate is unclear, and an air of mystery surrounds their alliance. Why, after all, do the Black Cat and Pirate eagerly traffic and kidnap an abandoned and unwanted blue puppy? Does the Pirate like little puppies? Do the Cat and Pirate run a puppy prostitution ring? The ambiguity of their relationship is depicted through animation techniques during the couple's cabaret-style duet. As they sing, in raspy baritone and plangent tenor, "You and I are so different / yet we are bound by intense friendship /

The pirate's word is sacred / We will be friends forever / … we belong together," their ink figures repeatedly merge, forming a big amorphous blot, and separate again. When individuated, the two dance while embracing and zestfully drinking beer, pouring barrels down one another's throats. Toward the end of the number the Pirate points a knife at the Black Cat, playfully threatening, "Do you want to lose your tail?" (Gamburg, 1976, 13:17), as the Cat giggles nervously and demurs. The bout of orgiastic drinking, mutual flattery, tango dancing, and sadomasochistic bonding ends with the pair falling asleep on top of one another. It would not be a stretch to say that the Black Cat and the Pirate occupy a queer time and space: They do not heed the clock, conventional morality, standardized spatial units, or body boundaries. They are outlaws who live by their own, unique code of ethics.

Just before the Black Cat and the Pirate burst into musical celebration of their union, a new character is introduced. He is the benevolent Sailor, a tenor of course, who wants nothing more than to "sail the light blue seas / help all those in trouble" and, more generally, to "do good deeds" (Gamburg, 1976, 7:01). The Sailor's love of traveling the blue (*goluboe*) sea instantly marks him as an ally of Goluboi shche-nok and a hero of queer temporality. The Sailor, moreover, is a sinewy 18th-century dandy type, singing in breezy and broad-voiced musical theater style while perched on a swan-shaped pink confection of a ship. Clad in epicene blue and pink Maca-roni fashion, complete with tricorne hat, butterflies, roses, and parasol, he is an embodiment of effeminate virility.

The well-meaning but naive Sailor is told about Goluboi shchenok's abduction by the wily Black Cat. The Sailor races to save the victim and is defeated when the Pirate unleashes a Sawfish that swiftly tears through the good seaman's rococo ves-sel and pastel bouquet. Now shackled with his would-be rescuer, the Puppy takes matters into his own hands, managing to turn the Sawfish against his captors and to free himself and the Sailor. The pair returns to the island where they are greeted by a three-part harmony chorus of "go-lu-boi" and welcomed into the dog community. Goluboi shchenok sings, "What else does one need to be happy / when a reliable friend is at one's side / If one is loved by everyone / it's not bad to be blue," and the Sailor picks up the vocal line, singing his theme song, "Sail the light blue seas / help all those in trouble" (Gamburg, 1976, 17:34). The two hold hands and dance together while the earth-toned dogs form a circle around them. Accepted and loved by their neighbors and each other, the Puppy and Sailor, one can only assume, live happily ever after.

~

With the Blue Puppy, I was born in the era of stagnation, the Soviet 1970s. I con-tinue to harbor and evoke something of its kitchen-table socialities, ubiquitous queues, and exuberant, Aesopian popular culture. Mikhail Gorbachev coined the term "stagnation" retrospectively, to draw attention away from Chernobyl and legitimate his reforms. The characterization was in many ways accurate. An impasse—at once temporal and rhetorical—was continually manifested in late socialist ideology, social formations, and cultural production. The eschatology that had underpinned Soviet life until the Thaw of the early 1960s had broken down by the Brezhnev period. The violent Stalinist past was once again relegated to silence, and communism was deferred indefinitely with the declaration of "developed socialism" by the Constitution of 1977. Those years now conjure images of dilapidated apartments, bare store shelves, and vodka-guzzling masses suffering from a lost belief in Bolshevism. But for me, Brezhnev's stalled and unfettered time held magical, reparative gestures that set the libido in motion.

The same censorship and economy of scarcity that immobilized bodies and warped official Soviet discourse also gave birth to a subversive children's culture that invited exultation in chronology-stopping spaces and nonreproductive corporeality. Perhaps the most dynamic and, finally, self-undermining feature of late socialism was its tendency to distort time and create moments of endless duration. Subjectivity and sociability are situated in and constituted through linear time; disrupt temporality and you disrupt gender, family inheritance, sexuality, and communist ideology. Stagnation produced not only queer time but also queer subjects.

~

The breast cancer diagnosis instantly merges me with Woman only to shatter brutally my feminine identification. By inflicting a wound in the Real of the body, cancer, paradoxically, robbed me of lack. It stripped me of reflexivity, reduced me to an object. I had difficulty imagining myself whole and unselfconscious, with ample space to feel, fantasize, and disavow mortality. To restore my sexuality and my ability to dream, I opted to cover the unbearable blankness of the missing breast. Against feminism and against queerness, I chose reconstruction.

~

"We made 21 slides from the tissue," my surgeon dryly reported at the post-op appointment. "Twelve of the 21 had cancer."

I pictured my breast, now referred to as "tissue," chopped into 21 pieces and then dissected, pressed, and dumped. Medical waste.

"It was all DCIS, high-grade. No cancer in the nodes. We got good margins."

She handed me a copy of the pathology report, and I gestured to my husband to gather my clothes. The brief meeting was almost over.

Then, in apparent slow motion, she offered a wry smile.

"I have to ask you something, I'm curious. Do you remember what you said right before you drifted off—before surgery?"

I was intrigued and mildly irritated by the question.

"No, I don't think so. I recall you there, by my side … and then I was in the recovery room."

"Do you remember me talking to you about a trip to Paris, sitting with your husband in a Parisian café? I was reassuring you."

"No. I have no memory of it."

She appeared genuinely surprised.

"When patients begin Propofol—it's part of anesthesia—we in the OR like to send them off with positive, good thoughts … We were trying to make you feel better because—"

"I'm not sure I follow."

"You were silent, lost in thought. I asked what you were thinking about. You looked at me and said, 'The Holocaust.'"

References

Auslander, L. (1996). The gendering of consumer practices in nineteenth-century France. In V. De Grazia & E. Furlough (Eds.), *The sex of things: Gender and consumption in historical perspective* (pp. 79–112). University of California Press.

Cleto, F. (1999). Introduction: Queering the camp. In F. Cleto (Ed.), *Camp: Queer aesthetics and the performing subject. A reader* (pp. 1–42). University of Michigan Press.

Entin, Y., & Gladkov, G. (1976). *Goluboi shchenok: Muzykal'naia skazka* [Blue puppy: A musical tale] [Audio recording]. Melodiia.

Gamburg, Y. (Director). (1976). *Goluboi shchenok* [Blue puppy] [Animated short]. Soiuzmul'tfil'm. Retrieved August 21, 2024, from https://www.youtube.com/watch?v=qKqtwkpCPTY

Lacan, J. (1992). *The seminar of Jacques Lacan: Book VII. The ethics of psychoanalysis, 1959–1960* (J.-A. Miller, Ed.; D. Porter, Trans.). W. W. Norton & Company. (Original lectures presented 1959–1960)

5

"... not without object"

A decade after a double mastectomy and several years after the discovery of a spinal metastasis that would eventually claim her life, queer theorist Eve Kosofsky Sedgwick (2003) wrote about her feeling of shame in the weeks following the 9/11 destruction of the Twin Towers:

> I had a daily repetition of an odd experience, one that was probably shared by many walkers in the same mid-southern latitudes of Manhattan. Turning from a street onto Fifth Avenue, even if I was heading north, I would feel compelled first to look south in the direction of the World Trade Center, now gone. This inexplicably furtive glance was associated with a conscious wish: that my southward vista would again be blocked by the familiar sight of the pre–September 11 twin towers, somehow come back to loom over us in all their complacent ugliness. But, of course, the towers were always still gone. Turning away, shame was what I would feel.
>
> (p. 35)

Sedgwick's example of shame is unusual, even surprising, and it is intended to be. It supports her argument that the affect does not ensue from transgression or prohibition (Sedgwick, 2003, p. 36). Shame, rather, is occasioned by a disruption in an identity-constituting circuit of recognition, a blank stare in response to a searching communication. The infant smiles at his mother, she doesn't mirror, and the infant cries. Shame buffets and marks me when my bid for identification fails to elicit a narcissistically gratifying image. I am deprived, ashamed when my gaze is unmet, and I have been made aware of a lingering desire to reconstitute the interpersonal bridge. I blush, "eyes down, head averted" (Sedgwick, 2003, p. 36). The unrequited message, the void—like the position of the analyst—harks back to infantile, erotic longings: I am dropped but nonetheless turned on, left wanting more.

I caught a glimpse of Eve on the main quad of West Campus when I was a sophomore at Duke University in the 1990s: the famous professor, harried and bald, with a scarf around her head. As a New Yorker, I too drew comfort from the Twin Towers. Their reassuring presence served as a compass and home base. Wandering downtown immersed in reverie, momentarily adrift, like Eve I would

DOI: 10.4324/9781003498582-6

glance southward, and their sight would gather me in a maternal embrace. The gap produced by the demise of the towers incited unease in me and other pedestrians, "a disappointment of expectations and a loss of familiar coordinates" (Copjec, 2006, p. 14). Sedgwick renders this response as the blazon of shame, "a bruise to her urban identity," a wound that is "not accompanied by any sentiment of rejection or abjection," but, rather, gives rise to "a feeling of solidarity with others" (Copjec, 2006, p. 14). And herein lies the central and oft-repeated paradox of shame: It is simultaneously social and profoundly isolating, "a movement 'toward individuation and toward uncontrollable relationality,' or social contagion" (Copjec, 2006, p. 14). It tugs both ways for it is the trace and evocation of the originary scene, the fault from which the Law and desire emerge.

Joan Copjec (2006) pays tribute to Sedgwick, correcting her "unfortunate error," the insistence that the shame she felt was not for herself but for the absent towers:

[Sedgwick] interprets the social sentiment as a feeling of shame for or on behalf of something other than herself. In so doing she gives shame an object, the missing edifices. The effect of this error was to permit a whole literature on shame to sprout within queer theory whereby queers take themselves as the despised objects of shame and in a second, compensatory movement convert the common trait of their abjection into a badge of honor and the basis of group feeling. Shame ... is here thought to bind individuals into a group by becoming that which they share: they form the group of all rejected or excepted from the larger group of the "normal." This disastrous misunderstanding can begin to be challenged by making it clear that the phrase "shame for" is, strictly speaking, a solecism. I feel shame neither for myself nor for others because shame is intransitive; it has no object. Shame is there in place of an object in the ordinary sense (though ... shame is [in Lacanian terms] "not without object" ... it concerns object a). To experience shame is to experience oneself not as a despised or degraded object, but to experience oneself as a subject. I am not ashamed of myself, I am the shame I feel.

(pp. 14–15)

Copjec, with Jacques Lacan, insists that shame is the principal affect of subjectivity. Here she does not contradict Sedgwick (2003), who explains that shame "attaches to and sharpens the sense of who one is," whereas guilt attaches to what one does (p. 37). Sedgwick also points to shame's relation to "visibility and spectacle" (2003, p. 36). The blush and its attendant turmoil are not so much caused by one's debasement or objectification by the other as by the sudden awareness of the part of oneself that is more than oneself—a visible and perceived aspect that one cannot control.

When encountering the chasm where the towers had stood in the weeks and months following 9/11, my heart would race and my chest would ache. I would experience anxiety, not shame. What, then, is one to make of Sedgwick's somewhat peculiar reaction—her feeling of shame "not especially for [herself] ... but for the hapless visibility of the towers' absence ... the shockingly compelling theatricality of their destruction" (Sedgwick, 2003, p. 36)? Was her reading of the affect an "unfortunate error," as Copjec claims? Can one really argue that Sedgwick's shame for the towers was misguided or illegitimate?

If we consider that the flattened towers might have conjured for Sedgwick the image of mastectomy scars, then we might understand her shame as self-exposure. For the voided vision of the Twin Towers echoed another rupture in the narcissistic circuit: the mirror's failure to return to Sedgwick her own, familiar bodily form. Shame for the "estranged and denuded skyline" (Sedgwick, 2003, p. 36), a figuration of Eve's amputated breasts, may in fact have been the blazon of a highly personal loss, now registered in downtown Manhattan for the world to observe. Eve's shame for the missing towers was also *she*.

~

"Good morning, welcome to MC! Is this your first time with us?"

Wrenched from an exceedingly private and singular state of terror, I was struck mute by the question. Was I at the right building?

I mustered a distracted reply as we rode the sleek elevator to Check-in:

"I'm here for a mastectomy."

I returned to Famous Cancer Hospital's Mastectomy Central three times. After a while, the greetings, boutique-hotel ambience, and upbeat tone began to make sense. MC is a state-of-the-art freestanding surgical facility with 28 well-appointed private rooms overlooking the East River. Upon arrival, a valet parks your car, and a concierge escorts you to the reception desk upstairs, where you and your caregiver are given clip-on tracking devices and informed of the amenities on offer. The next 8 to 18 hours, including pre- and postoperative care, are an onslaught of compassion and aesthetic solace. Nurses in smart hospital attire smile at you around the clock; members of the surgical team tranquilize with bedside lullabies. The lounge and other common areas resemble a Jonathan Adler showroom or upscale version of IKEA, only instead of Swedish meatballs, cinnamon buns, and particleboard furniture, you're likely getting a mastectomy, prostatectomy, or silicone implants.

The morning after surgery, patients are strongly encouraged to visit the Oasis, a well-lit café where shockingly good coffee and a continental breakfast await. If you ignore the hospital gowns and nonslip gray socks, the place feels like a bed-and-breakfast. Post-mastectomy, I was inexplicably euphoric as I ate my mini bagel and hardboiled egg in a mid-century modern easy chair. Other patients, too, appeared relaxed or animated—chatting with family members or gulping cereal as they perused the newspaper—not at all like people beset by pain, removed body parts, and life-threatening illness. Prior to discharge I was given a folder with exercise and drainage system instructions, a bag of pills, and a packet with pink surgical bras, gauze, pads, a prosthesis puff, and a travel-size magnifying mirror.

Every element of MC is contrived to manage and reduce shame. The handsome couches, soft lighting, friendly staff, and carefully arranged rooms all produce an atmosphere of middle-class normality. They reflect back a unified, serene, and recognizable self-image, veiling loss and enabling you, for moments, to imagine that you're enjoying a short stay at a spa. Within 24 hours, before you have a chance to fully assimilate—amid the comfort, attention, and commodity fetishism—that you have been robbed of a core part of your being, you are handed a goodie bag and sent home.

~

I came home the morning after surgery a cyborg, with a stuffed bra and a drain hanging from the right side of my torso. The drain tube had to be "milked," and the bulb's contents emptied into a container, measured, and logged twice daily. The whole apparatus would be removed, and my humanity would be restored when two things happened: the drainage amounted to less than 30 milliliters over 24 hours, and its color changed from deep red to tangerine and, finally, to a benign pale yellow. The nurses told me the process would take 1 to 2 weeks. The quantity and thickness of the serosanguineous fluid would decrease with each passing day. Unfortunately, my progress was not steady or linear. On some mornings the output climbed and my spirits fell. The stuff continued to pour out of me. At 3 weeks the drainage amount held stubbornly at 40 milliliters. The surgeon's office told me not to bother coming in for the removal. But there were patients to see and classes to attend. I could not return to work with a hose sticking out of my body, even if neatly pinned to the inside of an oversized sweater. A potential armpit seroma seemed a small price to pay. I told the plastic surgeon to yank the drain.

~

My husband helped with the bleak and increasingly mundane task of milking the drainage tube and emptying the bulb. Heroically, gently, he moved the bloody clots along with thumb and forefinger as he pinched the tubing close to where it entered my skin. Indifferent to his efforts, by noon each day, the bulb hanging from the pink ring of my surgical bra grew heavy with fluid and tugged painfully at the insertion site. Bruises formed across my swollen chest and the incision oozed. I was groggy and flushed from anesthesia and antibiotics. Still, my vanity triumphed. In anticipation of visitors in those early days post-mastectomy I put on makeup and padded my bra to approximate symmetry. I wore a billowing hoodie to hide the drainage system. Close friends came bearing casseroles, stories, and compliments. "You look like your old self! … You are handling this so well!"

I was in a narcotic fog and tired quickly, napping between visits. My son was at his grandparents', and I enjoyed the company of friends. I was not putting on an act: An exhilarated feeling prevailed initially, a manic defense, or plain relief that the surgery was over and the prognosis was good. While I was still under anesthesia, the surgeon had informed my husband that the lymph nodes appeared healthy. I would have to wait a week for the pathology report to receive definitive results, but I knew that Dr. G had "held the sentinel node in her hand" and determined it was cancer-free. I was soothed by the fantasy of her squeezing it like one of those rubber stress-relief balls. For nearly a week the surgeon's confident words and professional experience afforded reassurance.

But no news arrived on day 7, and my anxiety intensified. I started imagining that the pathologists were taking longer because they had noticed something anomalous; the slides had to be remade; unexpected and barely detectable cancers had been discovered. I phoned my surgeon's office daily, but she was too busy to take my calls: incommunicado, doubtlessly cutting off other women's breasts. I paced and messaged friends but found it impossible to speak directly about the source and magnitude of my anxiety. Privately, I attempted to parse it. I was terrified of needing chemo (really, any sort of adjuvant therapy). Chemo would make me grotesque and unlovable. I would lose my femininity, my hair, my patients, my sexuality; the look of recognition in my son's eyes; my charm. I would become an emblem of cancer, cancer anthropomorphized. Most important, I would lose time.

A mild-mannered surgical fellow and assistant to Dr. G returned one of my many phone calls. As I sobbed and perseverated about microinvasions, occult leaks, radiation, chemo, tamoxifen, and all kinds of worst-case scenarios, I heard the beep-beep of a microwave on the other end of the line. I glanced at the clock: It was almost 7 p.m. She was warming up dinner and catching her breath, probably after a long and taxing day. A surge of sympathy pierced my narcissistic preoccupation and then dissipated. I wanted the sleep-deprived and famished young doctor to tell me something she absolutely could not: that there was zero chance of metastasis, zero chance of occult invasion, zero chance of chemo. "Let's think this through," she reasoned between bites of defrosted lasagna: "If it's all DCIS, how could it travel to the lymph node? It's certainly possible that something got out but highly unlikely!"

On day 11, the call came. Staggering panic gave way to giddy relief in a flash. The oncologist's tone was jaunty: "Sorry for the delay! Our lab moved to a new building. It's all DCIS, nodes clean." The entire conversation lasted less than a minute. The post-op appointment had been scheduled, and there was little to discuss. All I needed to know at that juncture was that there was no invasive cancer. I laughed and danced a little and downed a shot of vodka in celebration. The relief was of a complicated sort: *Thank God they actually found it*, I thought.

~

Anxiety, Lacan tells us, "is the only affect that does not deceive" (1962–1963/2014, p. 116). That's because it is a signal, not of lack, but of *the lack of lack*. It is a signal, in other words, of "the failing of the support that lack [or limit] provides for the subject." Anxiety is not a signifier (Lacan, 1962–1963/2014, pp. 160, 218). Other affects and emotions are symbolic constructs because they can be directed toward the self; they can be thought. With sadness, grief, and love there is always some lack, a modicum of distance.

In the days leading up to the oncologist's call, at the peak of my anxiety, there was no possibility of opera and no space for tears. Virtually frozen, I awaited a decision about my fate. This wasn't the Romantic fate of Beethoven's Fifth Symphony or Verdi's quartet on the fortuitous stormy night ending in Gilda's murder. The latter are fate motifs drenched in signification and pathos, requiring narrative and virtuosic creativity, reflections on one's lot. Anxiety's relationship to fate, on the other hand, is primal. While sadness, resignation, and mourning concern past losses, anxiety is the anticipation of some event or sacrifice, an uncertain certainty: I am not sure yet what the Other wants from me, but clearly it wants *something* (Lacan, 1962–1963/2014, pp. 152–153). Anxiety, therefore, belongs to the register of the Real—the reality of castration—the formation and collapse of the subject. It is structurally similar to the uncanny, another confrontation with limit and potentiality—that which is beyond one's command, extrinsic, yet paradoxically intimate, indeed, so intimate as to be smothering. While Sigmund Freud claimed that anxiety, unlike fear, has no object, Lacan (1962–1963/2014) qualified that anxiety "is not without object," not an object in the colloquial sense but object *a*, the object of primordial loss (p. 131): the ineffable excess that cleaves to the subject, making her tremble, sweat, and gasp for air. This object *a*, this surplus jouissance, lends panic attacks their orgasmic appearance.

In the initial days at home following the mastectomy, shame and anxiety alternated until panic could no longer be stemmed. Then, after the arrival of the pathology report and the waning of anxiety, shame reemerged in full bloom. Friends visited less frequently, and my husband went back to work. I found time to cry, to scrutinize my reflection, to write and listen to music. I wept for my breast and for my freakish appearance. On short walks in my neighborhood, I suffered bouts of mild paranoia, imagining that passersby noticed the drain or my asymmetry. I was terrified of running into neighbors, colleagues, and former students. I became increasingly obsessed with the public domain, especially with what and how much could be seen or known about me by others. My body was no longer mine. It presented and spoke from a scene that I did not control, drawing negative attention from strangers. I peered in the travel-size mirror provided by Mastectomy Central and was unfamiliar to myself. I worried that family, friends, and colleagues would cease recognizing me, too.

When the drain was finally removed, I was fitted for a marginally more comfortable and supposedly sexier bra. The tissue expander in my chest received its first injection of saline. It would eventually be filled and replaced with a permanent silicone implant. But for the next several weeks, the site of my amputated right breast would house a small, hard, and aching stump.

I wore a prosthesis to maintain the semblance of recognition, so that my body wouldn't overflow and embarrass itself. By deceiving others, I felt less of myself, less ashamed.

~

Copjec pivots from Sedgwick's writings on shame to an argument about the shared foundation of shame and anxiety, and the relation of the latter to something loosely called "modernity." In doing so, she provides an overview of the ways Freud, Lacan, Søren Kierkegaard, Martin Heidegger, and Emmanuel Levinas variously conceptualized anxiety as the condition par excellence of secular, modern life. They looked beyond the romance of the nuclear family and lent the affect ontological import, connecting it to God and the Other, to faith and its loss. Modernity, explains Copjec (2006),

> was founded on a definitive break with the authority of our ancestors, who were no longer recognized as the founders of present-day actions or beliefs.

And yet this effective undermining of ancestral authority, though in certain respects freeing, confronted moderns with another difficulty: by rendering their
ancestors fallible, they had transformed the past from the container of already
accomplished deeds and discovered truths into a kind of repository of all that
was unactualized and unthought. The desire of past generations and thus the virtual past, the past that had never come to pass—was not yet finished—weighed
disturbingly on twentieth-century thinkers, pressing itself on their attention.

(p. 18)

The temporal rupture of modernity—a new relation to the past—put us face to face
with what Lacan calls "the desire of the Other." As moderns, we are not severed
from dead and long-silenced previous generations; we find ourselves haunted by
their enigmatic appeals. Our ancestors "do not address us in the present," as they
did before. They now address us as "expected, and far more still, as lost" (Lacan,
1962–1963/2014, pp. 152–153). What does this mean?

The Other, Lacan (1962–1963/2014) ominously declares, does not acknowledge
me *as here* (that would be far too easy, for it would allow me to break free of the
Other through conflict or violence) but, rather, "solicits my loss so that it can find
itself there again":

The Other puts me in question, it interrogates me at the very root of my desire
as *a*, as cause of this desire and not as object. And because this is what the Other
targets, a temporal relation of antecedence, I can do nothing to break this hold,
except to engage with it.

(p. 153)

For Lacan, anxiety is the feeling of being riveted to an unassimilable element that
nevertheless nominates me in my singularity, an element I neither can accept as my
own nor from which I am able to separate myself. Copjec (2006), too, underscores
that anxiety arises "from being connected to a past that, insofar as it had not happened, is impossible to shed" (p. 18). How can I disengage from something that is
yet to be actualized, "the condition which is not," a not-yet that amounts to my potentiality (Kierkegaard, 1980, as cited in Copjec, 2006, p. 21)? Before the modern age,

a subject's ties to her past were strictly binding, they were experienced as external, as of the order of simple constraint. One had to submit to a destiny one did
not elect and often experienced as unjust. But one could—like Job or the heroes
and heroines of classical tragedies—rail against one's destiny, curse one's fate.
With modernity this is no longer possible. ... We cannot distance ourselves sufficiently from the past to be able to curse the fate it hands us, but must, as Lacan
put it, "bear as jouissance the injustice that horrifies us."

(Copjec, 2006, pp. 18–19)

In Seminar X, we recall, Lacan insists that anxiety signals not the loss of an
object but precisely its overbearing presence, *the absence* of lack, that is to say,

the lack of distance between the subject and the Other, and between the subject and that which is Other within herself. Anxiety paralyzes and chokes when the subject's constitutive alienation in language and separation from the maternal body and parental desire (castration, in Lacanian parlance) unravels. As the symbolic dimension collapses, and with it the fantasy of our independence from the Other's will, "we are gripped by jouissance, the object-cause of our own actions that we nonetheless experience … as an alien object so suffocatingly close that we cannot discern what it is. … Anxiety [therefore] can be understood as the affect that registers our encounter with the death drive," the absolute dimension, or, potentiality as such (Copjec, 2006, p. 19).

Potentiality for the subject is the gaze, not sight but the capacity of sight. It is the voice-as-object rather than speech, the subjectivizing trace. It is not sound; it is the silence that enables sonic discernment and differentiation. This potentiality is not "at the behest of an autonomous will but attaches us, rather, to the ontologically incomplete past into which we are born," all that could have been done by us and by those who lived before us. Anxiety and its attendant jouissance are evidence and products of the subject's uniqueness and social link, "the affective result of our relation to ancestral desire" (Copjec, 2006, pp. 19–20).

Copjec emphasizes the historically situated nature of anxiety. But if we cast our attention to the affect's narrowly familial and intrapsychic dimension and back again to the more sweeping ontological perspective, it is immediately apparent that anxiety signals the undoing of the primary repression that structures the subject's autonomy. To be clear, this is not a reiteration of Freud's initial view that anxiety is the threat of the repressed returning. It is an elaboration of Freud's later understanding of anxiety as a signal of internal danger: the undermining of the illusion that my *I* occupies a third position, located elsewhere, external to me and the reflecting surface. Anxiety alerts me to the shrinking of the self-distance that allows me to experience myself, to be the master of my body and my actions. Anxiety marks my brush with the ever-pulsating libido, my eye sockets, my vocal cords, the undead foreign aspect, the surplus of self that structures my desire, Lacan's *a*, the object of the drive. Its eruption indicates that some force threatens to restore to me my potentiality, to make me once again, into an object.

Following her lengthy discussion of anxiety, Copjec (2006) turns to shame, another affect featuring a "non-actualized, unassumable object [that] sticks to us like a semi-autonomous shadow" (p. 21). Hewing close to Lacan and Levinas, she notes that while anxiety is a state of emergency, an imperative to escape into sociality—to find there some image of ourselves, a recognizable portrait that will bind our jouissance and give our desire direction—shame is a kind of secondary affect: It is a response to the other's observation of our potentiality, our object *a*. Put another way, shame is induced by the exposure of my otherness—my privacy and interiority—causing me to withdraw and conceal it once more (Copjec, 2006, p. 22). Ashamed, squirming, I hide "in order to protect and preserve that inalienable and yet unintegratable excess [that] designates me [undeniably]" (Copjec, 2006, pp. 25–26).

In mapping the relationship between anxiety and shame, Copjec (2006) points out that with the former affect, our self-distance and self-opacity "threaten to annihilate us totally," while with the latter, "the threat is aimed *at* this opacity whose exposure would, annihilate us. We therefore seek to preserve this opacity at all costs, even though its presence brings its own pain" (p. 26). Copjec's observation must be qualified, for a paradox emerges in Lacan's idea that anxiety is the manifestation of a certain overproximity: With anxiety, we are pained by our self-distance in so far as we cease to *have it*. No longer occupying unselfconsciously a comfortable distance from ourselves, *we become that very distance*. As our opacity—our gaze, our lived body—comes into view and moves nearer, it ceases to exist as a differentiated entity and merges with our being. Shame, therefore, is even closer to anxiety than Copjec allows, for both affects signal a divided subject's objectification, an existential danger to the ego.

What, then, ultimately distinguishes shame from anxiety, and why did I only experience shame fully once the panic had passed? Copjec's explanation is thoroughly convincing. We are seized by shame when the imperative of anxiety—*Escape! Flee!*—is replaced by another—*Hide!* Shame is a consequence and imperfect antidote to anxiety, its milder cousin: a meaningful action superseding the paralysis brought on by a surfeit of libido. The sentiment of shame is felt

> when in the exterior space of social existence, of public appearance, I suddenly appear in the flesh. I see not only the public images I ordinarily see, but alongside them, as if momentarily granted a slightly wider peripheral vision, the red patch of my own cheeks. I appear there in the flesh alongside—at a slight distance from—my own image as the gaze with which I look at the world appears in the world, gazes at me and locates me there at a remove from myself. *This* is the radical point: the gaze under which I feel myself observed in shame is my *own* gaze.
>
> (Copjec, 2006, p. 26)

Here it would be apt to recall Sedgwick's reaction to the absent Twin Towers, as well as the cardinal paradox of shame: It is both isolating and acutely social. It exposes our interiority, that which sets us apart, and makes it visible outside of ourselves, "as an event in the world" (Copjec, 2006, p. 27).

When I appeared in public after my mastectomy, I put on display not only my wounded body but also castration as such. I showed something of myself that gestured toward the loss of my mother's body, my birth and weaning, my disgust and longing for the maternal breast and for the body of my maternal grandmother: the plump hands and ample bust through which her desire poured out, an inscrutable desire that bore itself into my vulnerable ears and mouth and pint-sized chest. I circled Morningside Heights burdened by a drain and a prosthetic, my own trauma, as well as the weight of the trauma of my forebears—the violent inheritance of the never-completed Soviet project—the World War that killed my relatives,

Chernobyl, the legacies of genocide and the gulag, antisemitism, the forced choices of piano teaching and electrical engineering.

~

In traffic on the Brooklyn–Queens Expressway a week after 9/11, I saw the carcass of the Twin Towers for the first time. Once welcoming and majestic, they now rose from smoke, an unsightly twisted piece of steel, a silent scream. My heart pounded as I strained to assimilate the unbearable. On that occasion, it wasn't the absence of the World Trade Center but its ghastly remains that triggered anxiety. They conjured past injuries and potential destruction—the caving of memory, history, and sense—a stain anticipating future losses.

Eventually the towers' ruins were cleared away, and their footprints converted from a gaping hole into a solemn memorial to the victims. But what if one of the towers had stood? What would it have been like to see the North Tower without its southern counterpart? Would passersby have looked away, head averted and cheeks flushed, unable to integrate the altered landscape—the sole tower, bereft, stripped of its original meaning, transformed into a testament to its obliterated double—a memorial to the primordial loss? Would New Yorkers have felt twice the shame? Would they have borne witness to the split in themselves, their own unconscious and castration? With both towers gone, pedestrians gradually adjusted and ceased searching for the old skyline. After some years the towers' absence made possible a new consciousness and a new horizon of expectation. If one tower had remained, would we continue to experience a void?

The concept of originality took shape and acquired value only after the advent of mechanical reproduction, of exact copies. Similarly, the presence of one tower brings the loss of its twin into sharp relief; it invites the partial return of the gaze and the lingering hope of recognition. Even momentary forgetting becomes impossible. And so, if one tower had survived, what would we have done? We would have rushed to bury the corpse, erase the uncanny remainder; we would have covered it up with another presence, a double phallus. We might have rebuilt the second tower, made it larger, more ornate, with laser beams and spires and screens. What deluge of wealth, what immense resources of labor and capital would have been proffered to ensure our collective forgetting, to reduce the shame of origin and amputation, the disappointment of our unmet gaze!

~

The confrontation with cancer, an alien yet internal threat, brought me into direct contact with the potentiality of the Soviet past, my attachment to the unfathomable decisions of previous generations. Here Copjec's critique of Sedgwick resonates, for my shame could not be reduced to "an intersubjective relation" (2006, p. 27)—a stranger's quizzical look making me ashamed of my felt nakedness, my missing breast—nor was my shame caused merely by my being anchored to a drain or to a marred anatomy. Shame also sprang from memories of unanticipated encounters with my father's rage and my parents' opaque desire—the wish for something beyond a sickly daughter, electrical engineering, and immigration—desire that carried the burdens of abandoned utopia, transgenerational trauma, impending losses, and a wild yearning for freedom.

DCIS itself raises the problem of potentiality: Some argue it is not even cancer but precancer, as there is a good chance of it remaining forever in situ. Only about 40% of low-to-intermediate-grade DCIS will progress to invasive carcinoma. Even the high-grade variety might never penetrate the ducts, clogging them for a lifetime; alternately, it might seep out, stealthily, in an occult invasion.

Invaders did not sufficiently alarm Polina, my mother's aunt and namesake. When the Germans occupied Ukraine in 1941, she refused to leave. Like other Kyivan Jews who had lived through the more innocuous occupation of the First World War, she believed German soldiers to be civilized, fair, and "European," incapable of doing serious harm. My grandmother, who had fled east with Polina's oldest daughter Anna, returned briefly to Kyiv at great risk to her own life to try to convince her sister to join her in evacuation, to no avail. Polina was killed in Babi Yar with her twin toddler boys, shot, pushed into a ravine, and buried alive with almost 34,000 others.

References

Copjec, J. (2006). The object-gaze: Shame, hejab, cinema. *Filozofski vestnik*, *27*(2), 11–29.

Lacan, J. (2014). *The seminar of Jacques Lacan: Book X. Anxiety* (J.-A. Miller, Ed.; A. R. Price, Trans.). Polity. (Original lectures presented 1962–1963)

Sedgwick, E. K. (2003). Shame, theatricality, and queer performance: Henry James's *The art of the novel*. In E. K. Sedgwick (Ed.), *Touching feeling: Affect, pedagogy, performativity* (pp. 35–66). Duke University Press.

6

The Sarcophagus

Retired dosimetrist and nuclear disaster expert Alexander Kupny appears in the 2011 documentary film *Chernobyl's Heritage: The Zone*. He knows as well as anyone the Chernobyl Power Plant's "sarcophagus," the shelter constructed over the destroyed Reactor Unit Four: "It has become a part of his life, and they have become inseparable" (Bendarjevskiy & Maczelka, 2011, 47:43). A stolid British voice-over provides the relevant biographical data:

> Kupny was born on August 25, 1960, in Kazakhstan. His parents moved from Kazakhstan to the Urals in 1963 to work for the Beloyarsk Nuclear Power Plant. It was the 3-year-old boy's first contact with nuclear power plants. At the age of 18, Alexander worked at the construction of Reactor Unit Three, and at the age of 20 he started to work at the Beloyarsk Nuclear Power Plant itself: first as a troubleshooter for the equipment, then as a dosimetric measurer. At this time his father was promoted to the post of director of the nuclear power plant in Ukraine's Zaporozhye [*sic*]. In early 1986, Alexander left the Urals and went to work in the Zaporozhye Power Plant. A little later, in 1988, he decided to go to Chernobyl.
>
> (Bendarjevskiy & Maczelka, 2011, 47:55)

Kupny then takes over the narrating duties: "I worked in the Chernobyl Power Plant from 1988 to 2009." He began as a dosimetrist and retired as an instructor at the Education Center of the sarcophagus. For 10 years Kupny helped oversee the safety training of personnel contracted to work and operate machinery in and around the structure. He was part of a special squad that conducted dosimetric expeditions and took photographs and videos of its dark, labyrinthine bowels: "We were a unique team with comprehensive authority to visit [the sarcophagus] and all the spaces and corridors inside and explore new routes … where workers could venture with relative safety," recounts the unassuming Kupny. "It was at that time that I acquired intimate knowledge of the Object, though I first went there in 1988" (Bendarjevskiy & Maczelka, 2011, 48:49).

The sarcophagus, also known as the Object of Shelter or, more familiarly, the Object, is a colossal steel and concrete structure built in just 206 days in 1986 to

DOI: 10.4324/9781003498582-7

limit radioactive contamination of the environment. Locked inside its menacing Cascade Wall and rusty buttresses are 200 tons of radioactive corium, 30 tons of highly radioactive dust, and 16 tons of uranium and plutonium. Even more ominously, it contains large quantities of "nuclear lava," fuel that melted through the floor of the reactor building, seeped into its basement, and solidified. About 8 months after the accident, a remotely operated dosimeter measured its radioactivity at approximately 10,000 roentgens, a dose that would prove fatal after only minutes of exposure (Bendarjevskiy & Maczelka, 2011; Plokhy, 2018, p. 152).

Almost as soon as the sarcophagus was erected, an extensive catalogue of its problems emerged: Its walls were riddled with gaps and small cracks, letting in hundreds of gallons of rainwater and allowing radioactive particles to escape (Blackwell, 2012, p. 30). A 1996 article in *Ogonyok* magazine reported:

> The sarcophagus, [designed to last 20 to 30 years,] … was constructed in absentia, the plates were put together with the aid of robots and helicopters, and as a result there are [over 200 meters of] fissures. … Might the sarcophagus collapse? No one can answer that question, since it's impossible to reach many of the connections and constructions in order to see if they're sturdy. But everyone knows that if the Shelter were to collapse, the consequences would be even more dire than they were in 1986.
>
> (Alexievich, 1997/2005, p. 4)

By the late 1990s the sarcophagus had significantly deteriorated and was deemed irreparable due to astronomical radiation levels and the instability of the debris within its walls. The Ukrainian government held an international competition to design a second sarcophagus, and in 2017 the largely French-engineered, shiny New Safe Confinement was slid, on two huge rails and with hydraulic jacks, over the old structure. Many continued to speculate about the fate of the first, decaying Object and its hidden radioactive waste. Would it crumble into a giant heap of rubble? And would the new structure ultimately require another sarcophagus, and on and on, for generations, "a massive nesting sarcophagus doll funded by the entire world" (Blackwell, 2012, p. 31)? In August 2019, a plan to dismantle the original sarcophagus was announced. The demolition is being carried out remotely, by robot-operated cranes and carriages suspended from the arched roof of the new shelter.

~

Kupny is a soft-spoken, affable middle-aged man of attractive mien, with tinted glasses and a mane of brown curls. I watch him because he has had a boundary-shattering experience. He is among the few who have penetrated the sarcophagus: "As a dosimetrist I was always excited to see what was on the other side of the wall. I was interested in seeing the epicenter. I wanted to peep in, to go in and measure the high radiation, to feel what it was all about," he confesses with a coy smile. The voice-over discloses that Kupny often entered the sarcophagus surreptitiously, illegally, thanks to the winks and nods of security guards. He always went accompanied by a colleague so that if he needed anything—became trapped or fell—his partner would rescue him or call for help. "Valera and I [were often together]. We were very eager to learn, to know, and also to capture everything [on film]. This information is vital, and we will always need it" (Bendarjevskiy & Maczelka, 2011, 59:26).

Alexander and Valera, explorers: adventurers with a keen sense of history and mission. They recorded and photographed for the sake of something beyond themselves—for posterity—but also, one gathers, for their own, excruciatingly private pleasure.

Kupny narrates clips of the video he and Valera took inside the sarcophagus. The camera zooms in on a sepia-toned junk pile: scraps of metal, gobs of congealed fuel, sand, beams and rods thrown together. The images are grainy, with a basso continuo of crackle and dosimetric beeps, and a sprinkling of small white dots, "marks that radioactivity leaves on the digital sensor" (Bendarjevskiy & Maczelka, 2011, 1:01:52). Kupny calmly guides viewers through the postapocalyptic footage:

> There you can see the ruins of the control center ... this is a piece of nuclear combustion rod. ... You can see the total chaos inside ... all sorts of building materials. This is a piece of solidified nuclear fuel. And here we have a graphite rod! They say this room will be deconstructed, but to do that they have to know where things are buried. ... Here is one of the known locations of lavalike material—nuclear fuel—but there is much more of this, all over the reactor. It slowly falls apart and disperses.
>
> (Bendarjevskiy & Maczelka, 2011, 1:02:03)

These dosimetrist-filmmakers, these daredevil documentarians, are possessed by the epistemophilic drive. Despite obvious health hazards, they do its bidding: the work of unveiling, penetrating and cataloguing, of measuring and documenting all. "Fear is a very natural feeling," remarks Kupny. "I didn't have fear that prevented me from going inside. Rather, I was afraid of the unknown. People always fear what they don't know" (Bendarjevskiy & Maczelka, 2011, 1:02:24).

The voice-over elaborates Kupny's commentary on fear. Many famous Soviet scientists and nuclear engineers arrived in Chernobyl knowing "full well the risk; they had buried friends and colleagues." The first inspectors of the damaged reactor "ignored safety regulations and took off protective lead gear so that they could maneuver more easily in narrow spaces." They of course understood nuclear energy and its danger. Because liquidators were allowed to receive a specific, maximum dose of radiation, they removed and left behind their survey dosimeters in order to produce lower readings and be given the opportunity to return. The British narrator concludes that scientists' "jobs and their efforts to control the catastrophe meant more to them than their own lives" (Bendarjevskiy & Maczelka, 2011, 1:02:45).

Viewers are invited to feel the tragedy and heroism in the story of these highly educated, brave men. And yet, we sense immediately a certain jouissance—an excess of meaning—motives external to ethics and sense. Like Kupny, these nuclear scientists and engineers went to Chernobyl for reasons they could not completely fathom. They entered the sarcophagus in search of the sublime: paradise, the inconceivable, reunion with the lost object. "I was a pioneer discovering a new world," Kupny muses, "I wasn't afraid [about my health]. My curiosity, my desire to see with my own eyes what was inside helped me overcome my fear." He admits, "the sarcophagus, in the best sense, infects people. It attracts and pulls like a magnet." Kupny says he would go there again, but since the mid-2000s "there has been a push to stop illegal entries" (Bendarjevskiy & Maczelka, 2011, 1:03:57, 1:06:14).

The sarcophagus, like Andrei Tarkovsky's Room, is the heart of the Exclusion Zone. Stalkers flock there, to the Object, to realize their deepest wishes. They are impelled by an identification with the object, an urge to embrace its sheer thingness, emptied of meaning, to escape the Other's dizzying vacancy. Is their relation to the Object (and the object) a suicidal *passage à l'acte*? Repetition compulsion? An illness of mourning for a Soviet future, unfulfilled?

~

I found videos online of my plastic surgeon interviewed by a handsome woman of morning television fame. J. D. Forceps, MD, reconstructed her breasts after a preventive bilateral mastectomy. She is positively thrilled to rehearse her story and to see Dr. Forceps in a nonmedical setting. Dr. Forceps, radiant and self-assured, declares: "Reconstruction is a woman's choice. There is a federal law in place that entitles women to have insurance pay for reconstruction and any parts [*sic*] that have to do with the reconstruction, at any time."[1] My own, highly regarded Dr. Forceps, whom I share with attractive television personalities and countless others, informs women that they can get new breasts whenever they want, or not at all, and instructs them on how and where they might find qualified surgeons.

Years earlier, I was nonplussed to discover YouTube videos of my analyst giving talks about endometriosis patients. At annual conferences dedicated to the disease, he appears as an expert in matters of psyche and pain. Not just any pain, endometrial pain. My analyst administers preoperative care and counseling and gathers data and insight that he then dispenses to patients, nurses, and doctors. I imagined his other analysands poring over these banal videos with a mixture of shame, guilt, and bitterness. I made several attempts to watch one but always lost interest a quarter of the way through.

Both my surgeon and my analyst are preoccupied with women's suffering. What are they doing, these men, in my domain? What draws them there, over and over? Again, I wonder: What is this repetition, this recycling and recall? What or whom are they trying to mourn?

~

A Russian-speaking interviewer meets Kupny in the Chernobyl Nuclear Power Information Center, where there are photographs, diagrams, and a scale model of the Object of Shelter. Kupny makes sweeping hand gestures over the miniature sarcophagus and proceeds to name and disassemble its components: "Here we have the Counterforce Wall ... this is the western side. From the north is the Cascade Wall. This is the part you can see from the observation deck." He points to and strokes the top of the model. "These are called the Northern Hockey Sticks, and these are the Southern Hockey Sticks," Kupny says, touching roof panels that look nothing like hockey sticks. The pet names accumulate: "This here is called the Cathouse, and this is called the Doghouse" (Bendarjevskiy & Maczelka, 2011, 53:47).

One's impression is that the architects, builders, and engineers of the sarcophagus created more than a concrete structure; they immersed themselves, with considerable zeal, in the construction of fantasy and metaphor. They sought to domesticate their tomb, to shroud it in sentimentality. Just as the Hockey Sticks bear no resemblance to sporting equipment, the Cathouse and Doghouse share no discernable features with shelters for cats and dogs. The Object is, first and foremost, a love object.

"This is the light roofing," Kupny explains, gently removing it from the turbine hall. He had just unhinged the front wall to reveal a large part of the interior, its chaotic wreckage meticulously recreated. The core's radiation shield, a 2,000-ton lead plug catapulted into the air by the explosion, landed on its side and became lodged at the top of the core. Kupny notices that in the model the shield has been placed erroneously right side up and quickly repositions it. He then lifts another layer of the roof: "These pipes were on the Airplane Beams …" The interviewer is compelled to interrupt: "Why—What is with all these names?!" Kupny is dismissive. "Oh, who knows! The builders named them. … This one here is the Mammoth Beam … and this is the Octopus" (Bendarjevskiy & Maczelka, 2011, 56:38). When pressed about the origin of the names, Kupny insists that they are the official terms that appear in archival documents. "So many," he admits, and suddenly grows ebullient, recalling a bit of Chernobyl lore:

> There are other strange nicknames, too. For instance, there is the so-called Dosifey Staircase. I knew about it in 1988 but only recently, last year, learned the story behind [its naming]. I'd heard different versions … that it had been called that because of some construction worker or building engineer … but that's not true. It turns out that there was a man named Dosifey Stepa—I don't remember his patronymic, to be honest … Dosifey Shchepkov! He is a specialist in building materials, a veritable walking encyclopedia. When someone would ask him about the type of concrete used in the construction of such and such part of the Object, he would be able to tell the person exactly what brand was utilized, when and how, etcetera, down to the last atom. So, the Dosifey Staircase was built according to his blueprints, and he frequently used it.
>
> (Bendarjevskiy & Maczelka, 2011, 54:14)

I immediately associate to another Dosifey. In Modest Mussorgsky's 5-hour operatic masterpiece *Khovanshchina* (1881), the patriarch Dosifey is the fanatical leader of the Muscovite Old Believers, schismatics who believe that Tsar Peter's Western reforms have ruined the Orthodox Church and precipitated the apocalypse. Because the end of the world is near, and a love triangle threatens to overshadow the political drama, Dosifey's disciple Marfa convinces the old man and his other followers to join her in collective self-immolation:

We are betrayed, surrounded. There is nowhere to hide,
We cannot save ourselves.
Fate has bound us together
And ordained the hour of our death.
                                    (Mussorgsky, 1881/1992)

In most productions of this gripping last scene, the Old Believers, steered by Dosifey and Marfa, form a procession, mount their stake via the ubiquitous operatic stage prop—a ladder, or a staircase to nowhere—and sing a hymn as they go up in pyrotechnic smoke: "We have no fear, father. / Our faith is sacred before God and will remain unshakable" (Mussorgsky, 1881/1992).

Kupny's Dosifey is also a true believer, a relic, a Soviet holy fool. Legend has it that he would go to the ravaged reactor alone, with a small thermos and other modest provisions. "He'd always have with him a little something to drink and eat in case [debris] fell on him. ... *This man*," stresses Kupny, "*realistically understood* that he was going to a dangerous place, where he could *die*, where he might be buried under something. But at the same time, he went there with the deep conviction that two or three sandwiches would be enough to tide him over until someone found and rescued him." Ardently gesticulating, Kupny asks, "Do you see *what I mean*? The optimism is breathtaking!" (Bendarjevskiy & Maczelka, 2011, 55:39).

The filmmakers are incredulous of their subject's well-being. Alexander Kupny stands before them vibrant and intact. Given his frequent exposure to radioactive material, they are pressed to inquire about his health. Kupny is evasive. The interviewer seeks to make romance of his weary reality.

As I always say: My health problems are not unique ... I mean, who doesn't have health problems? They are the same as those of an average 50-year-old man. That is, I have no specific illnesses, at least *so far*, that could be linked to my work inside the Object of Shelter. *So far.*
                                    (Bendarjevskiy & Maczelka, 2011, 1:10:49)

Kupny was conceived and raised beside nuclear power plants. His parents worked in such plants their whole lives. For him, the gut of the sarcophagus is the primal scene, the parental bedroom. He goes there to "peep in," to dig deeper and deeper, to investigate the disaster, as well as more fundamental matters: *Why was I born? What is my purpose? What is at the bottom of it all?* These questions, unanswerable and invisible, "pull like a magnet." The Object is not *the object*, but its shelter, a surface representation of the drive to know and see all. Kupny imperiled his life and ignored fear for the chance to get to "the other side of the wall," to close the gap; to hear the crackle of the dosimeter and view the white dots on film.

The Object is a lure, and it is satisfaction; it is also a coffin. A thing concealing the Thing. There is nothing there but decaying waste, indifferent and immortal. Alexander Kupny, the legendary Dosifey, and the engineers and builders who warmly named the beams and walls returned repeatedly to the sarcophagus to conduct research, certainly, but also to continue the project their parents and grandparents had lived for and failed to complete. The epistemophilic drive and the death drive are one. Science is a cover for the inability to mourn.

~

Sebastián Lelio's 2017 film *A Fantastic Woman* testifies to the violent forms the search for knowledge can take, and to the centrality of mourning for subjectivity. The mesmerizing trans mezzo-soprano Marina Vidal, played by the mesmerizing trans mezzo-soprano Daniela Vega, has an adoring older boyfriend, Orlando (Francisco Reyes). They are in love; they celebrate Marina's birthday and discuss a trip to Iguazú Falls; they go dancing, return home, and have steamy sex. In the wee hours, Orlando wakes up in distress and collapses, it turns out, from an aneurysm. The frightened Marina rushes him to the hospital, but he cannot be saved.

Twenty minutes in and Orlando is no more. His death is sudden, unexpected and postcoital, a brutal cut in what appears to have been his sexual renaissance. He had not put his affairs in order, nor established a place for Marina in his will and within his family. The remainder of the film is about Marina trying to mourn Orlando, to attend his wake and funeral; to care for their dog, Diabla; to grieve and memorialize the fullness of the man she knew. In essence, to bury him. To do this she must be acknowledged by others as his partner and his beloved. She must be recognized as a woman—and as his woman.

Marina is continually thwarted. She is misgendered, assaulted, defamed, and dehumanized by Orlando's son Bruno (Nicolás Saavedra) and ex-wife, Sonia (Aline Küppenheim), and by hospital staff and law enforcement. The shared view is that Orlando and Marina's relationship is perverse and that she must be silenced and eradicated. Bruno and Sonia attempt to bully Marina into severing all ties to Orlando and their life together. They evict her from his apartment and bar her from memorial services; they try to seize custody of Diabla. The family goes so far as to involve the police, implicating Marina in Orlando's death. A female detective (Amparo Noguera) with a prurient interest in the case threatens to arrest Marina unless she reports to the Sexual Offenses Unit. Marina eventually complies and is forced to submit to a gratuitous medical examination. She is told to strip, waist down, in front of the investigators.

Virtually from the start, we understand that the main preoccupation of Marina's various enemies—Orlando's family, the detective, and the medical examiners—is the question of what is *down there*, between her legs. In a sense, it consumes Marina and Lelio, too, as both she and the film work hard to resist an easy solution to the issue of her sexual identity, an identity not reducible to genitalia. Despite (or because of) Marina's fortitude and statuesque beauty, viewers are made complicit in the many oblique and direct attempts to see underneath her clothes. Guided and enframed by the camera, they are implicated not only in the drive to know, urgently, what is not shown (whether Marina has had surgery or not); they are also invited to identify with the frustration, rage, and pain of others engaged in such a quest. Bruno and his thuggish friends kidnap Marina and viciously wrap her head in sealing tape, disfiguring her face. But she survives, unscarred and self-possessed. After carefully ripping and removing the tape, she walks the streets of Santiago, dazed yet without blemish. Though epithets like "chimera" and "monster" are hurled at Marina, she is indomitable, peering into the camera, close-up, in overproximity.

This is the fantastic Transgender Body: it throws all bodies into question. It is a scandal, like sex itself. It insists on heterogeneity and so ignites the pressing desire to resolve sexual difference and proclaim male–female complementarity. Trans bodies are violently attacked because people want to put an end to that which confuses, that which reveals the noncoincidence of truth and knowledge. "When I look at you," Sonia tells Marina, "I don't know what I'm seeing!" (Lelio, 2017, 47:40). Marina is a woman who gives the lie to Woman. Woman, she shows us, does not exist: She is necessarily fantastic. There are only women.

Resilient as she is, Marina has not achieved transcendence. She, too, is caught in projects of subjectification and her own illusory quests. At the beginning of the film, she appears as a phallicized nightclub performer singing a torch song for Orlando's gaze. A typical hysteric, she flaunts an "excess of visibility"—a stagey flat character—in order to maintain deception, to keep herself invisible (Copjec, 2002, p. 124). On the evidence, then, Marina, if not defined by a man, is a woman in pursuit of phallic significance. When Orlando dies, Marina's identification as a woman becomes linked to her ability to publicly mourn her lover, which, in turn, is dependent on inheritance, ritual, and naming, all in recognition of their love relationship. Until she bids Orlando a proper farewell, his apparition regularly surfaces: in the backseat of their car, in a nightclub, in the morgue. Orlando ceases to haunt Marina when she manages to get back Diabla and descend into an underground crematorium to view his body for the last time. A melancholic cycle is thereby averted.

But for much of the movie, Marina's future seems, at best, uncertain. In a reversal of film noir logic, the femme fatale goes sleuthing, too. Our stoic enchantress is not above needing to find out, to get to the bottom of things. During Marina's birthday dinner, Orlando tells her that he misplaced the tickets he'd bought for their trip. The bungled action, along with a key given to Marina at the hospital, becomes a parting message and creates a mystery, postmortem. To what door does the key belong and what will it unlock? Will Marina be able to go to Iguazú Falls, fulfilling Orlando's final dream for the couple? The key is an object of fascination for Marina until the penultimate, climactic scenes, when she figures out that it belongs to a locker at a sauna—the same sauna Orlando visited before meeting her on the night of his death. In a suspense-filled sequence, Marina courageously infiltrates the sauna's men's locker room. Anxious but determined, hair fixed in a ponytail, she undresses and wraps a towel around her hips, stripping in order to disguise herself. Finally, she opens the locker door. In two Hitchcockian tunnel shots, we first see Marina's gaze from inside, her face bordered by the locker doorframe. Next, we observe the interior of the locker from her point of view: it is empty, a deepening void. The answer is stark and absolute. There is no Other, except in fantasy. The sole truth is that there is nothing to find out. Marina has no choice but to walk away.

Jacques Lacan's notoriously difficult "sexuation formulas," thrown together in the 1970s during his 20th seminar, are depicted in a two-sided, four-part diagram with a masculine (left) side and a feminine (right) side. Men and women in this scheme are psychically determined structures that bear no relation to biology or anatomy. Sexual difference is fundamentally asymmetrical and rooted in a subject's position with respect to jouissance (the drive) and the Other (language, the signifier). On the masculine side, the logic is as follows: There is at least one x that is not submitted to the phallic function. For all x the phallic function is valid. This means that everyone is subjected to the signifying order, and to castration—everyone has had to give up what he has never had, that is, unlimited enjoyment—because there exists One who is not castrated: the mythical primal father, the Woman. Castration is the subtraction of something; it is a minus that is imposed by language and the social realm. There is always something I cannot express as a speaking being. And since I was born into language and into society, there was never a time I could express it: Even the baby's first cry immediately becomes a call *for something*, a cry to which meaning is attributed by caregivers. Each subject in his unique way transforms what he never had, the "minus one" of the Symbolic—into something one has renounced, or lost (Zupančič, 2017, p. 51). What does this logic imply for masculine-positioned subjects? Philosopher Alenka Zupančič (2017) offers an overview:

> The mythical One of exception (the One, which, by being "cut out" … provides the signifying *frame* of the inaugural minus) also constitutes the frame or the "window of fantasy" … through which the other can be desirable (as object-cause of desire). In other words: the formal structure that provides the signifying frame for the lack of the signifier, combined with the particular circumstances in which this "swap" takes place for a subject, determines the concrete conditions under which (and only under which) the Other appears desirable.
>
> (p. 52)

Masculine subjects can only know phallic jouissance, that is, sexual pleasure necessarily mediated by signification and fantasy.

The feminine side of the formulas is electrifying. It is precisely because castration allows for no exception that universal statements about women are impossible. Woman is the Other of Man (since the phallus is the signifier of Man), but Man is not the Other of Woman (there is no signifier for the essence of Woman). Woman, Lacan asserts, is "the Other, in the most radical sense, in the sexual relationship." She cannot be for herself the exception that proves the rule: "There is no Other of the Other," and, further, the nonexistence of the Other is inscribed in the Other. Speaking beings cannot know *all* not because of an inaccessible reality—an unreachable knowledge—but, rather, because there is a (constitutive) gap in knowledge itself. This is the unconscious. The implications are borne out by another claim: "Being the Other, … woman is that which has a relationship to the Other" (Lacan, 1972–1973/1998b, p. 81). Lacan's so-called feminine jouissance, or "Other jouissance," is the signifier of this inconsistency in the Other, this gap in knowledge. Zupančič (2017) again provides clarification:

> The emergence of the signifying order directly coincides with the nonemergence of one signifier, and at the place of this gap appears enjoyment [jouissance] as the heterogeneous element pertaining to the signifying structure, yet irreducible to it. … The enjoyment at stake … belongs to the unconscious (and its gap): not as repressed, but as the very substance of the missing signifier, which, as missing, gives its form to the unconscious. This also explains Lacan's emphasis … on the question of knowledge and its "limits": Can one know—and say—anything about this other, non-phallic enjoyment? No. … This other enjoyment cannot be the object of knowledge because it is a placeholder for the knowledge that does not exist. … Feminine jouissance is not an obstacle to the sexual relation but a symptom of its nonexistence.
>
> (pp. 53–54)

Even Marina, who endures so much societal resistance in laying claim to her specific bodily morphology and gender identity, must grapple with self-destructive repetitions premised on binary logic and the existence of Woman. She sees, finally, that the box is empty and there is no getting to the other side of it. There is no sexual rapport, no symmetrical relation between the sexes. What is more, the nonrelation of masculine and feminine "does not stop not being written" (Lacan, 1972–1973/1998b, p. 94). Every concrete invention designed to patch it up, every resolution of the non-rapport, instantly posits its own negation (Zupančič, 2017, p. 146, fn. 6). Each of us must figure out how to live in her body and with her drives. Just as there is no "trans experience," there is no defining feminine characteristic. There is only Marina/Daniela, her distinctive features.

A pivotal shot follows the crematorium visit and a brief scene of Marina jogging with her reclaimed Diabla. We see a side view of the heroine sitting naked in bed with knees slightly bent. The camera inches closer, enticing viewers with a potential revelation of the secret of Marina's anatomy. But then it cuts to a POV shot of Marina's face reflected in a travel-size round mirror covering her genitals. Having sought answers below the waist, the audience is chastened. Marina's face is in seamless correspondence with herself, and this correspondence completes her self-actualization and mourning.

One could well agree that subjectivity is located at the borders of bodily apertures, where eyes, mouth, and nostrils pass into gaze, voice, and smell. There is nothing to see, dear viewer, behind the small round mirror; nothing, at least, that will decide Marina's sex. But this is not the entire story. Marina has to mourn something besides Orlando. Perhaps the object of mourning is her former body: not her real, physical body, but the fantasied body, its felt surface and psychic representation. Perhaps it is the idea of her wholeness, or wholeness as such.

Shortly after the forced medical exam, Marina calls on her former voice teacher (Sergio Hernández) for a brush-up lesson and paternal tenderness. She comes to him, mostly, in search of love. The grizzled maestro receives Marina through a refusal. "You can't look for love," he insists, quoting St. Francis: "[He] doesn't say: 'give me light, give me peace, give me this, give me that.' He says: 'make me an instrument of your love; make me a channel of your peace'" (Lelio, 2017, 58:44). Marina learns that she must sing, not salsa or merengue, but high, like an angel. She must return to opera.

Lacan has something else pertinent to tell us about the feminine subject's relation to the barred Other, and it has to do with sublimation. His concept of sublimation diverges from the Freudian variant, at least as the latter is commonly understood. Sublimation in Lacanian teaching is not about substituting a more refined pleasure for a base, carnal one. Rather, it posits sublimation as the drive's *proper activity*.

> While the *aim* of the drive is death, the … positive activity of the drive is to inhibit the attainment of its aim … the drive *as such* is inhibited as to its aim, it is sublimated, "the sublimation of the drive through the inhibition of its aim" being the very definition of sublimation.
>
> (Copjec, 2002, p. 30)

Lacan (1964/1998a) says outright in Seminar XI: "Sublimation is satisfaction of the drive, without repression" (p. 165). But in Seminar XX, explains psychoanalyst Bruce Fink (1995), Lacan implies that feminine jouissance relates both to the Freudian variety of sublimation, where the drives are diverted toward the social and satisfied fully ("the Other jouissance"), and to his own, earlier formulation of sublimation: "the ordinary object elevated to the status of the Thing" (p. 115).

> The Freudian Thing finds a signifier … "God," "Jesus," "Mary," "The Virgin," "art," "music," and so on, and the finding of the signifier must be understood as an encounter, that is, as fortuitous in some sense. Apart from the imaginary satisfaction we may associate with religious ecstasy or rapture, or with the artist's or musician's work, there is nevertheless *a real satisfaction obtained* [emphasis added].
>
> (Fink, 1995, p. 115)

Fink's reading of Lacan suggests that sublimation is the feminine path "to the beyond of neurosis," providing consummate satisfaction of the drives. In iterations like religious ecstasy, or a "bodily, corporal jouissance," it is asexual, that is, not limited to sexual organs (1995, p. 120). This is Lacan's version of cure through love. It is also the primary theme of *A Fantastic Woman*.

Marina is changed at the conclusion of the film, and the metamorphosis has little to do with gender transition or new lovers. In the final scene, she arrives at a theater where she sings "Ombra mai fu," the opening aria of George Frideric Handel's

Serse (1738). A close-up of Marina reveals that she is wearing a tight-fitting gold key necklace. The object that once opened the door to a void is now repurposed— made golden and symbolic—and placed near her music-making throat. The original, real key proved useless, failing to provide information, and yet it cleared the path to the production of glorious vocal art.

Marina doesn't simply channel her libido into making music. She embraces the voice-as-object—its duality and in-betweenness—her own otherness. Lacan observed that the human voice bears a ventriloquistic quality: It is never simply mine, never a property of myself as a body. Because the voice escapes the mouth and has an independent materiality, it is always object *a*, an organ inside oneself that feels like a foreign intruder. The voice is also heard, taken in by others: It is an aspect of the social link. If vocalized speech is language, the domain of the Other, it is simultaneously a physical entity that exceeds the system of differences governed by the signifier. Utterance as carrier and product of a speaker's singularity—inflection, timbre, grain, and pure resonance—normally acts as a vanishing mediator destined to be subsumed by meaning. But operatic high notes, which make speech inaudible and shatter meaning, allow the singularity of the singer to float to the surface, revealing the voice as the locus of subjectivity. Marina's voice is in a dialectical relationship with sexual difference, redoubling and erasing it in merry-go-round fashion. She sings mezzo-soprano, the *fach* of *travesti* roles. And she performs an aria originally composed for castrati, using falsetto.

In an act of Lacanian sublimation, Marina assumes her body and herself. She accomplishes her act via the signifiers *key* and *opera*, and through singing. Genitals, sexual characteristics, are nowhere on the scene and, in any case, insufficient: they are imaginary, mere semblance. Marina's voice moves her away from objects, things, and penetration—the locker, the phallus, the questions of what is inside and underneath—and toward object *a*, the Thing, exchange, and receptivity. Marina acts by inventing, devising a unique way of using her voice (which is not fully hers) to become, in the words of her teacher, an instrument of others' love.

A Fantastic Woman writes the difference between perversion and sublimation. Marina is not a voice fetishist. She utilizes and elevates the voice as an object of lack. From a woman who hides through hypervisibility she transforms into a woman who loves by giving what she doesn't have.

~

Sound reproduction redefines rather than destroys the ritual value of a work of art. Record producers do not merely capture but also construct "live" performances. Music scholar Evan Eisenberg (1987/2005) recognizes this, declaring: "There is no original musical event that a record records or reproduces. Instead, each playing of a given record is an instance of something timeless. The original musical event never occurred; it exists, if it exists anywhere, outside history. In short, it is myth, just like the myths reenacted in primitive ritual." Studio recordings record *nothing*, Eisenberg provocatively writes, and recordings "piece together bits of actual events" to "construct an ideal event" (pp. 41, 89).

Just as Walter Benjamin's "aura" is the retroactive creation of mechanical reproduction, the "natural breast" is a byproduct of mastectomy. The "original" body, once identical with itself, becomes post-mastectomy the object of nostalgia. My transformation was meticulously documented by the plastic surgeon's office. Six views of my torso were photographed prior to the first surgery and at the conclusion of every post-op visit. Five times I stood bare-chested looking straight ahead; three-quarter view, side view, right and left. Click-click-click-click-click-click. Dr. Forceps has a record of his exemplary work. At the end of the reconstruction process, I requested a copy of the archived slides but failed to recognize myself in these acephalic shots, the uncanny residue of the Before. Mastectomy and reconstruction produce an idealized, presurgical body that resists depiction. It exists, if it exists at all, in the fantasy support of an elusive and circular drive. The remaining "natural" breast is lifted and reshaped to resemble the silicone forgery.

A cover-up! I opted for the misleading "immediate reconstruction." Even the initial breast implant surgery is really a two-step process. I awoke from the mastectomy with a tissue expander where my right breast used to be: an empty balloon-like plastic sac that had been inserted under the pectoral muscle. Over about 5 weeks, using a syringe, the sac was gradually inflated with saline to stretch the muscles and skin to a size larger than my left breast. The sac hardened, making the skin into an envelope that eventually would hold a slightly smaller and more supple prosthetic. My chest ached for days after each expansion, and by the end of the process I was in severe discomfort, especially at night. During the next, "exchange" surgery, which I was told would be "easy-peasy," the expander was removed and replaced with a silicone gel implant.

I started going to Dr. Forceps's office for expansion 3 weeks after the mastectomy. There was something highly satisfying about those appointments. They served a holding function. The staff pampered me and recognized my new body. I often became lightheaded after injections. Nurses assured me I could stay reclined as long as I wanted. They brought me water and graham crackers and chatted about how well I was doing. At Dr. F's the ordeal was reduced to appearance. A "good result" meant the best possible cosmetic outcome. Neither function and cancer nor pain and sexual pleasure were permitted on the scene. Form and symmetry, surface, and the gazes of others were primary concerns. *Can people tell the difference? Can I pass for a woman with two natural breasts? Will I be found out?*

"Look at you! You look great!"

"I would never know!"

"Here, adjust the bra like this … completely symmetrical!"

After a few saline fills, I attended an academic conference to which I had committed a year in advance. The trip from New York to Chicago, intended as a flight into health, was a mélange of nausea, gastrointestinal pain, and psychic suffering. It was a manic attempt at normalcy as well as a daring flirtation with exposure. Upon arrival at the conference hotel, I grabbed an empty table in the lobby and proceeded to edit my paper. Sentences formed on the screen, but my attention was elsewhere. I glanced up from my computer and saw familiar colleagues. Did my body appear diseased and misshapen? I wanted to hide, and yet I also yearned for affirmations of health and wholeness. Turning outward, I searched the faces of acquaintances for signs of warm recognition. Shame and guilt intertwined, aiming to undo each other.

Joan Copjec (2006) describes "anxiety as the sentiment of a negative capacity *to not be* which we flee by choosing social existence, where we appear not only to others but also to ourselves." One's own gaze and consequent shame are found in the "space of publicity" (p. 26). When I am ashamed, I am threatened externally but also revealed to myself. Copjec draws a distinction between shame and guilt, for the latter is an alternate response to anxiety:

> The … desire to brush aside barriers and veils arises through a specific … relation to our culture which we can call guilt. Common to the affects of anxiety, guilt, and shame is our sense of an inalienable and yet unintegratable surplus of self. In guilt this surplus no longer weighs on us as the burden of an unfinished past, but as the unfinished business of the present. The sentiment of our opacity to ourselves is disavowed and in its place arises the sentiment of being excluded from ourselves by exterior barriers. … The mechanisms of this conversion of anxiety into guilt are the social and ego ideals, which relieve us of the responsibility of having to invent a future without the aid of rules or scripts. Ideals give our actions directions, goals to strive for, and thus alleviate the overwhelming sentiment of anxiety. But because ideals are unattainable, by definition, the (bitter) taste of the absolute is still discernible in them through the experience of the elusive beyond they bring into existence.
>
> (2006, pp. 23–24)

We escape the absolute, a devouring ancestral quicksand, and run to the social sphere. But trouble arises when

> the realm of social appearance seems to offer a poor reflection of who we are, if in gaining an appearance we seem to lose ourselves. When among all the images of myself and others, I remain absent. When the cost of appearing in the world is the loss of my own gaze, of the "I" who sees myself in my public image, then the passion … associated with guilt is aroused: to break through the façade of appearances.
>
> (Copjec, 2006, p. 26)

I imagine Audre Lorde's judgmental glare. Guilty, I incant her arguments against breast reconstruction. Audre Lorde, driven by guilt, devastated by cancer, urged one-breasted women to reveal themselves, to see one another's truth and unite around their loss. Through visibility we would get beyond appearances. Audre Lorde, robbed of her right breast, did not countenance women nursing their lacks privately while their missing body parts were hidden in plain sight.

~

The first sarcophagus, elephantine and porous, was built mainly to hide radioactive materials. Wrapping the wound was more important than treating the infection.

Alexander Kupny warned in 2011 that inspections of the wrecked reactor had all but ceased. Internal dangers remained, but for decades they received scant attention. Such use of the Object was of course emblematic, both of Mikhail Gorbachev's initial handling of the accident and the Soviet modus operandi generally: Systemic problems had to be hidden, atrocities effaced, industrial catastrophes attributed to a handful of saboteurs. Symptoms arise and multiply after such repressions. Kupny understood but failed to know this.

Sigmund Freud wrote that repetition appears at the site of trauma: We repeat what we fail to remember. The psychoanalytic clinic is a space in which the compulsion to repeat leads to "acting out"; it is also the motor of transference. In the presence of the analyst, one is compelled to repeat so as to remember and work through traumatic events. Post-Freudians have elaborated these mechanisms: The trauma being repeated is not repressed but, rather, external to the realm of experience. For D. W. Winnicott (1974), an individual might live with unconscious anxiety over a breakdown that already has happened but not been experienced. The "need to experience" is for some "the equivalent of a need to remember" (p. 105).

But if psychoanalytic literature offers a too-neat division between the processes of repeating and remembering, "culture blurs them," offers Russianist Alexander Etkind (2013):

> On the stage of postcatastrophic memory ... repetition and remembering produce warped imagery, which combines the analytic, self-conscious exploration of the past with its reverberations and transfigurations. Spirits, ghosts ... and other creatures conflate reenactments with remembrances in creative forms that can be naive or sophisticated, regressive or productive, influential or isolated. What we usually fear is the uncertainty of the future, but we often imagine this future as a repetition of the past. ... If the suffering is not remembered, it will be repeated. If the loss is not recognized, it threatens to return in strange though not entirely new forms, as the uncanny. When the dead are not properly mourned, they turn into the undead and cause trouble for the living.
>
> (pp. 16–17)

Etkind the cultural historian is more interested in mourning than melancholia and trauma, for the latter already have received much scholarly attention and are not especially suited to historical investigation. Where trauma is unsymbolized and melancholia is contained within the subject, mourning is an address to the other. Mourning consists of attempts to remember, creatively work through, and make loss manifest in poetry, memorials, film, and other art forms. With this definition, Etkind concludes that Soviet mourning was warped: "In matters of mourning, Freud based his distinction between the healthy and the sick on the subject's ability to acknowledge the reality of the loss. But this distinction did not work well in the terrorized Soviet Union" (2013, p. 17).

The deadly incarcerations of the Stalinist 1930s were not fully worked through for a number of reasons: The gulag was a product of state violence (and the state controls public mourning), the division between perpetrators and victims was far from clear, and mourning the persecuted eventually became entwined with the mourning of communist ideals. Improper burial and recognition of the dead, and consequent unfinished mourning, generated a culture replete with specters and uncanny monsters. The unpaid debt to the unburied, in turn, produced a strange temporality: Russia's present is inordinately flooded by the past. In the absence of proper monuments or sufficient memory making, history haunts Russia, propelling its politics and shaping its narratives with an immediacy and force unknown in the West.

The Chernobyl catastrophe presents such a mixture of repeating and remembering that resists dialectization. Its central monument, the sarcophagus, invites a compulsive epistemophilia, the spawn of the death drive. Kupny's and others' repeated quests for truth and knowledge are also attempts at mourning: They are ritualized, sacred, and interminable. But to mourn that which is hidden, unseen is a laborious task. The radioactive waste must be excavated, scrutinized, documented. Radiation-related and "natural" deaths must be distinguished and catalogued.

It was the regime's secrecy that gave rise to Chernobyl's human-made catastrophe, and secrets are what drive its pilgrims. The cover-up is thereby remembered and repeated. "Like a magnet," the sarcophagus pulls to itself the voyeur, the scientist, the researcher. But the truth of Chernobyl will never be known, and its dead will never be counted. The full breadth of the devastation cannot be represented. The sarcophagus is a cover-up of a cover-up, the crypt of the sublime object, a trauma excluded from time and experience.

That the Chernobyl disaster was ignited by nuclear energy is in itself a trauma transmitted across generations. Nuclear power plants had been the bright hope of the Soviet Union, symbols of conquered nature and the building of a new world. Now post-socialist descendants swim in their own and their parents' shit, unable to drain it away. In the words of Kupny's father: "We've been liquidating [the accident] for 25 years now. My son, my grandson, and my great-grandson will all be liquidating, and this will continue until all the strontium, cesium, and plutonium decay," that is, for thousands of years (Bendarjevskiy & Maczelka, 2011, 1:11:24).

~

The recently erected sarcophagus, the New Safe Confinement, is a smooth semicircular structure, a 303-foot arch of burnished steel. Breast-like and obscene, evocative of the first part-object, it is an uncanny monument to originary loss. This monstrosity—this nippleless breast that conceals the initial Object and its lethal radioactive loot—cannot but induce repulsion and awe.

Philosopher Ray Brassier (2007) universalizes the notion of trauma as real but not experienced. In his reading of "Beyond the Pleasure Principle," where Freud (1920/1955a) discusses the death drive as the return to the inanimate, Brassier explains that repetition is driven by the originary traumatic occurrence: Again, this is not an experience but rather a scar or trace that *conditions experience as such* and constitutes the subject's capacity for experiencing something as "traumatic." The objective nature of trauma, in other words, creates the subject of the unconscious, enabling psychic life. The separation of organic interiority from inorganic exteriority is achieved at the cost of the death of a piece of the organism:

> This death, which gives birth to organic individuation, thereby conditions the possibility of organic phylogenesis, as well as of sexual reproduction.
>
> Consequently, not only does this death precede the organism, it is the precondition of the organism's ability to reproduce and die. If the death drive *qua* compulsion to repeat is the originary, primordial motive force driving organic life, this is because the motor of repetition—the repeating instance—is the trace of the aboriginal trauma of organic individuation. … The death drive is the trace of this scission: a scission that will never be successfully *bound* (invested) because it remains the *unbindable* excess that makes binding possible.
>
> (Brassier, 2007, pp. 237–238)

My wound is dressed, but the scar remains. I stuff it into a bra—and still, there it is, attracting attention in its negativity. I return again and again to Famous Cancer Hospital for injections of saline. The replacement mound grows while the trauma screams silently. How can I mourn the surface of my former body when the fissure is in the Real? There are no public rituals, no funeral, and no grave to visit. The premastectomy body is gone, chopped up. How does one mourn a body part, especially the breast, the mythic lost object—an object always already lost, prior to memory and prior to experience?

Note

1   I have chosen not to cite the video as it would reveal the identity of my plastic surgeon.

References

Alexievich, S. (2005). *Voices from Chernobyl: The oral history of a nuclear disaster* (K. Gessen, Trans.). Dalkey Archive Press. (Original work published 1997)

Bendarjevskiy, A., & Maczelka, M. (Directors). (2011). *Chernobyl's heritage: The zone* [Film]. Urania Cinema. YouTube. Retrieved June 14, 2019, from https://www.youtube.com/watch?v=l-nvfu9QA8k

Blackwell, A. (2012). *Visit sunny Chernobyl, and other adventures in the world's most polluted places*. Rodale, Inc.

Brassier, R. (2007). *Nihil unbound: Enlightenment and extinction*. Palgrave Macmillan.

Copjec, J. (2002). *Imagine there's no woman: Ethics and sublimation*. MIT Press.

Copjec, J. (2006). The object-gaze: Shame, hejab, cinema. *Filozofski vestnik*, *27*(2), 11–29.

Eisenberg, E. (2005). *The recording angel: Music, records and culture from Aristotle to Zappa* (2nd ed.). Yale University Press. (Original work published 1987)

Etkind, A. (2013). *Warped mourning: Stories of the undead in the land of the unburied*. Stanford University Press.

Fink, B. (1995). *The Lacanian subject: Between language and jouissance*. Princeton University Press.

Freud, S. (1955a). Beyond the pleasure principle. In J. Strachey et al. (Eds. & Trans.), *The standard edition of the complete psychological works of Sigmund Freud* (Vol. 18, pp. 1–64). Hogarth Press. (Original work published 1920)

Lacan, J. (1998a). *The seminar of Jacques Lacan: Book XI. The four fundamental concepts of psychoanalysis* (J.-A. Miller, Ed.; A. Sheridan, Trans.). W. W. Norton & Company. (Original lectures presented 1964)

Lacan, J. (1998b). *The seminar of Jacques Lacan: Book XX. On feminine sexuality: The limits of love and knowledge, 1972–1973* (J.-A. Miller, Ed.; B. Fink, Trans.). W. W. Norton & Company. (Original lectures presented 1972–1973)

Lelio, S. (Director). (2017). *A fantastic woman* [Film]. Fabula; Komplizen Film.

Mussorgsky, M. (1992). *Khovanshchina* [Album recorded with the Kirov Opera and Orchestra, St. Petersburg, Valery Gergiev, conductor]. Philips. (Original work published 1881)

Plokhy, S. (2018). *Chernobyl: The history of a nuclear catastrophe*. Basic Books.

Winnicott, D. W. (1974). Fear of breakdown. *International Review of Psycho-Analysis, 1*(1–2), 103–107.

Zupančič, A. (2017). *What is sex?* MIT Press.

7

A Dialogue on Loss

Love Letters to Audre Lorde

Audre Lorde died of metastatic breast cancer on November 17, 1992. In September of that year, she agreed to a filming of what would be her last poetry reading, in Berlin. Lorde is gaunt; her voice is thin and hoarse. I wince at each raspy word uttered sotto voce, each clearing of the throat; at the abundant energy expended and the pain endured. Audre Lorde, author of "A Litany for Survival," is dying. Her liver swells with cancer as her body shrinks. It is difficult to watch her struggling to be audible in the intimate, parlor-like setting. I contemplate the courage, the fortitude necessary to sit upright at the table, her giant notebook before her, amid vases of flowers, smiling and hospitable. Off-screen applause follows the reading. I am not alone with Audre, it turns out. She apologizes for her voice, devoid of its former splendor: "I'm sorry it isn't better today, but I hope you could hear the love with which I shared these" (Audre Lorde in Berlin, 2018, 26:08). We could, kind Audre, "black lesbian feminist mother lover poet" (Lorde, 1980/1997, p. 24).

~

In 1977, at 43, Lorde had a cancer scare. A tumor was found in her right breast, biopsied, and determined to be benign. A year later, during a self-exam, she discovered a lump in the same breast. This time the biopsy revealed a malignancy, and she underwent a unilateral mastectomy at Memorial Sloan Kettering on September 22, 1978.

The Cancer Journals was published 2 years later. The collection includes journal entries that begin 6 months after her mastectomy and "extend beyond the completion of the … book." The journal fragments "exemplify the process of integrating this crisis into my life," Lorde explains (1980/1997, p. 8). She also intersperses speeches, essays, and reminiscences that argue vehemently against breast reconstruction, calling it a "pretense," an "empty comfort," and an "atrocity" (Lorde, 1980/1997, pp. 58–59, 62, 70).

~

I do not forget cancer for very long, ever. That keeps me armed and on my toes, but also with a slight background noise of fear. … Visualizations and deep relaxing techniques … help make me a less anxious person, which seems strange, because in other ways, I live with the constant fear of recurrence of another cancer. But

DOI: 10.4324/9781003498582-8

fear and anxiety are not the same at all. One is an appropriate response to a real situation, which I can accept and learn to work through ... the other, anxiety, is an immobilizing yield to ... namelessness, formlessness, voicelessness, and silence.

(Lorde, 1980/1997, p. 12)

Dear Audre:

I was a year older than you when I was diagnosed, at 45. My mammogram was also in September, and now I associate the fall with anxiety, which can feel like falling forever. I too thought of banishing the well-intentioned, concerned friends recommending "mindfulness" exercises. Where was my mother, why couldn't she hold me? My mother had never experienced a suspicious mammogram, serious illness, general anesthesia, surgery of any kind. A perverse erasure of generational boundaries! Suddenly I am older than my mother; I am my mother's mother! I am sick, while she is innocent of existential threat. I might die first. I, too, am a parent. My young son might lose his mother. Audre, I wish I could take away your fear and mine, and the anxiety, the dread of death and things unknown. I would cradle you and myself, and we would sing drowsy duets with serenity and love.

I want to write about the pain ... of waking up in the recovery room, which is worsened by the immediate sense of loss. ... The euphoria of the 2nd day, and how it's been downhill from there. ... I'm so tired of all this. I want to be the person I used to be, the real me.

(Lorde, 1980/1997, pp. 23–24)

Dear Audre:

You are still you! That's what my friend Kate said to me as we crossed the street on a raw December night. The overfilled expander in my chest felt cold and heavy, an intruder pulling at me from the inside. I was sore, silently crying, estranged from myself, and Kate's words buoyed me. You are still you. I also was euphoric on the second day; then began the arduous work of mourning.

The pain of separation from my breast was at least as sharp as the pain of separating from my mother. But I made it once before, so I know I can make it again.

(Lorde, 1980/1997, p. 24)

Dear Audre:

The above lines follow your reflections on the difficulty of making meaning of cancer:

I could not write about the outside threats to my vision and action because the inside pieces were too frightening. This reluctance is a reluctance to deal with myself, with my own experiences and the feelings buried in them, and the conclusions to be drawn from them. It is also, of course, a reluctance to living or re-living, giving life or new life to that pain.

(Lorde, 1980/1997, p. 24)

What you say is true in analysis, and it is my searing truth even as I write these words. Weaning, separation, accepting castration—acknowledging that our speech cannot capture all, and that it exceeds and embarrasses us, that our mothers cannot protect us, cannot save us from mortality—are breathtakingly epitomized in losing one's breast. The repetition, the reliving of the primordial loss, is agonizing.

There is also the matter of sexual difference. We become sexed beings, not-whole, in infancy, as we cry out for nourishment and love and are met with the breast's periodic absence. In utter dependence, we lean upon the self-preservative drives and encounter the unconscious of our primary caregivers, the unfathomable. This mythical anaclitic flourish inaugurates a lifetime of translation and retranslation, repeated attempts and failures to understand sex and death. For these insights I thank Sigmund Freud, Melanie Klein, and Jean Laplanche; and Lana Lin, a brave filmmaker and academic, a cancer survivor and fellow one-breasted woman who preceded me in paying tribute to *The Cancer Journals* with an inspired Kleinian reading.

Klein's theory and your poetry mesmerize, but also disturb and intimidate me. Audre, you evoke Klein at her most literal and revolutionary, across time and culture, arm in arm in your explorations and your fury and courage. Steadfast, you and she conquered worlds you were not supposed to enter.

As I waited ... for my first biopsy, I had grown angry at my right breast because I felt as if it had in some way betrayed me, as if it had become already separate from me and had turned against me by creating this tumor. ... But on the day before my mastectomy I wrote in my journal [that] ... the anger I felt for my right breast last year ha[d] faded. ... My breasts have always been so very precious to me. ... And I think I am prepared to lose [the breast] now ... because I really see it as a choice between my breast and my life, and in that view there cannot be any question. ... And yet if I cried for a hundred years I couldn't possibly express the sorrow I feel ... the sadness and the loss.

(Lorde, 1980/1997, pp. 33–34)

Dear Audre:

At moments I too was angry at my breast. I also pitied and cried for it as for a mother or daughter. I had an accommodating good breast and an attacking bad breast, and the latter had to be eliminated. The amputation was necessary to preserve my nurturing good object, that is, myself. But after the initial crisis and mastectomy, in a time of reflection, I so regretted the hate I'd felt toward my fair and unsuspecting breast, and I wept for the deep and irreparable wound. I dreamed of restoring to my left breast her dear friend and sister, so that she would not be bereft and alone: "Non morir, mio tesoro ... Oh mia figlia!" And now, years later, I grieve because memories fade and new ones aren't in the making. I can no longer recall vividly my right breast's appearance, the pleasure it brought me, the sensation of feeding my son.

The absence of the maternal breast gives rise to persecutory feelings, aggression stimulated by hunger and other forms of discomfort, projected and introjected, and projected again, palpable aches mistaken for menacing external enemies. Occasionally, especially around the anniversary of the diagnosis, I have fantasies of breaking into pieces, rotting internally, the toxins erupting on my skin. I got rid of my bad breast but not its psychic counterpart, and it retaliates from within and from without, in the guises of my mother and my superego—*I* against myself.

"Look at me," she said, opening her ... jacket and standing before me in a tight ... sweater, a gold embossed locket ... provocatively nestling between her two considerable breasts. "Now can you tell which is which?" I admitted that I could not. ... I ached to talk to women about the experience I had just been through, and about what might be to come, and how were they doing it. ... But I needed to talk with women who shared at least some of my major concerns and beliefs. ... And this lady, admirable though she might be, did not. "And it doesn't really interfere with your love life, either, dear. Are you married?" ... I didn't have the moxie or the desire or the courage maybe to say, "I love women." ... [A] groundswell of sadness rolled up over me that filled my mouth and eyes almost to drowning.

(Lorde, 1980/1997, pp. 42–43)

Dear Audre:

It is too easy, perhaps, to deride the woman from Reach for Recovery who visited you in 1978. Her ecstatic exhibitionism, her assumptions about your sexual preferences, her flamboyance and implicit urging to wear a prosthesis—to get on with it already—betray the systemic misogyny, sexism, and homophobia that, as you put it, "had allowed her a little niche to shine in" (Lorde, 1980/1997, p. 42). But even in 2018, with the copious lip service paid to reconstruction being "a woman's choice," the myriad support groups, and the Famous Cancer Hospital's "breast surveys" diligently completed at every plastics appointment, the loss of my breast was consistently reduced to an aesthetic matter. Who in the cancer zone would discuss the loss of sexual pleasure, the erogenous parts of my body? Who would help me live with the numb blankness on the right side of my chest? And why did my plastic surgeon, the esteemed Dr. Forceps, address only my husband when he spoke of improving the appearance of the scar? "I'll fix that, don't worry," he assured the other man in the room. More than 40 years after your clarion *Cancer Journals* there is so much work still to be done.

I looked strange and uneven and peculiar to myself, but somehow, ever so much more myself, and therefore so much more acceptable, than I looked with that thing stuck inside my clothes. For not even the most skillful prosthesis in the world could undo that reality. ... Prosthesis offers the empty comfort of "Nobody will know the difference." But it is that very difference which I wish to affirm, because I have lived with it, and survived it, and wish to share that strength with other women. If we are to translate the silence surrounding breast cancer into language and action against this scourge, then the first step is that women with mastectomies must be visible to each other. For silence and invisibility go hand in hand with powerlessness.

(Lorde, 1980/1997, pp. 44, 62–63)

Dear Audre:

You are a braver and truer feminist than I. I did not have the courage to forgo prosthesis, and to spare myself three additional surgeries! I was afraid of living without an implant, afraid of being asymmetrical—of facing the demise of my breast with daily dollops of visibility and shame, more shame than I could bear. I'd rather feel guilty than ashamed. I chose body ego over ego ideal. Joan Copjec claims that shame and guilt are varying responses to anxiety: to prefer guilt is to prefer exposing others to exposing oneself. But, Audre, aren't you, too, escaping into guilt? In calling on fellow one-breasted women to show themselves, in pursuing identity politics as a vehicle for your social ideals, you transform the blazon of shame into a battle cry, you turn it outward, denying yourself and others a private space to mourn. I admire you. I worship you even as I yearn to destroy in a conflagration of envy your project of making us visible to one another, of celebrating the terrifying experiences that bond us as women. Choosing "reconstruction," I question my love of women, unsure if I am on the side of difference or the leveling superego, whether I am yielding to the pull of the past—the violence of history—or moving forward into a better future. The distinction between shame and guilt breaks down along with my confident identifications.

When I mourn my right breast, it is not the appearance of it I mourn, but the feeling and the fact. But where the superficial is supreme, the idea that a woman can be beautiful and one-breasted is considered depraved, or at best, bizarre, a threat to "morale." ... I must separate ... external demands about how I look and feel to others from what I really want for my body, and how I feel to my selves. As women we have been taught to respond with a guilty twitch at any mention of the particulars of our own oppression. ... A mastectomy is not a guilty act that must be hidden ... to protect the sensibilities of others.

(Lorde, 1980/1997, pp. 66–67)

Dear Audre:

We choose, but we never choose freely. Our autonomy is thrown into question, and the *I* is drained of identifications in the zone of illness and cancer. You probably experienced this privation when you came to a medical appointment without a prosthesis and were told, "it was bad for the morale of the office" (Lorde, 1980/1997, p. 60). What cruelties, what barbarity for the sake of care and psychological well-being! There are many such moments. You write: "In order to keep me available to myself, and able to concentrate my energies upon the challenges of those worlds through which I move, I must consider what my body means to me" (Lorde, 1980/1997, p. 66). You say, and you are right, that we are offered prostheses and implants so that others will feel comfortable and "will not know the difference," but we sure as hell know! Reconstruction is largely about the "external demands about how I look and feel to others," and we must separate that from our own desires. But, Audre, we internalize the voices and gazes of others, so how can we, how can I, distinguish fully between external and internal demands? I have betrayed you, "black lesbian feminist mother lover poet."

Please forgive me, try to understand me. I cry for my right breast, which has not returned in silicone form. And for the psychic breast, my first object, which was once my mother's and part of me, always and eternally lost. I mourn it when I mourn my amputated breast. The prosthesis does nothing to tranquilize the pain or quell the sadness. If only I'd had the strength, the moxie, as you say, to go one-breasted. I would not have to put up with the constant sensation of a foreign object in my body. But the other's gaze that views one-breasted as "bizarre" is incorporated. When I look in the mirror, I see myself from an external, third position. In my mind's eye I am an object. I gaze upon myself looking at myself, walking on the street, among others. And now I imagine something not-whole that will never be whole (though, it never was). Instead of my beautiful, supple, indolent breast, I see a rigid and perky breast-manqué. I cannot agree that those who reconstruct fool themselves. Women are not gullible; we know that reconstruction is, at root, a fallacy, misogyny even, and yet we go ahead. And we survive.

I'd give anything not to have cancer and my beautiful breast gone, fled with my love of it. But then I guess I have to qualify that. ... I wouldn't give my life. ... I wouldn't give ... the children, or even any one of the women I love. I wouldn't give up my poetry, and ... I wouldn't give up my eyes, nor my arms. So I guess I really do have to be careful that my urgencies reflect my priorities. ... At times, I miss my right breast, the actuality of it, its presence, with a great and poignant sense of loss. But in the same way, and just as infrequently, I miss being 32 ... knowing that I have gained from the very loss I mourn.

(Lorde, 1980/1997, pp. 78–79)

Dear Audre:

Your breast or your life? It's the latest in a series of forced choices. The first was between jouissance and language, the pleasure principle and the reality principle. Now, another lose–lose situation. I choose life. Again, I choose language. I would not give up my eyes or arms either. Nor my writing, nor opera, nor the people I love.

You are still you! But what does this mean, really? Am I more than a collection of selves? At 32 I was a graduate student struggling to find "my own voice." At 45 I was a writer, a mother, an analyst, a lover, a friend. Cancer instantly made me into a body to be intruded upon. Jean-Luc Nancy (2008) wrote about his heart transplant, a manifold ordeal of medicalization and incremental loss: "The *I* ends up being nothing more than a fine wire stretched from pain to pain and strangeness to strangeness. One attains a certain continuity through the intrusions, a permanent regime of intrusions" (p. 169). My body props up the illusion of the continuity of self. When I am disillusioned through forced choices, what happens? I lose my sense of body as possession. The *I* becomes a placeholder, tinnitus between resounding leitmotifs: checkups, surgeries, imaging, and blood tests.

Audre, you arouse me with the idea that surviving entails more, or less, than picking up the pieces of my shattered *I* and putting them back together. I pay attention to the divisions, lapses, and lacks, and I write them into being.

I miss my breast and the pleasure it brought. And I miss your voice, Audre, but at least you left us your songs.

References

Audre Lorde in Berlin. (2018, March 21). *Audre Lorde—The complete last reading in Berlin* [Video]. YouTube. Retrieved August 12, 2024, from https://www.youtube.com/watch?v=Uo7TcxauHqw

Lorde, A. (1997). *The cancer journals* (Special ed.). Aunt Lute Books. (Original work published 1980)

Nancy, J.-L. (2008). *Corpus* (R. A. Rand, Trans.). Fordham University Press.

8

Queer Temporalities

At Famous Cancer Hospital (FCH), every second counts. Every moment is extraordinary, everlasting, and witnessed. With a cancer diagnosis I fall through a crack in reality. The future is shrunken and obscured. The past, once narrated with conviction, is instantly eclipsed by a terrifying imminence. This state of affairs—the collapse of diachrony—is only bearable inside the hospital, with its gently affirming mauve walls, floral furniture, and whispering staff. "You're in good hands … You have all the time you need," the nurses express with their smiles, kind glances, and shuffling feet. When I leave the undulating, saturated present of FCH to rejoin the bustling, inattentive social world, I am struck by the absolute incommensurability of these two temporalities. Dislocated and dazed, I am forced to think the nonrelation between hospital time—palpable, savored, shimmering, and expanded—and the vapid, invisible time of the putatively healthy: wasted, killed, gained, borrowed, stolen, and, yet, ultimately, taken for granted. Time moves through the able-bodied, unnoticed. Alain Badiou says that in order to convey this sort of radical heterogeneity—the nonrelation precipitated by a shattering event, say, a political revolution or a cancer diagnosis—one must first write the relation that preceded it, not with the self-assurance of an autobiographer retelling her fully understood past, but, rather, with the curiosity and invention of a foreigner in her own land. Only after the relation is told, can the nonrelation be staged and interrogated (Badiou, 2005/2009, pp. 1–26).

~

My interest in "queer time" preceded my preoccupation with the temporality of illness, the presentism regnant at FCH and in the cancer zone. Prior to 5-year survival rates there were deadly 5-Year Plans and, later, the languid Soviet stagnation era, constructed *nachträglich*. In making the Brezhnev period the subject of my second book, I chose, without yet knowing it, the Before of the Event, the latter being what Badiou (2005/2009) defines as the rupture of Law, the "break of an established natural and social bond" (p. 15). Stagnation, the harmonious order retroactively birthed by the Chernobyl catastrophe, became the queer utopia of my childhood. I studied animated films and musicals of that period, arguing that depictions of atypical life paths born of unusual friendships and loves facilitated real-world explorations of transgressive, boundary-crossing fantasies and usages

DOI: 10.4324/9781003498582-9

of time. More controversially, perhaps, I suggested that Brezhnev-era cartoons' particular voices, musical language, embodiment—and the positioning of the spectator alternately in the role of the child and the psychoanalyst—made available a queer potentiality. Gaps, magically intimate spaces, and disfigured time were performed within the diegetic frame as well as instantiated by the film-as-intrapsychic object, inviting spectators to play with the tatters of late socialism and improvise new truths.

~

In 1976 Audre Lorde sojourned 2 weeks in the Soviet Union as an American observer of the African-Asian Writers Conference sponsored by the Union of Soviet Writers. There she produced a travelogue that later became "Note From a Trip to Russia," the lesser-known opening essay of her lauded collection *Sister Outsider*. Much of the Russian trip was spent outside Russia. After several days in Moscow, Lorde traveled to Uzbekistan, first to the capital Tashkent and then to Samarkand. The official Soviet tour agency Intourist predictably curated Lorde's itinerary to ensure that the Black American poet observed only the fabled Soviet "friendship of peoples." While the Russian guide and interpreter, the "attractive large-boned" and affable "Helen" (Elena?), evaded what I imagine were Lorde's delicately phrased questions about antisemitism, tersely saying "that there were Jews in government," she did show off the Central Asian outpost of Soiuzmul'tfil'm, the state-run animation studio where Lorde mentions watching "several children's cartoons which handled their themes beautifully, deeply, with great humor, and, most notably, without the kind of violence that we have come to associate with [American] cartoons" (1984/2007, pp. 2, 12).

Lorde might not have been aware that children's records and animated films were essential elements of Soviet popular culture that engaged publics of all ages. Their veiled political satire and Aesopian messages had a wide reach: It was a commonplace that genres like animation, puppet theater, and musical sound recordings were innovative because they were subject to less censorship. The studios of Soiuzmul'tfil'm were nests of *shestidesiatniki* (the 1960s generation) and their sympathizers, dissenting voices whose strident Thaw-era demands for "socialism with a human face" found more introspective and oblique expression in the 1970s (Losev, 1984, pp. 193–216; Pontieri, 2012). Lorde wasn't tipped off (alas!) that Brezhnev-era Soviet animation was a quintessentially queer domain of social and cultural critique. Ideological and sexual nonconformists with shattered lives and criminal records gravitated toward children's cultural production when other forms of paid creative work were barred to them (N. Beshenkovsky, née Chervinskaia, personal communication, 2015; Beumers, 2008, p. 161; Nikolaieva, 1996, p. 379).

Lorde remained preoccupied with Russia upon her return to the United States, dreaming about Moscow for weeks. In one dream she is "making love to a woman behind a stack of clothing in the [GUM] Department Store in Moscow." The woman becomes ill, and Lorde seeks medical attention, begging a "matron upstairs" for help in getting her lover to the hospital for brain and kidney scans. When the omnipotent mother figure assures her that all medical treatment will be available and free, Lorde is incredulous until she remembers that she is in Russia (Lorde, 1984/2007, p. 1).

Lorde could not have realized that the Russia trip and her subsequent dreaming would encompass the Before of the Event. A year later she would face a life-altering cancer diagnosis.

~

The phrase "queer temporality" was coined by Stephen Barber and David Clark in their 2002 introduction to a volume devoted to Eve Kosofsky Sedgwick, by then the doyenne of queer theory. Commenting on Sedgwick's work, they suggested that queer identity is rooted in aberrant relationships to time, a disorientation of temporality that emerges from several phenomenologies, including queer childhood, queer kinship and sex, and from the AIDS epidemic—the necessity of an expanded and voluptuous present in the face of a diminishing future (Barber & Clark, 2002, pp. 1–53). For her part, Sedgwick, an AIDS activist confronting cancer, suggested a connection between queerness and nonlinear modes of time in her 1991 essay "How to Bring Your Kids Up Gay: The War Against Effeminate Boys." There she introduced us to the "protogay child," the child whose existence too often was wished away by parents and therapists hoping for a "nongay outcome" (1991/1993a, pp. 154–164). Denied a present, created afterward from a past that never was, the protogay child—perhaps the ultimate ghost in the nursery—does not grow up in the usual sense but awaits his erasure and retrospective birth, or his future haunting. In "Tales of the Avunculate," published a few years later, Sedgwick charted for the gay child a "non-oedipal" course: spaces and relations forged with uncles and aunts whose nonconforming sexualities and life trajectories functioned as alternatives to the law of the biological domestic father, offering pleasures and futures lacking within the conventional nuclear family (Sedgwick, 1993c, pp. 52–72). "'Artistic' Uncle Harvey, 'not the marrying kind' Cousin David ... and Aunt Estelle and Aunt Frances, sisters who slept in the same room for most of their eight decades," carved out in the sterile zone of heteronormative family hygiene and rule-bound religious observance, nonreproductive space and time, protracted and twisted to accommodate imaginative detours and utopian moments of budding queer desire (Sedgwick, 1993c, p. 63).

Although queer temporality as a concept and mode of experience was from the start thought together with queer childhood, the figure of the child remained on the margins of queer studies until Lee Edelman's controversial and instantly classic book *No Future: Queer Theory and the Death Drive*, published in 2004. With irreverence and flair, *No Future* utilized Lacanian psychoanalysis to aim critical fire at the politics of "reproductive futurism," the conceptual children in the name and for the protection of which we are constantly called to sacrifice the present. The child, in Edelman's work, is the antiqueer: the fantasmatic object that promises imaginary wholeness and enables discursive unity by screening out the unreachable Thing—or the disavowed constitutive lack in the heteronormative order. *No Future* exhorts queers to turn away from the political spectacle of cooing White babies, arguing that such a politics always excludes the queer and, indeed, is constituted through the queer's abjection. Children are not *our* future.

Edelman (2004) told queer theorists and all outcasts to "fuck Little Orphan Annie," look askance at the wide beckoning eyes of Tiny Tim, and, more grandly, reject the impossible neoliberal queer variant of reproductive futurism: same-sex marriage, gay adoption, surrogacy, and so on. Instead, he challenged queers to occupy the politically unthinkable position assigned to them by the sociopolitical order (a position they cannot, by definition, escape anyway) so as to undo it from within: to embrace negation, masochistic enjoyment, and the ruthless work of the death drive (pp. 29–31, 41–42).

After the appearance of Edelman's book, the unthinkable happened. The temporally troubling queer child became visible in popular culture and political debate, not only as a scare image to be feared by "normal" adults or a pathological adolescent to be cured by therapists but also as a sympathetic victim: the target of homophobic bullying at school; the suicidal trans teen needing support and recognition; the beneficiary of international adoption or puberty blockers afforded by understanding parents; the one for whom it would eventually "get better." Initially alongside and perhaps in reaction to Edelman's controversial intervention, and in response to the return of the repressed queer child in public discourse, Jack Halberstam and others in queer studies began treating the figural queer child as the spark for imaginative exploration in the political sphere and a vital source of new affective modes and social alternatives (Halberstam, 2011; Muñoz, 2009/2019; Stockton, 2009).

Halberstam (2005) was among the first to grant the idea of queer time an extensive elaboration, attributing it, like Sedgwick, to the AIDS crisis, which forced an "emphasis on the here and now" and "an erotics of the compressed moment" (p. 2). In Halberstam's view, queer temporality is a mode of time deeply invested in the present, undoing narrative and expanding the potential of the moment; it is at odds with futurity and generational thinking. Dissociated from a national historical past, inviting cathexis of the transient and contingent, it means for some living in drug-induced "rapid bursts," or with the malleability and chimeric imprecision of Salvador Dalí's melting clocks (Halberstam, 2005, p. 5).

Later, Elizabeth Freeman in *Time Binds* (2010) described queer time as nonsequential—a warped chronology—contrasting it to *chrononormativity*, defined as "the use of time to organize individual human bodies toward maximum productivity" (p. 3). And José Muñoz (2009/2019), in *Cruising Utopia*, drew on Martin Heidegger and Ernst Bloch to conceptualize queer time as *ecstatic*: "a horizontal temporality that allows one to step outside oneself, to comprehend a temporal unity which includes the past (having been), the future (not yet), and the present (making present)" (p. 186). With the notion of ecstatic time, Muñoz emphasized queer potentiality: "a mode of nonbeing that is eminent, a thing that is present but not actually existing in the present tense" (2009/2019, p. 9). Somewhat differently from Halberstam and against Edelman, he viewed "queerness" primarily as the near future, the *not-quite here* that inspires hope and critical investment in utopias. Muñoz, contra Edelman, made the simple point that "racialized kids, queer kids, are not the sovereign princes of futurity" (2009/2019, p. 95), and it is for them that we must imagine a "not yet," a queer temporality that enables them to grow up and to become fully realized subjects.

Despite Edelman's call for the queer refusal of the child and the entire symbolic order it signifies, and precisely because of the ways "protogay" children and queer adults torque time, the child quickly became that thing queer theorists could not *not* talk about. In fact, queer theory, psychoanalysis, childhood studies, and the public discourse surrounding the child seemed increasingly to be converging. Theorist Kathryn Bond Stockton (2009), for one, explored childhood as a queer, nonlinear time of "sideways growth," a swollen temporality that permits children not simply to grow *up* in one continuous vertical movement but to expand horizontally, incorporating sensations, emotional connections, and experiences (masochistic scenes, violent impulses, and seductions, for example) later disavowed by the retroactively conceived, figural child. In her book *The Queer Child: Growing Sideways in the Twentieth Century*, she not only asked how gay children play with the asynchronicity of their queer, publicly impossible, and deferred identity but also looked at the undeniable strangeness of all children. Stockton took apart the implied Whiteness and middle-class privilege even of the polymorphously perverse and onanistic psychoanalytic child (the child queered by Sigmund Freud) to illuminate other models of "dangerous children": the child queered by innocence, the child queered by color, the child queered by money, the grown homosexual seen as a child, and the gay child made ghostly, unavailable to itself, by legal and parental misrecognition (Stockton, 2009). Stockton's work in particular lent legitimacy to my academic study of late socialist children's culture, freeing me in 2010 to interpret Soviet animated films and fairy tale audio recordings through the unexpected lenses of queer theory and psychoanalysis.

~

What can one make of the apparent dialectical synthesis of the child and the queer? Over a decade ago, the It Gets Better antibullying campaign was widely criticized for perpetuating the myth that gay, White, cisgendered children would "get more normal" in adulthood: achieve financial success and find acceptance, love, community, family, and so on. Now, at least in the United States, trans children and their supportive families are commanding media attention and shaping the discourses of transgendered agency and embodiment.

Is the queer child a newly created object or an old one, refound? More to the point, is the figure of the queer child the latest fetishistic invention or has it been there all along, the specter shadowing both Edelman's fantasmatic child and the adult queer? Psychoanalysts know but too often forget that it was Freud who introduced the queer child when he located perversion in infancy and posited an adult genital sexuality gradually achieved through a fusion of narcissistic, oral, and anal pleasures. In the *Three Essays* (1905/1953f), Freud famously suggested that homosexuality was regressive, that it meant getting stuck at a primitive, "pregenital" stage of development. But another strain in his thought universalized perversion and lamented the libidinal sacrifice required by "normal" adult genitality.

It was from this Victorian understanding of psychosexuality that the idea of the ever-threatened and threatening child emerged, a child at once innocent of fully realized sexual knowledge and the seedbed of abnormality, a potential victim of corrupting adult perversion and the pervert haunting each of us. The impeccable childhood requiring protection at all cost, the childhood structuring citizenship, therapeutic optimism (and hopefulness as such) results from the disavowal of both psychoanalytically normalized, ubiquitous queerness—that is, perversion—and the psychically mature queer.

Though Edelman's *No Future* has been exhaustively critiqued and in important ways superseded, it remains exemplary in its merger of psychoanalysis and queer theory, and in its identification and use of the congruence between the two fields. Edelman conceived queerness and the queer as figurations of the blind force of the drives that both structure and disrupt the workings of the Symbolic, meaning everything from politics to social arrangements and culture broadly defined. To add conceptual support to this claim, he drew on Jacques Lacan's notion of the *sinthome*, a neologism designating the idiosyncratic way each subject manages the Real (unruly drives) by knotting it with the Symbolic (language) and the Imaginary (the body ego). If the *sinthome* is senseless and radically contingent, it also anchors each subject in the symbolic order and guarantees her consistency (Lacan, 1975–1976/2016). Created at the place of the lack in the Other, the *sinthome* also functions as a limit to the psychoanalytic cure. The end of analysis for Lacan is the "identification with the *sinthome*": an acceptance of the fact that one's identity— and one's very being—is fixed by a random, undecipherable, and self-created signifier (Verhaeghe & Declercq, 2002, pp. 59–83). Edelman recursively created his own neologism, *sinthomosexuality*, the permanent condition of the queer qua *sinthomosexual*. Like the procedure of the psychoanalytic cure, the figure of the *sinthomosexual* works perpetually to undercut the fetishistic child through whom mortality is disavowed, exposing the arbitrariness of fantasmatic, or "imaginary," identity. The queer-as-*sinthomosexual*, then, will always be perceived as a danger to the social order, even as affluent gays and lesbians increasingly marry and adopt children—and become domesticated through campy media depictions.

My discussion of the intersection of queer studies and psychoanalytic theory takes as its starting point precisely this element of Edelman's argument, for the unseemly *sinthomosexual* and his *sinthomosexuality* also comprise the great scandal of psychoanalysis, where they appear as none other than the Freudian baby and infantile sexuality. The embarrassment of Freud's infantile sexuality is not so much that children are sexual beings, for example attaining pleasure unrelated to nourishment from breastfeeding (though that, too, has generated its share of outrage), but that sexuality can operate independently of biological and symbolic support: Infants' sexual organs are not yet fully functional and children have no means of making sense of their sexual feeling (Zupančič, 2017, p. 8). Still more disconcerting, infantile sexuality does not become completely contained by biology and culture in adulthood. It persists throughout the subject's life, amorphous and enigmatic, eluding both her symbolic capacities and the exclusive purview of reproductive organs.

Despite its sustained use of psychoanalytic theory, *No Future* missed the opportunity to reveal the inherent queerness of childhood: the *sinthomosexual* baby veiled by the innocent figural child. Fifteen years later, and in the context of the recent eruption of media coverage surrounding LGBTQIA+ (especially transgender) youth, it behooves queer theorists to redouble their engagement with psychoanalysis. Psychoanalytic theory doesn't simply offer the insight that drive sexuality, denatured and perverse, arrives prior to innate, hormonally based sexuality. Psychoanalysis also imbricates sexuality and the unconscious. With primary repression, the infant becomes the point of convergence for drive and "instinctual" sexuality, a convergence that produces the sexual as the fissure in being: irreducible, confounding, and inassimilable.

~

In Freud's writings, sexuality is coterminous with primary repression. The temporality of the unconscious is a queer temporality! Already in his 1895 manuscript "Project for a Scientific Psychology," Freud gestures toward the two nonlinear temporal logics implied by *Nachträglichkeit* through the case of Emma. When Emma was 8 years old, Freud narrates, she entered a small grocery store, where a shopkeeper grabbed her genitals through her clothes. She soon returned to the store, and the man touched her again. At the time, Emma was too young to understand the incident as sexual and did not register it as traumatic (as her return to the store suggests). After puberty and with full awareness of the meaning attributed to sexual arousal, the 12-year-old Emma walked into a different store alone and fled after noticing two clerks laughing together and imagining they were ridiculing her attire. The second incident reawakened the memory of the first, giving it a new, traumatic significance: It prompted "a sexual release," anxiety, repression, and symptom formation. Emma no longer recalled the occurrence of groping but developed an acute fear of going into shops unaccompanied. Freud here shows the forward movement of "deferred action"—an ambiguous, prepubertal sexual experience that has the potential of being viewed later from the perspective of the grinning, adult "seducer"—as well as the retroactive movement of postpubertal interpretation or, more radically, *invention* of the first event as trauma, in the *après-coup* (Freud, 1895/1953d, pp. 352–359).

For Jean Laplanche (1998), the concepts of *après-coup* and (infantile) sexuality are closely related, as he underscores the second meaning of *Nachträglichkeit*, that of "retroactive revision," the subject's ongoing attempts at completing initially failed translations: meaning production that pulls apart and redirects toward itself previously introduced, undeciphered signifiers. Post-Freudian accounts of child development, notes Alenka Zupančič (2017), tend to downplay or elide the repression constitutive *of* the sexual (and not merely performed *upon* it). But in Laplanche's theory, infantile pleasure is sexual because it is compromised *from the outset* by "enigmatic signifiers," the unconscious and sexually inflected messages of caregivers intruding on newborns in their first contact with the world (1998, p. 10). These messages, subject to repeated efforts of translation, are enigmatic not only for children but also for the adults generating them. The point worth stressing here is that infants' pleasurable experience is sexualized through the encounter with the unconscious of adults. In this "primary seduction," Zupančič (2017) clarifies, infants confront not a *surplus* of "mature" genital knowledge (incomprehensible to young children and hence difficult to translate) but an *absence* or *minus*, a missing part in the solicitations of the Other (p. 11). The unconscious comes to us from an external source and an ontological negativity or failure that also constitutes sexuality. And childhood is queered in other ways, too. For adults, it is the site of the crime, as it were, the spatiotemporal dimension of shame and confrontation with difference: the acquisition of that which is more than ourselves, of that which cannot be known. It is unsurprising, then, that trans children have become the primary and most emotionally charged arena in battles over gender identity, science and medicine, feminism, and LGBTQIA+ rights.

~

My love for a childhood spent in the stagnant Brezhnev era is impervious to sense, unless cast as a fascination with queer temporality. I wax nostalgic at the candid and lyrical way Yurii Norshtein's 1975 animated short, *Ezhik v tumane* (*Hedgehog in the Fog*), renders the experience of Soviet stagnation, making transparent its dilemmas and affects, and its ultimate dialectization. The plot is eloquently simple: The narrator informs us at the beginning that the Hedgehog and the Cub meet every evening, sit on a log under the broad sky, sip tea, and count stars. Before them looms a house with a chimney that provides a convenient boundary between their respective domains: on the right are the Cub's stars, and on the left, the Hedgehog's. For an unspecified and unmeasurable duration, the relationship between the Cub and the Hedgehog is contained in this innocent and circular temporality, unburdened by conflict, accident, and change. Their routine is so predictable, in fact, that the Hedgehog can rehearse verbatim the Cub's words in anticipation of their nightly encounter. As the Hedgehog makes his way to the Cub's house, he compulsively recites the dialogue that structures all their meetings: "I'll tell him I've brought raspberry jam, and he'll say: The samovar has cooled off—we'd better put some … what are they called? … Juniper twigs! … in the fire" (Norshtein, 1975, 1:34).

The phrases are incanted as if they possessed magical, transformative properties. Words are *things* without referents; they enact rather than signify. The Hedgehog and the Cub live in a world with no objects in the psychoanalytic sense: no distance between word and deed necessitating a bridging metaphor, no fantasy mediating reality, and no love. They form a sealed dyadic unit, completing one another. But then something happens. A third area appears, a rupture in the tie between the two characters. One day, on his way to the Cub's place, the Hedgehog comes upon a thick and mysterious Fog where a silent white Horse resides. The Horse stirs his interest, and a question forms in the Hedgehog's mind: "If the Horse lies down to sleep, will it choke in the fog?" (Norshtein, 1975, 1:55). He is lured into the Fog by its enigmatic aspect, and once submerged, an abyss opens between him and the Cub, a tear in the dyad, and with it a yawning lack, curiosity, and desire. The Hedgehog temporarily forgets about the Cub and their routine and seeks meaning. He wonders, refusing to turn away when opacity threatens and answers do not emerge. We are provoked to feel his anxiety in unexpected and violent orchestral outbursts and his captivation in the woodwinds' broad and sustained melodic lines. Eventually, the Hedgehog makes his way back to the Cub, but he does not truly return. For the Hedgehog, at least, the purity of their repetitions, dumb and beautiful, cannot be recaptured: "The Cub talked and talked, and the Hedgehog thought, 'Isn't it wonderful that we are together again.' And also ... he thought about the Horse ... 'How is she doing there ... in the fog?'" (Norshtein, 1975, 9:31).

Ezhik v tumane, on the one hand, performs stagnation (or, at least, draws our attention to its performative dimension): The Hedgehog and the Cub construct their intersubjective reality by uttering, indeed monotonously repeating, the signifiers assigned to their respective roles and deeds: stars, "juniper twigs," raspberry jam, and so forth. The very act of enunciation makes the Hedgehog and the Cub what they are, granting them a fixed and confining place within the symbolic order. On the other hand, the film invites identification with the Hedgehog's disorienting experience in the Fog. By means of exaggeratedly loud or echoing sounds—crunches, whistles, creaks, tinkles, and whispers—that seem both to displace and draw one into intimate association with the Hedgehog's moving body, as well as crosscutting and tight close-ups that undermine a "focused and objective point of view" (MacFadyen, 2005, p. 165), we gain an idea of what it feels like to live in isolated compliance, to occupy a particularly vexed stance toward desire.

Ezhik v tumane also illustrates the impossibility of a return to wholeness after the intrusion of a third term or figure, and psychoanalysis has much to say on this topic. The fundamental insight behind Freud's Oedipus complex, and, later, D. W. Winnicott's "transitional phenomena" and Lacan's dual processes of "alienation" and "separation," is that sacrifice is integral to subjectivity. Even before the "paternal metaphor" or thirdness-as-language intrudes upon the mute pleasures of infants and their primary caregivers, weaning and loss take place. When infants are forced to separate from the maternal dyad, they cede a piece of the body they mistook for their own. A part that once belonged to the infant now bears an attribute of the Other and begins to circulate *out there*. The infant constructs a fantasy around this primary loss and its marker, an object carrying something it once possessed, that eventually becomes Lacan's object *a* (Lacan, 1972–1973/1998b, pp. 53–78, 174–186, 203–229; Winnicott, 1971/2005, pp. 1–34, 51–86).

A crucial point for Lacan is that object *a* is not the object of desire or desire as such but is its *cause*: It determines how one's desire is structured. Through elaboration of fantasy, divided subjects become fixated on particular manifestations of object *a*, which pull the strings of desire, as it were, choreographing its movement. Object *a* defies apprehension and can only be sensed momentarily in a tone of voice, a scent, a gaze, a fleeting sensation—memorials to a primordial loss. It is located in people and things that exert a power of fascination, propelling the subject to yearn, seek, and fail again and again to fill the constitutive lack. Object *a*, finally, is construed by Lacan as the void around which the drive endlessly revolves (1972–1973/1998b, p. 242).

In *Ezhik v tumane* object *a* appears at a pivotal moment as the voice of Someone, the experienced but unseen amorphously bodied creature that saves the Hedgehog's life and brings him back to the safety of the Cub's friendship. Having wandered far into the Fog, the Hedgehog stumbles and *plunk*, "I'm in the river. Let the river carry me along," he decides. The Hedgehog "sigh[s] deeply and begins to drift with the current." He hallucinates the Horse in a whirling starry sky as the Cub vainly calls "Hedgehog!" in the distance. We are enveloped, with the Hedgehog, by the sounds of the river and the onomatopoeic whisper of a tinkling piano. He thinks, "I'm completely soaked. I'll drown soon." But then, the narrator informs us, Someone from the water's murky depths touches his hind paw: "'Excuse me,' says Someone without making a sound, 'Who are you and how did you get here?'—'I am Hedgehog. I fell in the river.'—'Then sit on my back. I'll carry you to the shore'" (Norshtein, 1975, 7:18). A flourish in the string section indicates a sudden shift in mood and perspective. Someone remains immersed in darkness, but the Hedgehog now sits up, firmly supported and moving through the river with purpose. He is accompanied by an ambulatory pulse of dotted rhythms from a determined oboe. Its repetitive melody and progressive upward pitches signal the resumption of linear movement, a way out of the confusion of the Fog and the swirl of the night sky. Upon reaching shore, the Hedgehog thanks Someone. "Don't mention it," a voice replies (Norshtein, 1975, 8:31).

Here we witness the voice-as-object *a* at work, its interstitial quality and status as a border concept: the elusive object-voice, a silent mediator of body and language. In the film, Someone appears to be an indeterminate and free-floating agency that "speaks without sound" (Norshtein, 1975, 8:00). Are we to assume, then, that the voice we hear, to which only viewers and the Hedgehog are privy, inhabits his mind alone and belongs to him? But what do we make of the humplike body that carries the Hedgehog to shore, which seems also to give the voice shape and presence? Someone is both part of the Hedgehog and not. It exists between and within two places: under the law of speech and its linear dotted eighths and in an underwater, preverbal territory of aimlessly circling tones. When the Hedgehog enters the Fog, he opens a space for desire, its eternal movement and consequent fantasizing. The Fog is not yet meaning but its promise. It establishes a placeholder for the Hedgehog within the Symbolic. Eliciting questions without responses, breaking up habitual modes of thought and identifications with utterances, the Fog inserts silence—a fissure—between speech and action. It undermines the performative and shifts to the constative.

When the Hedgehog falls into the womblike river and contemplates submitting to its reassuring flow, he flirts with a restoration of a prelinguistic time prior to the fragmenting experience of the Fog. But he soon realizes that repairing the wound, merging with the river, would mean drowning, a certain death. It is at this moment that the Hedgehog finds Someone, his object *a*. He hooks onto it, and it saves him from being devoured by the current, directing him to the other shore where he resumes old rituals, but not entirely. Like a true object *a*, Someone circulates among the mOther, the self, and the signifier, preserving the integrity of each field while, paradoxically, cutting through and disturbing all three, ensuring that temporality will never be stagnant or circular, forever caught in mindless repetition. When our hero returns to the Cub, who is still in the same place, stupidly imitating speech rather than using language, one wonders if the naive pact of counting stars now seems slightly embarrassing to the Hedgehog. As the Cub prattles, his traumatized spiny companion stares blankly into the distance, thoughts elsewhere. Between the Cub and the Hedgehog now intervenes the memory of the Horse and the Fog.

~

Most commentary about *Ezhik v tumane* in the Soviet period and since attributes the film's popularity to a transparent sentimentality, its purpose of "investigat[ing] the psychology of human feelings." It was heralded, writes literary scholar David MacFadyen (2005), "as an especially successful work in its reduction of a folkloric tradition to the essence of a pure spatiotemporal freedom, one of express relevance and application to children's development" (pp. 164–165). After perestroika it was deemed by some an ecstatic withdrawal from public life, "revolutionary" in its "dissolution in the world of desire" (MacFadyen, 2005, p. 170). For me, the importance of *Ezhik v tumane*, like much other late Soviet children's culture, lies in its depiction of queer time, or what anthropologist Alexei Yurchak (2006) less provocatively calls "citational temporality" (pp. 60–76).

In his influential *Everything Was Forever, Until It Was No More*, Yurchak (2006) draws on J. L. Austin and Gilles Deleuze and Félix Guattari to make several compelling arguments about late socialism. His first and most generative insight is that a "performative shift" occurred within Soviet "authoritative" (official) discourse after the loss of its "master," Joseph Stalin. Because the *vozhd'* (leader) positioned himself as the only legitimate external editor of communist discourse, his death resulted in the hypostasis and increasing irrelevance of the discourse's constative meaning. By Brezhnev's time, authoritative discursive space acquired a citational temporality because party speeches, Komsomol reports, and *Pravda* articles could only refer to earlier official statements or hint at future events. Without a master to authorize fresh language and ideas, late Soviet discourse looped back on itself, producing a simulacrum: immutable, repetitive, and without individual authors. A point unexplored by Yurchak but particularly important for me is that a performative shift not only conditioned Brezhnev-era stagnation but also staged it linguistically. Stagnant authoritative discourse, in other words, inevitably performed stagnation itself.

Another, ensuing argument of *Everything Was Forever* is even more resonant to my queering project. Yurchak (2006) contends that because communist rhetoric was stripped of external referents after the Stalin era and mattered less for its veracity than for the quality of its expression, surprising connotations eventually were attached to familiar symbols and tropes. While authoritative discourse remained fixed, spectacularly reproducing itself, newly formed publics unrecognized by the regime arose and flourished within "deterritorialized" spaces: Words, places, and regularized practices evacuated of their original meaning by the performative shift came alive again (pp. 1–157). The realm of the Hedgehog (and of animation more broadly) was one such "deterritorialized" space, and psychoanalytic and queer theories permit its deeper examination.

Just as the uncanny material presence of the object-voice for Lacan poses a resistance to symbolization but also serves as the vehicle of speech, for the Hedgehog, the voice of Someone (a psychoanalyst?) and, for viewers, the film itself offered a path beyond the citationality of the purely Symbolic, on the one hand, and preoedipal paradisal ignorance, on the other. *Ezhik v tumane* indeed "allow[ed] emotional participation" (MacFadyen, 2005, p. 156)—instantiated the experiential dimension of stagnation—and pointed to an escape, one that was not simply a retreat to the Cub, that is, an apolitical private life (a commonly heard cliché about the Brezhnev years), but an invitation to explore temporality and its libidinal flow. The film ultimately demonstrates the ways repetition (the drive) can be revolutionary, as it is the very act of returning to juniper twigs and star counting that initiates enduring transformation. The Hedgehog will only know the impact of the Fog when he encounters the Cub again: the flatness of his speech, the rigidity of his tasks and pleasures.

We come, then, to what is perhaps the unwitting message of Norshtein's work: one transcends stagnation by reproducing it. This insight of *Ezhik v tumane*—that change is only possible through repetition—anticipates Yurchak's and my conclusions about the post-Stalin era: Stagnation as citational temporality, as interminable recycling, enabled tectonic changes (Yurchak, 2006, p. 282). Stagnation was crucial to the collapse of communism not only in the forms of economic depletion and popular cynicism but also as an experience of time and space. The shift from a teleological linear time to a queerly citational temporality amid more subtle alterations within the cultural environment—the socioeconomic background, so to speak—quietly opened an ideological gulf that produced Chernobyl and its fallout, a spark leading 5 years later to the catastrophic breakdown of the old order. Like the Hedgehog who changes as a result of his post-Fog return to the Cub because he cannot repeat what was once repeatable innocently, Soviet audiences could no longer be fully immersed in and merely *act out* stagnation after watching and listening to it on screen and records.

~

FCH is the sensual abundant mother who satisfies my longing for a prelapsarian childhood. Her routinized ministrations weave a circular temporality, concealing the nothingness of death. Abandoning FCH means reentering the linear time of adult desire, with its inevitable blows and cuts, as well as its retroactive effects, trauma and pain induced *après-coup*.

The cancer hospital is a phallic mother to its patients. Who else will give shelter and succor to the castrated, terror-stricken casualties of chemo and surgeries, stripped of hair, sexuality, and basic humanity? Where the oncologist subtracts, she immediately reconstructs. She is prosthesis and hope.

~

Socialist construction can be queer, especially when its would-be agent is the pinched soprano of a girl in Wonderland. Like in the "Song About Plans" from *Alisa v strane chudes* (*Alice in Wonderland*), a musical adapted from Lewis Carroll's

1865 story and recorded by Melodiia in 1977. The Soviet Alisa sings: "Even if one has talent / So as not to disturb, ruin, / So as not to wreck but build, / So as to increase in size, to double, to triple / One needs a very precise plan" (Vysotsky, 1977). The state-run record label made a strange choice: It released a children's story with music and lyrics composed by Vladimir Vysotsky, a famous dissident bard and political satirist whose alcohol and heroin addictions would lead to his premature death at age 42. Queerer still, Vysotsky's Alisa yearns for a "plan" redolent of the linear time of 5-Year Plans, inexorable progress toward communism, and the construction of the New Man, while the English Alice, as every Carroll scholar knows, resigns herself to a Wonderland where time alternately freezes, dissolves, becomes personified and unruly (Rackin, 1991, pp. 54–55). The fracturing of time and bodily morphological changes lead to a loss of subjectivity in Carroll's story. "How queer everything is today! And yesterday things went on just as usual. I wonder if I've changed in the night?" ponders Alice after several bouts of growth and shrinkage (Carroll, 1865/2010, p. 17). She desperately attempts to reconstitute her previous, surface-world psychic integrity by reciting the rote schoolhouse knowledge upon which it depended: multiplication tables, rhymes, and various other lessons. But when aboveground epistemologies confront Wonderland's incoherent meaning system, they are exposed as equally arbitrary and illogical. Alice's recitations and rememberings are altered through iteration, producing a jumble of signifiers in search of signifieds. "Who in the world am I?" she asks herself (Carroll, 1865/2010, p. 17).

Of course, virtually every interpreter of *Alice* also notes that the seemingly nonsensical children's books by "Lewis Carroll," the pseudonym of the mathematician, deacon, and photographer Charles Lutwidge Dodgson, both express and parody late 19th-century modernity: rapid technological developments, an increasingly mechanized and fast-paced mass society, tectonic demographic and political changes, unprecedented consumerism, and a bourgeois cultural life transformed by the ever-impinging, volatile market (Haughton, 2006; Hollingsworth, 2009; Holquist, 1992; Rackin, 1991, pp. 3–11). In the chapter "A Mad Tea Party," the March Hare, Mad Hatter, and Dormouse eternally move from one chair to the next around a circular tea table, engaging in disjointed banter while time stands still, vengeful and recalcitrant after an ugly quarrel with the Hatter. "Ever since that, he won't do a thing I ask. It's always six o'clock now ... always teatime," mournfully explains the Hatter (Carroll, 1865/2010, p. 57). The representation of time as an offended subject pokes fun at the real-world perception of "time's infinite, orderly, impersonal and autonomous nature," exposing it as a contingent fiction with "no binding claim to existence" (Rackin, 1991, p. 55).

The initial dissonance of a Brezhnev-era *Alice in Wonderland* dissipates when one recognizes the social and cultural similarities between the mid-Victorian English experience and Soviet everyday life in the 1970s (Kobrin, 2007). Late socialism had not given rise to a bourgeoisie facing threats to its power in culture and politics, nor was the Soviet Union in the throes of swift secularization and challenge from new ideologies and mass movements. But the Brezhnev years certainly witnessed an increasingly consumerist and fragmenting society contending with Western cultural influence, an expanding empire in need of constant maintenance, a reimagining of temporality prompted by the announcement of "developed socialism," and, arguably, spiritual and ideological crises (Fürst, 2021; Raleigh, 2012; Siegelbaum, 2008; Smolkin-Rothrock, 2011; Zhuk, 2010). One can appreciate how the Mad Tea Party in stalled time might have resonated for Soviet audiences in 1977, exquisitely connoting frustration with ever-breaking appliances, the boredom of queues, and stagnation itself. In Wonderland, as in late socialism, the performative dimension in discourse prevails, while constative meaning is more difficult to locate. The frequent shout "Off with their heads!" from the bloodthirsty Queen of Hearts at the slightest provocation or infraction (or for no apparent reason) becomes less terrifying for Alice once she realizes that no one in the kingdom is ever really executed, and, in fact, the subjects are "nothing but a pack of cards" (Carroll, 1865/2010, p. 96).

Vysotsky's musical adaptation relies on Nina Demurova's somewhat fanciful translation of *Alice* (Carroll, 1967/1978), the recitative following closely the structure of Carroll's text. Yet, two striking features distinguish the late Soviet version from the original. First, Vysotsky's *Alisa* is conceived like a Winnicottian transitional space, presenting listeners with several obvious and meaningful paradoxes requiring hermeneutic feats to unearth in Carroll's version. Early in the musical we grasp that its narrative elements are both part of a girl's imagination, a fantasy under her full control, and a series of arbitrary events that happen to her. Alisa is simultaneously an active participant in a Wonderland of her own creation and a product of the text; a narrating author not unlike Carroll and also Alice Liddell, for and about whom Dodgson wrote his books. She is a reader, a character in someone else's story, and a textual effect inciting amused confusion, desire, and play in the listener.

The Soviet *Alisa* illuminates such paradoxes through the imposition of three successive narrative frames on Carroll's tale: An omniscient narrator first addresses the audience, then becomes Charles Dodgson conversing with Alisa, and ultimately transforms into the bird character Dodo (Dodgson's nickname), who enters the story to shepherd Alisa through Wonderland, appearing and disappearing at just the right moments to ensure her adventures continue to intrigue but never feel too dangerous. Finally, Vysotsky himself sings a few of the songs, impersonating several characters in camp fashion. In doing so he simultaneously acts as an inner voice constructing an alternate narrative; an object-voice incarnating human affect, the cause of desire; and a reference to an extra-fictional personage who brings well-established cultural meanings to an otherwise nonsensical story.

The formulation of *Alisa* as a transitional, and transferential, space enables for listeners an exploration of especially difficult, emotionally knotted themes in late socialism. It also explains the second, related feature unique to Vysotsky's adaptation: the lyrical style of the music and its sharp contrast to the lighthearted tone of the story. The original *Alice in Wonderland* obviously is not a musical tale, and the dramatization of any prose work tends to make it, well, more dramatic. Nevertheless, one cannot fail to notice the discrepancy between the cheerfully self-parodying libretto and the weighty emotional burden Vysotsky placed on it through the songs. The expressive power of these musical interventions captivates me today as it did in Soviet kindergarten. I wish to account for the intimate and extraordinary spaces the musical referenced and instantiated, to resurrect a ruined civilization. As the narrator Dodo informs us in the opening arioso, in Wonderland "there are no borders, it isn't necessary to swim, run, or fly. / Access isn't difficult, no one is denied entry. / To find oneself there one needs only to desire it" (Vysotsky, 1977).

~

Winnicott (1971/2005) described transitional phenomena much like he characterized playing, as a potential space, an "intermediate area of *experiencing*, to which inner reality and external life both contribute" (p. 3). In the first months of life, the infant exists only in a dyad with its mother, a protected state of hallucinatory omnipotence and utter dependence. Eventually, a third field emerges, a neutral illusory world in which the infant, possibly through a relationship with a transitional object such as a blanket or teddy bear, and from the safety of its mother's unobtrusive love, confronts radical alterity and takes a crucial step toward true relating: the recognition of oneself and others as subjects with distinct internal worlds (Winnicott, 1971/2005, pp. 2–8, 10–20).

Transitional space lies between "the me and the not-me," reality and fantasy: The infant participates in both concurrently, experiencing internality and externality free of strain and without challenge. The transitional object has materiality and is acknowledged by the infant to be part of its physical world, a discovered "not-me" possession. Yet, it is also an extension of the infant's internal life, its omnipotent creation. The "baby creates an object but the object would not have been created as such if it had not already been there" (Winnicott, 1971/2005, p. 95). Winnicott insisted that the paradox of the transitional object, and transitional relatedness more generally, must be left unresolved so that meaning and metaphor can be forged. Transitional phenomena produce all creative impulses and subjectivity itself. They comprise the originary field of culture to which we retreat and from which we draw comfort and inspiration as adults: art, music, religion, and so forth (Winnicott, 1971/2005, pp. 18, 71–76, 95–96).

The caring presence essential to transitional phenomena is Winnicott's "good-enough mother," who, thoroughly preoccupied with meeting the newborn's needs, provides a "holding environment" in which its still unformed and fragile self can be contained. She mirrors the infant, recognizing it and relating to its internal state, while the infant utilizes mirroring to organize its own perceptions, to see itself as an Other produced by an external gaze (Winnicott, 1971/2005, pp. 95, 149–152). During a mythical pre-subjective period, the mother sustains the newborn's illusion that the surrounding environment is an extension of itself, under its magical control. She proffers the object of newborn's need so immediately and intuitively that it never experiences a gap between desire and satisfaction. At a later stage, through gradual failures in maternal adaptation, weaning is achieved. Only after the infant has experienced an unproblematized correspondence between external reality and its own capacity to create can it make creative use of the world. The mother figure, for her part, remains good enough by failing the infant, thereby allowing it entry into the transitional area of play, the matrix of the imagination that eventually enables full separation (Winnicott, 1971/2005, pp. 15–18).

Winnicott believed that love and play are central to psychoanalytic psychotherapy. He conceived analytic treatment as a holding environment, a place of trust and safety that serves a reparative and enlivening function for those who were deprived of proper maternal care. The analyst patiently withholds (but reliably keeps in mind) interpretations, allowing room for the analysand to play and create her own knowledge. The analyst, in other words, strives to fill the barren emptiness left by the nonrelating parent and provide the security and magical intimacy necessary for the formation of a desiring subject (Winnicott, 1971/2005, pp. 63–68, 76–86, 94–96; see also Guntrip, 1977/1994, pp. 364, 366).

In *Alisa v strane chudes*, framing devices—the therapeutically enigmatic narrator Dodo most directly—point to and hold together a series of paradoxes, reversals, and metonymic progressions the heroine faces. Richard Feldstein's (1995) Lacanian reading of the Carroll books suggests that Alice loses her identity in Wonderland and must bind herself to a master signifier, that is, a quilting point unifying the symbolic field, in order to reestablish her place within it, "to make sense of the nonsensical dimension confronting her" (p. 150). Alisa is never quite so adrift in the queer time and space of the Soviet *strana chudes*. In the absence of a master signifier, amid pandemonium and stark contradictions, an avuncular, or, perhaps more precisely, a masculine-maternal, narrative voice penetrates and soothes, prompting both Alisa and the listener to playfully examine the impasses of late socialism and imagine a more enchanted life, brimming with possibility.

~

Before the fall into Wonderland and shortly after a half-sung, half-spoken monologue by the narrator, we meet the plaintive Alisa in A minor, Vysotsky's and the heroine's signature tonality. Despite her girlish altitudinous voice and references to scenes of play, we intuit from Alisa's initial lethargic hopelessness and later capacity for strident pining that she is no innocent:

I'm terribly bored, simply exhausted
And thoughts intrude, making me anxious.
I wish someone would invite me somewhere,
A place I could see something extraordinary!
But what precisely—I truly don't know.
I get lots of competing advice:
"Read a while!"—I sit down and read.
"Play a while!"—I play with the cat.
And, still, I am awfully bored!
Sir! Please take Alisa with you!
I would like so much, so much I would like
Somehow, someday to leave the house

And suddenly find myself above, in the depths—
Inside and outside—where everything's different!
(Vysotsky, 1977)

Alisa dreams with the open-heartedness and resiliency of a child, yet her interior life is the site of the kind of a deadening boredom and richly drawn melancholia that could result only from adult experience. And what is that experience? She is trapped in, forbidden to depart, a domestic space, a land, let's venture, not unlike the Soviet Union. Its architecture is so rigid and dulling of imagination that she must rely on another, a kind wayfaring Sir, presumably foreign, to take her away to a place she cannot picture, to do and see things she cannot conceive. In the penultimate stanza, sudden modulations in the music suggest Alisa's vulnerability and agitation, conveying the high stakes entailed in departure, even in fantasy: "Let the house erupt in commotion, / And let punishment threaten, I am ready to meet it! / I close my eyes and count to three. / What will happen, what's next? I worry terribly" (Vysotsky, 1977).

Alisa longs for an abroad, a not-here. She wants to pulsate with dynamic aliveness, promiscuously traversing time and space: to be inside and outside, above and below. She seeks to erase borders, explore and embody fluid structures while remaining integrated and secure in the presence and under the gaze of the Other. Alisa addresses a phantasm, a Sir who is absent yet there (inside her?), desiring with and through the Other's desire. Anxious foreboding consumes her, menacing violence intimidates, and she must risk everything. But as danger is invoked, a poignant intimacy is created, too, an offering to the listener of intensely private suffering delivered in the fragile, arresting voice of a child. The song as much demonstrates as invites such an intimacy, and even while chaos is announced in the last stanza ("Everything's confused in the midday heat"), order is restored musically as we return home to A minor.

Are we, then, to understand Wonderland as an iteration of what Yurchak (2006) calls the "Imaginary West"—an imagined extraterritorial space hatched within Soviet borders by the socialist project itself—a kaleidoscopic "internal elsewhere" (pp. 158–162)? Yes, but not only. The transitional phenomena of Wonderland are also an "external here," a here made strange, the Soviet Union seen from an English girl's perspective. To complicate matters further, Alisa's Englishness is drawn with satirical emphasis and thereby exoticized as well. Her song is followed by an exchange among Alisa, Dodo, and the speedy White Rabbit, running late with pocket watch in hand. Alisa remarks on the watch with surprise, and the Rabbit replies in nervous staccato, "An excellent watch, with an alarm! Oi-ei-ei, already late! Goodness, how uncivilized! English rabbits can't stand being late!" (Vysotsky, 1977). The Englishness of the characters (needing no mention in Carroll's version) is here an excess to be lampooned and denaturalized, and made unstable, too, by various un-English, decidedly Russian traits and statements: for example, the Mouse's lecture on Peter the Great rather than the Norman conquest in the Pool of Tears episode, and, more fundamentally, the heroine's Russified name. Places and characters marked Soviet are treated with ironic distance as well, heightening the feeling of simultaneous externality and internality, East and West, home and abroad.

Tempting as this reading is, Vysotsky's musical portraits are never fully without historical pathos, rarely unmoored from Soviet themes, sounds, and gestures. This historicity is conveyed in several percussive and militaristic songs, especially the march accompanying the processional entrance of the Court (really a deck of playing cards) near the conclusion of the story. The musical number is the centerpiece of a supremely ironic scene: Alisa, after much vexation, has finally realized her most ardent desire in Wonderland and gained entry into the Garden. Instead of an idyll, however, she finds a near-psychotic realm governed by the heartless whims of an irrational Queen of Hearts (whose restrained low-pitched commands sound more like those of a Soviet party official than a Victorian hysteric) and an inert King, a thoroughly confused and ineffectual father, or failed master signifier. In the Garden, like everywhere else in Wonderland, there is no anchoring point unifying language, and Alisa has reached the nadir in her descent into chaos, or what she calls a "muddle." The symbolic order has so disintegrated that there ceases to be a division between inanimate and animate things. Geese and turtles are being used for mallets and balls in a game of royal croquet. The turtles crawl away and the geese bend their necks, making playing by the rules impossible. In short, the Law is dead, or never existed. And yet the marching guards swear to obey it in the person of their leader, prostrating themselves:

> Gallantly and tightly, we closed ranks,
> Like bullets in a clip, like cards in a deck.
> The King is among us, we're proud—
> We parade with enthusiasm before our people (*narod*)!
> Fall with your face down, down—
> You are given that right …
> No, the people (*u naroda*) don't have a difficult role:
> To fall on their knees—never a problem!
> The King answers for everything,
> And if not the King, well then, the Queen!
> (Vysotsky, 1977)

There is much satirical content in this song, even if we leave aside that the participants in the singing procession are flat and made of paper. Invoking "rights" before a nonexistent Law, the royal subjects are not only slavish; they are pure performance, unattached to any meaningful referent. The line "If not the King, well then, the Queen!" should be understood in all its absurdist sarcasm, since the former is a bumbling idiot and the latter acts solely on caprice.

But there is also a haunting seriousness here, and it emanates from the undeniable impression that the Soviet Union is the target of the satire. First, the word *narod*, rooted in a rich Russian historical and philosophical tradition, lends gravity and meaning to otherwise cartoonish, free-floating figures like the King and Queen. Second, Vysotsky's hoarse baritone, enunciating each word with deliberate pace and his usual mixture of passion, irony, and bitterness, immediately communicates a long chain of distinctly Soviet associations informed by his many similar-sounding outlaw and war-themed songs. And third, the very appearance of Vysotsky's heroic persona, which breaks through and surpasses the nameless character he is performing, transports the listener into the Brezhnev-era everyday: countless solitary or, more likely, communal experiences of listening to Vysotsky's voice on distorted cassette tapes in someone's kitchen. It is a voyage into feeling; an archive of friendship, sentimentality, and anguish; private confession amounting to a breach in the Wonderland story, a complete abandonment of its emotional and sonic palette.

The garden scene, therefore, achieves two effects. On one hand, it renders a late socialist space with a fractured ideological field due to a disabled master signifier, anticipating Vladimir Lenin's degraded status in the 1980s and foreshadowing the collapse of the Soviet Union (Yurchak, 2006, p. 74). On the other hand, Vysotsky's musical interlude, like his other Wonderland songs, acts as a nodal point that binds meaning. His well-known personality occupies an exceptional position with respect to the symbolic field of Wonderland and introduces a new organizing principle that recasts all other signifiers in relation to itself. With the introduction of Vysotsky's highly evocative voice, the listener draws away from a hallucinatory tale and toward the magic place of her own interiority and memory making, thereby reterritorializing affects, fantasies, and myths that have been displaced or made illegible by self-referential and adrift discursive structures. It is also at this moment that Alisa begins to "outgrow" the tale, her size (and humanity) increasing with mounting frustration over its incomprehensible messages and arbitrariness. She eventually grows so large that the tale "bursts" and Alisa reenters reality, knowledge, and relatedness. She exclaims, "Oh, how good that the story ended! So much confusion and disorder! Finally, I am in a place where I know everything and everyone knows me" (Vysotsky, 1977). Vysotsky appears, therefore, as another narrative frame. With Dodo and Alisa, too, he provides the evenly hovering attention of a Winnicottian good-enough mother or analyst, helping to create a transitional space between the me and the not-me, where novel and invigorating experience can emerge.

Transitional phenomena also appear at an earlier moment in the story after Alisa drifts off to sleep and plunges to the bottom of a narrow tunnel, landing on a pile of autumn leaves. She asks Dodo if he laid them down especially for her, knowing she would fall and ensuring a soft landing. "No," he replies, at once denying and asserting authorship, "you're the one dreaming the story, and I am narrating it to you." Alisa then spots the White Rabbit, chases after and loses sight of him, and winds up in an unusually long, lonely hall with hanging lamps and many locked doors.

Luckily, Dodo is nearby to offer a "perhaps" or some other oracular response to her queries. "Probably this is where toys go when they get tired of us," Alisa opines. "And why is this place—A Very Strange Place?" she asks her dependable companion. "Because all other places are too normal. There must be at least one very strange place," Dodo declares in fading voice and vanishes for a time, reminding Alisa of his invisible presence with an occasional titter ("he-he") while she braves her next adventure (Vysotsky, 1977).

If *Alisa v strane chudes* is constructed as a transitional space, what is the transitional object therein? Is it Charles Dodgson as Dodo, or the smile of the Cheshire Cat, who accompanies Alisa on several later adventures? Or is Dodo, rather, the maternal figure who presents objects? Or an analyst impersonating the good-enough mother? Winnicott (1971/2005) observed that the transitional object is fated to be de-cathected and abandoned: not because it "goes inside" or because the "feelings about it undergo repression. It is not forgotten, and it is not mourned. It loses meaning, and this is because the transitional phenomena have become diffused ... over the whole cultural field" (p. 7). Perhaps it is the tale itself, then—the diegetic events of Wonderland—that constitutes the transitional object. Alisa, we recall, outgrows the story, becoming estranged from and breaking through its maddening circularity. We might consider, finally, that the transitional object left behind, unwanted and unmourned, is socialist official discourse and its master signifier.

~

Vysotsky sings two ballads in the Mad Tea Party scene. The first, "A Song About Offended Time," is a meditation on queer time, the predicament of stagnation. It begins slowly and repetitively, with eight Gs, all eighth notes: "Lift the theater curtain by its edge— / What old and heavy stage wings. / This is what Time was like previously, / So regular—take a look, Alisa!"

A scene is framed for me, the listener, the proscenium representing representation itself. I have perspective now, distance from myself. I can see myself *over there*, with others in linear time, "But [then] happy people watched the clock, inattentively / And cowards slowed down Time, purposely / Clamorers rushed Time, urging / The lazy killed Time, without purpose,"

> And the wheels of Time
> Wore down from friction—
> Everything on earth is ruined by friction ...
> And then Time was offended—
> And the pendulum of time stood still.
> And midnight never struck.
> Everyone waited for noon, but it never arrived,
> Look what sort of time is upon us—
> So anxious—look, Alisa! ...
> Grease the wheels of Time—
> Not for the sake of reward,

But because friction hurts it so!
It isn't wise to offend Time,
It's bad and dull to live without Time.
                    (Vysotsky, 1977)

Vysotsky is accompanied by a harpsichord, an archaic instrument of the Renaissance and Baroque periods. This is not a nostalgic song, however: It is about being trapped in the past, or simply stuck, external to linear time. Nor is it an ode to chronology, to progress and its attendant notions of futurity. It seems, rather, a lament on the difficulty of coping with historical time, a story of anxiety and conflict, of time worn down by abuse and the burden of expectation. And yet, the ballad is hopeful, too, recommending a compassionate "greasing" of the wheels of time; and intimate, creating a sense of closeness through gently sung and almost whispered phrases, a message shared in sweet secrecy.

The second ballad borrows musical material from previous Alisa songs. It shares their tonality and abounds in melodic echoes. This leitmotivic quality, reinforced by the ballad's textual similarity to the inaugural musical number, "Song of Lewis Carroll," points to the interconnectedness and fluidity of narrating duties among Alisa, Vysotsky, and the Carroll-Dodgson figure:

Much is uncertain in this strange land—
It's possible to get entangled and lost …
It even gives one the creeps
To picture what can happen:
What if a gap appears and a leap is necessary?
Will you get scared, or jump bravely?
Ah? Eh … That's how it is, my friend,
That's the whole point.
In Wonderland, like everywhere,
Good and evil exist,
Only here they live on different shores.
Paths present all sorts of stories,
And fantasies run wild on shaky ground.
                    (Vysotsky, 1977)

Vysotsky here repeats Alisa's theme of risk in the face of fear, the necessity of a heroic leap into the unknown, the sort that establishes one's mettle and self-understanding. Bravery, an ethical stance, "good and evil on different shores," at once evoke Cold War–era discourse and authorize transgression. One might need to jump across a boundary, over an abyss and, like Alisa, on the count of three, eyes shut, trembling with anticipatory dread and pleasure, await an ecstatic shift in sensibility, place, even bodily shape. Both songs seem to promise something beautiful, even utopian, the potentiality in playfulness and free association.

At this point one might counter that hope and futurity are alien to Wonderland. Alisa experiences only exasperation there and yearns to reestablish an epistemological foundation, to be on firm ground with regard to knowledge and identity. This of course is true, but it is not Wonderland that provides comfort, prophecy, and enchantment. The utopian impulse originates in a more quotidian, relational realm, in the bonds uniting the voice and listener, Vysotsky and *I*, analyst and analysand. Between us is a private and expansive temporality, a space of transference, play, and yearning.

~

Once you've fallen into the chasm of the Event, it is tempting to remain there indefinitely, to embrace its stretched temporality. I am not prepared for afterwardness. FCH, all-powerful mother, took away my breast. The cancer hospital is both agent and repository of my loss, the best archive and storyteller, the only true witness of my suffering. Who else can possibly know and bear my moments of utter dependency?

In exchange for my breast, I received longevity. And, so, I must say goodbye to a body part and to the cancer zone, which is more difficult than one might imagine. I clamber out, acquire a modicum of distance, conceptualize the problem of the Event. This is analysis. This is survival. To venture out in recursive movements, just enough to gain perspective, with titrated anxiety.

I deceive myself a little when I claim fidelity to the Event. I trace its formal structure. My body anchors me—positions me at the border between inside and outside—so that I can think the exception, removed from its original circumstances. The Event is mapped and reactualized for satisfying perusal. But there is always an unthought aspect, a frightening rem(a)inder.

~

I return to my childhood Melodiia records, brought with care to Brooklyn from the Soviet Union in 1979. My very personal relationship to their stories and songs is echoed in my academic work. This cannot be disguised, and it cannot be otherwise. I am not especially interested in proving historical facts. My claim, necessarily partial and speculative, is that late Soviet children's records and animated films attracted a vast audience of adults because they, like the Winnicott's good-enough mother or analyst, presented queer worlds within transitional spaces and created the conditions for playing (Winnicott, 1971/2005, pp. 1–34, 51–86). In other words, they did not merely illustrate Winnicottian play or transitional spaces; they also embodied, summoned, and enacted them through and within narrative frames.

Marion Milner (1952), the preeminent theorizer of play who influenced Winnicott's thinking, explained that "the frame marks off the different kind of reality that is within [psychoanalytic session] from that which is outside it, [facilitating] … the full development of that creative illusion that analysts call the transference" (p. 182). Relating transference to the Winnicottian play framework, psychoanalyst Michael Parsons (1999) writes:

> Transference is sustained by a frame [where] … truth and illusion are inextricably mingled. … The therapeutic value of transference does not depend on

resolving the illusion but on accepting its paradoxicality. Although there is a close relation between the play frame and transference, they are not … the same. Where transference is concerned, what the paradoxical frame sustains is not its manifestations, but the possibility of doing analytic work with them.

(p. 875)

Playing, Parsons (1999) reminds us, is serious business. When we play, whether within the analytic session or in the real world, we try out various possibilities in the safe territory between fantasy and reality. We weigh our options and act out potential outcomes. Where the infant uses its transitional object, individuals and publics might use cultural products—spaces of play and illusion—to figure out how to affect their environment, to seek the new and bear the loss of the known while maintaining hope (Parsons, 1999, pp. 871, 878).

Vysotsky's evocative baritone elicits a transference in the listener. His voice erupts from his throat with force and fury, as if breaking out of prison or the womb. Vysotsky's voice cannot tolerate being inside of him any longer. It must fashion itself ex nihilo and engineer an escape. With each strained breath it vaults through the air and enters my ears, transporting me to a glorious world, conferring to me a powerful agency, the capacity for self-exposure and emotional risk.

As *A Fantastic Woman* demonstrates, the voice, freed from speech and meaning, is the key to subjectivity and transsubjectivity. It carries and shares all that is beautiful, fragile, and loving, a yielding and porous *I* that the listener's body can appropriate. "Not every diva origin is traumatic," writes poet and self-proclaimed opera queen Wayne Koestenbaum (1993/2001), "but the conviction 'I will sing!' begins with a primary alienation and unhappiness. I am locked up; *voice* is the key to the prison door, but it is also part of the prison, the body I am shut inside" (p. 87). I absorb the liberated voice, but it belongs neither to you nor me, not to internal nor external reality.

"Any staging of desire," muses Koestenbaum (1993/2001), "involves the comeback sentiment, [Freud's] uncanny: the long-hidden treasure (a body part, a lover) rises once more to consciousness. So when a desire first comes to mind it is really a return" (p. 130). In adulthood I find meaning in Vysotsky's *Alisa*. I am moved, agitated when my fingers graze the familiar terrain of its material form, the cardboard record sleeve. I encounter again its musty odor, the smells and primitive feelings of the Soviet Union. Nonetheless, I am busy making sense. As a child I listened to *Alisa* wrapped in queerness—a not-yet refugee status—drinking its sounds without comprehension, receiving love through the silent singularity of a voice. Vysotsky returns to me now a messenger, bearing knowledge and understanding.

~

In analyzing cartoons and musical tales, I follow an established subfield within literary studies at the intersection of psychoanalysis and children's culture. The Carroll books have been subject to numerous psychoanalytic readings (Coats, 2004; Israel, 2000). Psychoanalysts and children's authors have been in dialogue for many decades; most famously, Alexander Alan Milne's *Winnie-the-Pooh* (1926) inspired Winnicott's transitional object (Kidd, 2011, pp. 49–52).

One might well ask: What, if anything, makes stagnation-era children's culture unique? Does the queerness of Vysotsky's *Alisa* really present a stark contrast to that of Carroll's *Alice*? Can one maintain that Entin's *Goluboi shchenok* is any queerer than Arnold Lobel's *Frog and Toad*? And is the queer temporality occasioned by Karlson's arrival in Boris Stepantsev's animated adaptations (1968, 1970) of Astrid Lindgren's Karlsson-on-the-Roof stories (1955, 1962) truly different from the temporal and aesthetic shifts within Dr. Seuss's *The Cat in the Hat* (1957)? Queerness and subversion arguably are integral to figural children and animation across cultural and historical contexts. Halberstam (2011) reflects on the commonalities between childhood and the nonhuman characters of contemporary American animated films, arguing that both can signal and embody anarchistic revolt. Halberstam also points to the "potential queerness of all allegorical narratives of animal sociality" and calls for "creative anthropomorphism" in animated film (fantastical beasts that stage communitarian uprisings, for example) through which it might be possible to "invent new models of resistance ... in reference to other lifeworlds, animal and monstrous" (2011, pp. 46, 47, 51).

I reply with a straightforward observation: *Goluboi schenok*, *Ezhik v tumane*, and *Alisa v strane chudes* functioned differently because in the context of late socialism they were both products and producers of nonconformity. Like the Blue Puppy and the Fog, Wonderland acted as a transitional object that loosened the relation between the listener and the established sociopolitical order. When *Alisa* itself operated for its audiences as a syncretic universe—a Victorian 1970s Soviet Union in which authoritative discourse was subverted, satirized, and made mutative—it converted the hypostasized signifiers of late socialism into transitional phenomena, that is, into objects of creative play and soon-to-be discarded bridges to separation and individuation. Melodiia and Souizmul'tfil'm enabled Brezhnev-era citizens to dream a new habitus and ideology at a time when untempered playing and irony were becoming increasingly difficult. While opportunities for paradox diminished in post-Thaw Soviet authoritative discourse and printed fiction, animation and musical adaptations of children's tales shaped fantasies and made space for subjectivity.

~

"Queer time" was first and foremost a political project. For its exponents, queer temporality served not only to communicate and theorize the experiences of ephemeral socialities but also to mobilize them politically, bringing queer time into being. The writings on queer time thus offered plans for political becoming, utopias-in-formation. Freeman (2010) proposed the idea of "temporal drag," a type of queer performativity that works against contemporary forms of pastiche by operating as a "stubborn identification with a set of social coordinates that exceed one's own historical moment" (p. 60). Temporal drag is a mode of performance that instantiates anachronism, reviving disavowed and forsaken affects. In Halberstam's work, queer time affords opportunities for embodiments and subcultures that defy naturalized capitalist logics of punctuality, efficiency, and productivity and thrive "outside the frames ... of [the reproductive] family, longevity, risk/

safety and inheritance" (Halberstam, 2005, p. 6). Muñoz ended *Cruising Utopia* with an improbable rhetorical leap from Heideggerian ecstatic time to the drug MDMA, suggesting "taking ecstasy with one another, in as many ways as possible" as a means of effecting a timeless, queer collectivity. He linked the erotic and the sacred in the hope of inspiring a "fuller, vaster, more sensual, and brighter" political act (Muñoz, 2009/2019, p. 189).

Such a politics is of great use in the psychoanalytic clinic, illuminating essential features of the analytic process. What is transference, after all, if not an instance of queer temporality? In his book *Psychoanalysis and Deconstruction*, Jared Russell utilized the work of psychoanalyst Dana Birksted-Breen, reminding us that the dual processes of free association and the analyst's reverie permit fantasizing that transports the past into the present and expands the latter, creating a reverberant temporality, or ecstatic time, in the Heideggerian sense. The analytic session, paradoxically because of its set hour, its predictability, is not so much timeless as temporally elastic: Within the frame, the analysand's productions cut across periodizations and generational distinctions, dislodging meanings and recombining signifiers (Russell, 2019, pp. 71–86). Indeed, symbolization itself involves a movement forward and backward through time, a certain detachment and fluidity between memory and perception. In the analytic hour, when such temporal fluidity also gestures forward, toward the near future, it becomes the temporality of desire and the motor of the analysis. As Birksted-Breen explains:

> The characteristics of the [analytic] setting with its strict boundaries in time and space demarcate a particular temporality inside the boundaries, not so much atemporality or timelessness, it seems to me, as a *bi-temporality*. A specific temporality is given by the analytic pair who will speak of past or present. But whether the analyst chooses to interpret now *or* then, the time within the analytic setting is always now *and* then. The essence of psychoanalysis lies in that double register.
>
> (2016, p. 183)

Like the unconscious, time opens and collapses in the analytic hour in accordion-like fashion, and past and present seem not to follow but to conceive each other. The session belongs to a pulsating, ecstatic nonchronological temporality that promises a more ample subject—ahead of herself and with others—radically singular and connected relationally across temporal zones.

~

Muñoz (2009/2019) argued that queer performances like drag and voguing transmit queerness through fleeting gestures, movements, and soundscapes: a wink, a subtle twist of the hip, a tilt of the head, an accented remark, a thumping house music beat. Drag legend Kevin Aviance's spastic, genderfuck dance moves. Justin Vivian Bond's campy degeneracy. Those aspects of queerness, passed among performers and spectators, are left on the dance floor, on stage, at the club. And yet, traces remain in the felt experience of participants, in muscle and sense memory, the lingering materiality of performance. Muñoz built an archive around such "ephemera," evidence that could not easily be integrated into straight, aboveground life and written history. Muñoz explained:

> Ephemera comprise the temporary, the discardable, the gestural, the residual, at times the imperceptible. ... Think of ephemera as trace, the remains, the things that are left hanging in the air like a rumor. I [am] making a case for a hermeneutics of residue that looks to understand the wake of the performance. What is left? What remains? Ephemera remain. They are absent and they are present, disrupting the metaphysics of presence.
>
> (2009/2019, pp. 69–71)

In much the same manner, at the end of an analysis, one might ask: What remains? Psychoanalysis is the impossible profession, writes Mladen Dolar (2006), precisely because it is "carried only out *viva voce*, in the living voice, in the living presence of the analysand and the analyst. Their tie is the tie of the voice (analysis by writing ... will never do)" (p. 123). Like subjects of queer studies, the psychoanalytic act offers little to those who insist on traditional forms of research and evidence. The talking cure as vocal queer performance, nonetheless, also leaves a trace.

Dolar (2006) develops Lacan's ideas about the object-voice, its paradoxical "ex-timate" quality that troubles the opposition between inside and outside. Were we to apply Muñoz's hermeneutics of residue to the analytic session, we would find, or speculate about, ephemera: the medium of speech, the silent object-voice that cuts through sentences, syllables, and phonemes, making babble of our carefully crafted meanings. "This is not His Master's Voice," writes Dolar (2006, p. 124). It is not, in other words, the acousmatic maternal voice heard by the fetus in the womb, nor the command of God or the superego, but, rather,

> the impossible voice to which one has to respond. It is the voice that does not say anything, and the voice that cannot be said. It is the silent voice of a call, an appeal to respond, to assume one's stance as the subject. One is called upon to speak, and one would say anything that happens to come into one's mind to interrupt the silence, to silence this voice, to silence the silence; the whole process of analysis is a way to learn how *to assume this voice*. It is the voice in which the linguistic, the ethical, and the political voices join forces, coinciding in what was the dimension of pure enunciation in them.
>
> (Dolar, 2006, p. 124)

Psychoanalysis is therefore a fundamentally queer temporal act. Its traces and libido-carrying gestures—its ephemera—allow subjects to reach back into the past and perform leaps forward, invoking bygone eras and bisexual positions in order to achieve a more unique and capacious subjectivity.

Queer temporality is vexing, confusing: Is it curse or savior? It is the psychoanalytic session; it is the cancer zone; it is opera and drag; it is Soviet stagnation.

Its deviant and spatial properties bend gender, permit new bodily forms. Queer temporality elongates moments of enjoyment and safety, paradoxically conditioning risk and movement. Such qualities—not fully capturable, invisible—help explain why the stagnation era became for many an object of nostalgia after the collapse of the Soviet Union. And why I depict it lovingly. I return there again and again, and investigate, from the point of view of a child.

But one cannot stay indefinitely in queer temporality, which is the slowing and bracketing of time, not its freezing. Queerness is about stretching moments and sucking them dry. To avoid melancholic identification with one's illness, to value risk as sublimation rather than as destruction, one must eschew reification: Queer time is not a thing, it is a process. Eventually, I am forced to depart from childhood's Neverland and take inside transitional phenomena so as to play; so as to live.

References

Badiou, A. (2009). Thinking the event [in dialogue with S. Žižek]. In P. A. Engelmann (Ed.), *Philosophy in the present* (English ed., pp. 1–48). Polity. (Original work published 2005 in German)

Barber, S. M., & Clark, D. L. (2002). Introduction. Queer moments: The performative temporalities of Eve Kosofsky Sedgwick. In S. M. Barber & D. L. Clark (Eds.), *Regarding Sedgwick: Essays on queer culture and critical theory* (pp. 1–53). Routledge.

Beumers, B. (2008). Comforting creatures in children's cartoons. In M. Balina & L. Rudova (Eds.), *Russian children's literature and culture* (pp. 153–171). Routledge.

Birksted-Breen, D. (2016). *The work of psychoanalysis: Sexuality, time and the psychoanalytic mind*. Routledge.

Carroll, L. (1978). *Prikliucheniia Alisy v strane chudes; Skvoz' zerkalo i chto tam uvidela Alisa, ili Alisa v zazerkal'e* [Alice adventures in Wonderland; What Alice saw on the other side of the looking glass, or Through the looking glass] (N. M. Demurova, Trans.). Nauka. (Original translation published 1967)

Carroll, L. (2010). *Alice in Wonderland*. Tribeca Books. (Original work published 1865)

Coats, K. (2004). *Looking glasses and Neverlands: Lacan, desire, and subjectivity in children's literature*. University of Iowa Press.

Dolar, M. (2006). *A voice and nothing more*. MIT Press.

Edelman, L. (2004). *No future: Queer theory and the death drive*. Duke University Press.

Feldstein, R. (1995). The phallic gaze of Wonderland. In R. Feldstein, M. Jaanus, & B. Fink (Eds.), *Reading seminar XI: Lacan's four fundamental concepts of psychoanalysis; The Paris seminars in English* (pp. 149–174). State University of New York Press.

Freeman, E. (2010). *Time binds: Queer temporalities, queer histories*. Duke University Press.

Freud, S. (1953d). Project for a scientific psychology. In J. Strachey et al. (Eds. & Trans.), *The standard edition of the complete psychological works of Sigmund Freud* (Vol. 1, pp. 281–391). Hogarth Press.

Freud, S. (1953f). Three essays on the theory of sexuality. In J. Strachey et al. (Eds. & Trans.), *The standard edition of the complete psychological works of Sigmund Freud* (Vol. 7, pp. 123–246). Hogarth Press. (Original work published 1905)

Fürst, J. (2021). *Flowers through concrete: Explorations in Soviet hippieland*. Oxford University Press.

Guntrip, H. (1994). Confronting the critics on the reality of psychodynamic experience. In J. Hazell (Ed.), *Personal relations therapy: The collected papers of H. J. S. Guntrip* (pp. 371–398). Jason Aronson, Inc. (Original work published 1977)

Halberstam, J. (2005). *In a queer time and place: Transgender bodies, subcultural lives.* New York University Press.

Halberstam, J. (2011). *The queer art of failure.* Duke University Press.

Haughton, H. (2006). Alice's identity. In H. Bloom (Ed.), *Lewis Carroll's Alice's adventures in Wonderland* (pp. 193–203). Chelsea House Publishers.

Hollingsworth, C. (2009). Improvising spaces: Victorian photography, Carrollian narrative, and modern collage. In C. Hollingsworth (Ed.), *Alice beyond Wonderland: Essays for the twenty-first century* (pp. 85–100). University of Iowa Press.

Holquist, M. (1992). What is a Boojum? Nonsense and modernism. In D. J. Gray (Ed.), *Alice in Wonderland* (pp. 388–398). W. W. Norton & Company.

Israel, K. (2000). Asking Alice: Victorian and other Alices in contemporary culture. In J. Kucich & D. F. Sadoff (Eds.), *Victorian afterlife: Postmodern culture rewrites the nineteenth century* (pp. 252–287). University of Minnesota Press.

Kidd, K. B. (2011). *Freud in Oz: At the intersections of psychoanalysis and children's literature.* University of Minnesota Press.

Kobrin, K. (2007). Chelovek brezhnevskoi epokhi na Beiker Street: K postanovke problemy "pozdnesovetskogo viktorianstva" [Brezhnev-era man on Baker Street: Toward the question of "post-Soviet Victorianism"]. *Neprikosnovennyi zapas, 53*(3), 147–160.

Koestenbaum, W. (with Kushner, T.). (2001). *The queen's throat: Opera, homosexuality, and the mystery of desire.* Da Capo Press. (Original work published 1993)

Lacan, J. (1998b). *The seminar of Jacques Lacan: Book XX. On feminine sexuality: The limits of love and knowledge, 1972–1973* (J.-A. Miller, Ed.; B. Fink, Trans.). W. W. Norton & Company. (Original lectures presented 1972–1973)

Lacan, J. (2016). *The seminar of Jacques Lacan: Book XXIII. The sinthome* (J.-A. Miller, Ed.; A. R. Price, Trans.). Polity. (Original lectures presented 1975–1976)

Laplanche, J. (1998). *Essays on otherness* (J. Fletcher, Ed.; L. Thurston, Trans.). Routledge.

Lorde, A. (2007). *Sister outsider: Essays and speeches.* Crossing Press. (Original work published 1984)

Losev, L. (1984). *On the beneficence of censorship: Aesopian language in modern Russian literature.* O. Sagner in Kommission.

MacFadyen, D. (2005). *Yellow crocodiles and blue oranges: Russian animated film since World War II.* McGill–Queen's University Press.

Milner, M. (1952). Aspects of symbolism in comprehension of the not-self. *International Journal of Psycho-Analysis, 33*(2), 181–195.

Muñoz, J. E. (2019). *Cruising utopia: The then and there of queer futurity* (10th anniversary ed.). New York University Press. (Original work published 2009)

Nikolaieva, M. (1996). The "serendipity" of censorship. *Para*doxa, 2*(3–4), 379–386.

Norshtein, Y. (Director). (1975). *Ezhik v tumane* [Hedgehog in the fog] [Animated short]. Soiuzmul'tfil'm. YouTube. Retrieved August 25, 2024, from https://www.youtube.com/watch?v=ThmaGMgWRlY

Parsons, M. (1999). The logic of play in psychoanalysis. *International Journal of Psychoanalysis, 80*(5), 871–884.

Pontieri, L. (2012). *Soviet animation and the Thaw of the 1960s: Not only for children.* John Libbey Publishing.

Rackin, D. (Ed.). (1991). *Alice's adventures in Wonderland and through the looking glass: Nonsense, sense, and meaning* (1st ed.). Twayne Publishers.

Raleigh, D. J. (2012). *Soviet baby boomers: An oral history of Russia's Cold War generation* (1st ed.). Oxford University Press.

Russell, J. (2019). *Psychoanalysis and deconstruction: Freud's psychic apparatus.* Routledge.

Sedgwick, E. K. (1993a). How to bring your kids up gay: The war against effeminate boys. In E. K. Sedgwick (Ed.), *Tendencies* (pp. 154–164). Duke University Press. (Original work published 1991)

Sedgwick, E. K. (1993c). Tales of the avunculate: Queer tutelage in *The importance of being earnest.* In E. K. Sedgwick (Ed.), *Tendencies* (pp. 52–72). Duke University Press.

Siegelbaum, L. H. (2008). *Cars for comrades: The life of the Soviet automobile.* Cornell University Press.

Smolkin-Rothrock, V. (2011). Cosmic enlightenment: Scientific atheism and the conquest of space. In J. T. Andrews & A. A. Siddiqi (Eds.), *Into the cosmos: Space exploration and Soviet culture* (pp. 159–194). University of Pittsburgh Press.

Stockton, K. B. (2009). *The queer child, or growing sideways in the twentieth century.* Duke University Press.

Verhaeghe, P., & Declercq, F. (2002). Lacan's analytical goal: *Le sinthome* or the feminine way. In L. Thurston (Ed.), *Re-inventing the symptom: Essays on the final Lacan* (pp. 59–83). The Other Press.

Vysotsky, V. (1977). *Alisa v strane chudes* [Alice in Wonderland] [Audio recording]. Melodiia.

Winnicott, D. W. (2005). *Playing and reality.* Routledge Classics. (Original work published 1971)

Yurchak, A. (2006). *Everything was forever, until it was no more: The last Soviet generation.* Princeton University Press.

Zhuk, S. I. (2010). *Rock and roll in the Rocket City: The West, identity, and ideology in Soviet Dniepropetrovsk, 1960–1985.* Johns Hopkins University Press.

Zupančič, A. (2017). *What is sex?* MIT Press.

9

Prosthesis

My first preoperative appointment with the plastic surgeon was about a week before the mastectomy. I had been told by the oncologist's nurse that pictures would be taken and that I would receive more information about reconstructive surgery and the various breast implant options. I imagined that the pictures would aid the surgical team in finding a match for the healthy left breast and that the plastics technicians were artists requiring photographs from which to construct a likeness of the doomed right breast. Another consumerist fantasy: There would be a vertiginous catalogue of implants of various sizes, shapes, colors, and textures. After agonizing deliberation, I would be allowed to take home several preferred samples, like fabric swatches from a furniture store. A collector's dream: a cornucopia of commodities, arousal and embarrassment, the drama of choice. Reconstruction—Dr. Forceps and his plastic universe—would be a prophylaxis against loss, the best possible fit for my new body, a glimmer of optimism in an otherwise dismal situation.

The letdown was staggering. There was no dazzling array of products, no master designer obsessed with precision and customer satisfaction. The pictures were solely for the purpose of documenting the Before, later to be coupled with After shots. Like the legion of intrusive FCH "Breast-Q" surveys chronicling the "psychosocial and physical impact" of my reconstruction, the pictures were a record of the surgical department's work, assembled for the staff and, presumably, for future patients. The archive was not for me.

Suddenly I became an object in a keenly personal story. The size of the implant was barely discussed and, in any case, predetermined by the measurements of my chest wall and left breast and by tissue elasticity. Despite much hype about newly developed reconstructive possibilities and honed surgical techniques, my "options" were distressingly crude and limited.

"Here, hold this one, see how it feels." Dr. Forceps handed me the saline implant.

I squeezed the lifeless prosthesis and placed it on the table.

"Now, check this one out—this is the one filled with silicone gel."

"It's softer!"

Staring at the two implants, now side by side, I struggled to manage my disappointment. Both resembled water balloons, pathetically amiss.

DOI: 10.4324/9781003498582-10

"Most women choose silicone implants because they're more supple—they feel more like natural breasts than saline implants."

"But then, why would anyone choose saline? What's their advantage?"

Dr. F shrugged, appearing genuinely puzzled.

"Mostly older women choose the saline implants. They are less likely to tear, easier to maintain. Some women just want to get it over with and forget about it."

"And what about those 'gummy bear' implants I keep hearing about? You're not offering those?"

"Mmm, you're referring to the textured implants. They are more natural looking, teardrop shaped, not round. Quite popular for a while. But recent studies have linked them to a rare form of non-Hodgkin's lymphoma. It's very low-risk, Google it … It's just that now patients are asking me to take them out. Some are worried about the rare cancer. Others are unhappy because the textured implants are firmer, not as soft as the round silicone implants. Although they look more natural, they don't feel as much like fatty breast tissue—"

"But the lymphoma—"

"The lymphoma occurs, like, 1 in 500,000 and is associated mainly with textured implants. Very rare. And it's contained in the fluid surrounding the implant. Completely curable—we just remove it!"

He fidgeted sheepishly, wishing to change the subject.

"You don't have to make these decisions now. You can decide after the expander is in—you'll have weeks to think about it."

Further discussion about implants was deferred, and the rest of the appointment consumed by explanations about expanders, drains, and potentially chronic post-surgical pain. My attention shifted from aesthetics to prognosis.

~

When I first learned I would need a mastectomy, I was told about two or three "autologous reconstruction" options. These are surgeries in which a breast shape is sculpted from tissue (excess skin and fat, and sometimes muscle) that is transferred from another part of your body. The resulting "breast" has little, if any, sensation, but does age and change size with the rest of you. It also lasts a lifetime, unlike an implant, which typically needs to be replaced in 10–20 years.

Despite such advantages, I determined pretty quickly that autologous surgeries were not right for me. First, I did not have enough tummy fat for the outcome I desired. The idea of taking tissue from my inner thighs, buttocks, and abdomen was too overwhelming. So many opportunities for infections and hematomas! A second, related reason I balked: the prospect of spending 8–12 hours under general anesthesia and up to 8 weeks recovering from multiple-site surgery. I considered my 4-year-old—and my patients. Also, there was cancer, my top priority.

At the time of my exchange surgery (the swapping of the tissue expander for silicone gel), placing the implanted prosthesis over the pectoral muscle was not an option at FCH. But very soon such "prepectoral" surgeries were routine. When I complained at a yearly checkup that I constantly had a foreign-object sensation in my chest and that my reconstructed breast collapsed like a limp marionette every time I bent forward or flexed my pectoral muscle, the surgeon suggested that placement of the implant over the pectoralis would fix the "animation deformity" and chronic discomfort. I was chagrined that such techniques had not been available several surgeries before. I did not want to be cut open again.

Dreams of necrotic limbs in hospital beds and dissected corpses recurred. I have an alien body inside my chest, and as it prods my muscles from a most intimate and unreachable place, I wish it gone, along with the soreness. The skin covering the implant is a different matter. I run my fingers over its doughy, cold surface and feel almost nothing, as if touching another. If the uncanny is "extimate," as Jacques Lacan termed it, the fading interstice between animate and inanimate, belonging neither to the interior nor to the exterior—a foreignness frighteningly visceral— then the silicone blob under my flesh is its consummate representative. Is it me or not-me? Dead or alive? Friend or killer?

~

The "gummy bear" cohesive gel implants were recalled by their maker, Allergan, at the request of the FDA in 2019 (Santanelli di Pompeo et al., 2022, para. 25). Dr. Forceps stopped using them after finding that 1 in 800 in his practice developed breast implant–associated anaplastic large cell lymphoma (BIA-ALCL), a rare type of non-Hodgkin's lymphoma that sets up shop in the scar tissue encapsulating the textured implant.

~

At virtually every expansion appointment I was asked whether I wanted mastopexy (a lift) and mammoplasty (a reduction) of the contralateral breast during the exchange surgery, "for symmetry, to match" the perkier implant. I was certain that I did not wish to lose any more breast tissue, and to this day I do not understand why a reduction was pushed. I was less sure about the lift. I wanted to see first how I would look and feel without it, whether I could tolerate the asymmetry. The plastics team assured me that I could delay my decision until the nipple reconstruction in about 4 months. With that procedure I could opt also to have a "revision"— minor abdominal liposuction and fat grafting—to give the reconstructed breast a fuller, "more natural" appearance.

The exchange surgery was not as "easy-peasy" as Dr. F had promised. I did not tolerate the anesthesia well and spent many hours nauseous and in pain. The nurses and paraprofessionals at the famed Mastectomy Central seemed less delightfully attentive, even callous, and the same-day discharge was brutal. While the "permanent" implant was lighter and softer than the overfilled and inflexible tissue expander, it was nonetheless obtrusive, a palpable mass; not what I had been led to expect.

I removed the surgical bra and faced the prosthesis. It was so high on my torso that it gave the impression of originating at the base of the neck. Below, on the left, my remaining breast struck me as deflated and lonely, its nipple downcast. Still more unsettling than the asymmetry was the appearance, the bald thingness, of my new "breast." It looked nothing like its deceased counterpart. In fact, it did not resemble a breast. The semiglobular mound lacked a nipple and featured a horizontal, bisecting scar, like a closed mouth. It suddenly occurred to me that I had been better able to recognizable myself before the reconstruction. This latest postsurgical encounter with my specular image was more disturbing, uncanny. What had been the point?

Urgent questions arose. How would I make this mound mine? How would I shed the uncanniness, internalize not only what I had lost but, also, what I had gained? The prosthesis could not remain a sarcophagus. It had to be domesticated, loved; it had to be possessed, libidinized, made an object of fantasy. Is this what mourning my body would be about—the (re)making of an object through ownership, disappearance, and detachment? For the body in the mirror to belong to me again, the extimate had to release its grip: an object, *the* object, had to form, and fall away.

~

"Prosthesis" achieved academic currency in the late 1980s and has since journeyed far and wide in ever-multiplying metaphoric transfigurations. Its "opportunism" is well documented, as are its many usages across all manner of interdisciplinary subfields and hybrid genres (Smith & Morra, 2007, p. 2). One finds prosthesis in its robust and bloated versions in posthumanism, the history of science, film studies, critical theory, cultural studies, visual art and design; and in its narrower, concrete sense in disability studies, crip theory, psychoanalysis, autotheory, and creative nonfiction. Prosthesis has grown so encumbered by associative chains and—yet—so susceptible to metonymic flight that volumes on the topic suggest a critical reinterrogation of its material *and* metaphorical bases, as well as its "phenomenological … and embodied nature" (Smith & Morra, 2007, p. 3). Only queerness, perhaps, rivals the prosthetic's capaciousness and promiscuity. Prosthesis can be language, writing, memory, the voice, cigars, a wooden leg; it might also be culture, the animal, the human, technology, planet Earth. It is the mingling of the universal and the particular.

"Man has become a prosthetic God," proclaimed Sigmund Freud in *Civilization and Its Discontents*, having endured 33 surgeries and 10 prostheses (1930/1961a, p. 101). In 1932 alone, Freud consulted with his surgeon Hans Pichler 29 times (Lin, 2017, p. 29). Freud's smoking motivated much of the fussiness over his prosthetic jaw. It had to be right at the palate edge with optimal occlusion so that he could get the most out of his cigars. Smoking for Freud was an unsubstitutable source of pleasure that also facilitated writing and other intellectual activity. Like the cigar, his jaw prosthesis was a conduit of both vitality and grave illness, a testament to the entanglement of the life and death drives.

David Wills (1995/2021), in his genre-defying tour de force *Prosthesis*, a primal scream, "both thesis and theater of prosthesis" (p. xv), tells us that the word initially appeared in English in 1553. "Borrowed directly from the Greek," prosthesis denoted "the addition of a syllable to the beginning of a word." It was not until 1704 that prosthesis acquired its more recognizable meaning in John Kersey's revision of Edward Phillips's *Dictionary*: "the replacement of a missing part of the body with an artificial one" (Wills, 1995/2021, p. 218). Theorists have exploited this double, bitemporal sense of prosthesis—an extension or augmentation as well as something "placed before"—in attempts to think that which cannot be thought: the indiscernible articulation of nature and culture, the fading transfer from internal to external; an originary cut, the differential, ontological negativity, the *unbehagen* in culture, the hole in reality, sex, *geschlecht*, the trace, not-all, ephemera. The life-lessness haunting real life. The potentiality of the dead. Wills (1995/2021) writes:

> "Prosthesis" necessarily refers to two contradictory but complementary opera-tions: amputation and addition; and then, of course, the animal and mineral, living or natural and artificial, and so on. There is nothing that is simply or singularly prosthetic; it has no originary integrality. ... "Prosthesis" includes his and mine, my father's wooden leg and this prosthesis as text.
>
> (p. 133)

Like its conceptual siblings—queer temporality, primal repression, the uncanny, the extimate, object *a*, the Real—prosthesis aims to portray a fleeting and unutter-able operation, a temporal suspension and undecidability that nonetheless stirs and decides radically:

> Although there is no decisive moment that inaugurates prosthesis—its idea and structure—any given prosthesis will all the same be marked by a coming down of a decision, the diagnostic sentence, a prelude to the surgical falling of the ax.
>
> (Wills, 1995/2021, p. 149)

When we speak of prosthesis, we often invoke the liminal, the interstitial, the in-between. But the prosthetic really is not locatable. It oscillates between absence and presence; it twitches and slips through cracks in language and embodi-ment, the detritus of metonymy and metaphor, the hollow of the gaze. Prosthesis is not *of* the corporeal, but it is borne by it. This dynamic connection to the body is important. Wills refers to prosthesis as transfer itself, and as "*translation* ... a move-ment or spacing of and into difference" (1995/2021, p. 12). Is pain translatable?

Wills (1995/2021) begins his book with a two-page sentence. Next, a memory or an archive of memories of his father washing the dishes, leaning over the sink on his elbows and reciting Virgil, the same line over and over—"The hoof strikes the dusty plain in a four footed rhythm"—trying to distract himself from a phantom pain in his amputated leg, to preempt a spasm, shifting from the prosthetic steel leg to the warm, living one and back again, rocking gently from side to side, wincing and incanting (p. 3). Wills goes on to formulate:

> From earthbound gallop to quadrupedantic flight, from leg of flesh to leg of steel, it is necessarily a transfer into otherness, articulated through the radical alterity of ablation as loss of integrity. And this otherness is mediated through the body ... carried by the body. ... But it doesn't just carry itself; it carries a

self that is divided in its function—walking, carrying. Before it begins to carry anything external to itself it bears that effect of its own internal scission. Thus it is the otherness that the body must carry in order to move that begins—and a first-person adjective is now ready to bear it—this our prosthesis.

(Wills, 1995/2021, p. 12)

Where does the prosthesis end and my body begin? What is *mine* and what is *ours*? Is the prosthetic edge in the scar tissue encapsuling silicone; in the fat transplanted from my abdomen and injected beneath my skin and over the implant; in the transferred fat that became necrotic, a subcutaneous nodule of dead tissue? Is my borne otherness the inherited unconscious; or the "precipitate of abandoned object-cathexes" (Freud, 1923/1961b, p. 29), the residue of losses—cuts accrued over time? What are the limits of the hallucinated body? Where does ideal ego translate into the untrammeled Real?

~

If D. W. Winnicott is right and there is no baby without the "environment-mother," is prosthesis the mother or is it the baby? Winnicott asked that we not try to figure it out. The mother's opaque signifiers that she herself does not comprehend (because they are her unconscious) enter the baby. The baby receives these signifiers, foreign messages, and enters into identifications with them. The foreigners are welcomed since there is room at the inn, an emptiness awaiting their arrival, the body's orifices. Maybe, then, the maternal breast is the prosthetic, or it is breast milk, the medium of transfer from nipple to mouth, a translation into otherness?

All attempts at translation fail, a little. There is something of the maternal breast that is more than the breast, and less, the supplement that nourishes and the absence that frustrates. The breast appears and disappears, a satisfying mnemic image forever linked to the very pain it is conjured to alleviate. The moment of hunger, of desire is this alchemy, a mixture of agony and pleasure signaled by a memory trace of something invariably missing. Sex, sexual difference, all difference, bear an originary scar, the mark of mortality and the human's inability to fully assimilate it. The first satisfying object is also the hostile object. Prosthesis is both cause and remedy, subtraction and doubling.

The baby starts with a minus. It knows only *the* breast, not two. The object is always singular, always misrecognized. One breast, one nipple at a time, installs itself in the baby's organism. From within this fracture in vision and sense, through prosthesis, the baby gradually internalizes the two-breasted mirrored image of her mother, becomes a feminine subject with ties to other "women." The one-breasted woman is uncanny, frightening and shameful, for she is the mother-baby, the repressed pre-relational relation that shadows and dislocates subjecthood.

~

Posthumanist discourses employ the figural prosthetic to shake up tired hierarchies and binaries: "The prosthesis is not a mere extension of the human body; it is the constitution of the body qua 'human,'" writes philosopher Bernard Stiegler (1994/1998a, pp. 152–153). What does it mean to say that the category of the human is a byproduct of prosthesis, that it "shares the evanescence of the commodity and of spectacle … a type of dream flickering across a 'paralytic' entropic surface of mechanical reason" (Matviyenko & Roof, 2018, p. 18)? On first blush the suggestion that the mechanized world precedes the human might seem whimsical, the stuff of science-fiction horror. One way to understand the proposition is through the lens of Lacan's teaching, which posits that human drives are constituted in an encounter *with* civilization and not merely tamed *by* it, as some readers of Freud would have it. Drives are not reducible to biology; they are anaclitic derivatives of bodily needs and "an 'excess in advent' of technology or generalized technicity" (Matviyenko & Roof, 2018, p. 18). Freud certainly did not consider the matter settled, for even if the human had "become a kind of prosthetic God," sublime through technological extension, his "auxiliary organs" had "not grown on to him, and still give him trouble at times." Modern man "is not happy in his Godlike character" (Freud, 1930/1961a, p. 101).

The temporal being, contend Martin Heidegger's critics and followers, originates with the exteriorization of memory through orthographic writing and recording, through archives and the consequent dialectic between inside and outside (Derrida, 1995; Stiegler, 1994/1998a). Humans do not think themselves human before they become interested in time and its passing, in mortality and the anticipation of death. We're all on the clock, someone else's clock, alienated from ourselves through technological prosthesis, ecstatically preceding and ahead of ourselves, looking back, creating memories for deferred contemplation, "mythological moments of fore- and after-thought" (Wills, 2007, p. 250). Technology qua prosthetic tools that humans have utilized in writing, processing, tracking, preserving memory—from the stylus to the smartphone—initiates a spatiotemporal disjunction, the uncanny "becoming-space of time and the becoming-time of space" (Wills, 2007, p. 256). Technological developments thus inevitably bear questions about temporality and contribute to a discursivity of speed: instant or delayed, fast or slow, before or after.

Stiegler (1996/1998b) tells us to be suspicious of technological immediacy. His thesis is that "technical time" is not continuity and connection achieved through speed but, rather, its opposite: originary breakdown and dislocation. Speed, in fact, is the very disarticulation of time and space. Televisual and cinematographic technologies might trumpet "real time"—immediate retransmission of recorded images—but "electronic transmission [really] occurs within a confusion in which what happens and the happening itself are destroyed in their coincidence" (Stiegler, 1996/1998b, p. 124). Neither "real time" nor Facetime is free of technological intervention, of prostheticity. And yet we, children of Romanticism, continually celebrate their transparency, equating spontaneity with authenticity and privileging both via the fantasy of personal autonomy.

~

"Immediate breast reconstruction" veils prosthesis. It obscures weeks, months, sometimes years of corporeal definition and dismantling, chronic discomfort, grief and anxiety—a hermeneutics of pain and elaborate ensembles of care. Immediate reconstruction is neither immediate nor reconstruction, but, rather, a mirage hiding "relations among people, machines, and practices," social and biological transfer and deferral, the "conceptual and practical labor" (Sterne, 2003, p. 219) of preparing and adapting to shifts in corporeality.

Reconstruction is billed as an antidote or alternative to the prosthetic breast form that is attached externally, inside a bra and under clothing. But prosthesis technology is precisely what permits reconstruction and, more fundamentally, the idea of the body as an "entity" with a surface and an "outside" (Wills, 2007, p. 258). A pocket must be forged under or over the pectoral muscle before silicone gel can be implanted. The skin is cut and stretched over time, making space. After the implant is inserted, encased in scar tissue, the contralateral, "natural" breast is lifted, sculpted, and tattooed to "match" the copy in a bidirectional mimetic process. Almost seamlessly prosthesis transforms from an ersatz supplement into an aesthetically superior growth necessitating adaptation.

What is resisted and often denied by the discourse of breast reconstruction, therefore, is the prosthetic mutability of bodies, the differentiating and self-dividing effects of technicity; that the pristine human organism never was—that it is but a trace left by proleptic and retroactive translation. Prosthesis is and is not part of me—the queer part, "animation deformity"—an aspect that extends and mutilates simultaneously, confounding my bodily boundaries.

~

Roman Kachanov's four *Cheburashka* stop-motion films (1969–1983), easily the most popular cartoon serial produced in the Brezhnev years, rendered every Soviet child an initiate of queerness. The tetralogy is principally about the relationship between Gena, a lonely crocodile bachelor who seeks friends, and Cheburashka, an animal (or is he a toy?) of ambiguous species, age, and gender affiliation. From the start, Cheburashka embodies, effects, and performs a radical unknowability. In the first installment, he arrives at a produce store in a crate of oranges with no name, clothes, or other identity markers and is promptly taken to the zoo. After some fuss and inquiry, the zookeeper explains to the store clerk that Cheburashka cannot be accepted because he is "unknown to science" and nobody can figure out "where to place him" (Kachanov, 1969, 2:49). Part monkey, part bear, possibly neither, Cheburashka defies categorization: He simply does not fit. Gena's search for "cheburashka" (a nickname related to the word "topple" invented by the store clerk) in an encyclopedia yields only a dumb gap somewhere between the city Cheboksary and *chemodan* (suitcase).

Cheburashka, too, fails to solve the riddle of his own identity. Characters ask repeatedly about his species in the initial episode, and each "who are you?" elicits from him an unperturbed "I don't know." One might expect that such unintelligibility and ignorance would disable Cheburashka, make him the object of ridicule, social exclusion, judicial action, perhaps even medical scrutiny and scientific experimentation. But nothing of the kind happens. Cheburashka is quite subjectivized and self-possessed, unfazed by his biological indeterminacy. He gains the respect and love of Gena and everyone else he meets, helps build the House of Friendship, and, in general, seems comfortable in his own skin. In fact,

Cheburashka's "unknowing" enables him to evade regimes of truth and injurious ideological interpellation (Sedgwick, 1988/1993b, pp. 23–51). In a totalitarian society, Cheburashka is free.

Freer, in any case, than Crocodile Gena, who, working in a zoo "as a crocodile," believes in his immediate identity with himself. When we first meet Gena, he is a crocodile in essence—biology, occupation, public and inner realms—in seamless unity with his symbolic mandate. Gena's inability to achieve a mediated distance toward himself is evidenced by his difficulty in spelling "crocodile" while composing a flyer announcing his quest for friendship. Gena easily writes the rest of the announcement and demonstrates literacy by reading signs and newspapers. In the last installment, *Cheburashka idet v shkolu* (*Cheburashka Goes to School*; 1983), he even sends Cheburashka a telegram. But because Gena views his crocodile-ness as an inherent property, he has trouble formulating it discursively, as a symbolizable fantasy construction. Sitting in a zoo enclosure, his red coat and white shirt hanging on a tree branch, the eponymous hero of the inaugural *Krokodil Gena* (1969) has being but no subjectivity. It is arguably through his friendship with Cheburashka that Gena gradually acquires a space between *what he is* in the signifying network and his imagined self. Upon meeting the adorable misfit, Gena leaves his post at the zoo for other pursuits: He builds a playground, travels, and battles a polluting factory manager. Witnessing Cheburashka's alienation from the symbolic order—and his self-actualization despite, or precisely because of, failures internal to the process of interpellation—Gena too becomes a subject.

Yet the matter of Gena's subjectivity becomes more complicated when approached from the perspective of queer aesthetics. As a crocodile who wears human clothing in "real life" and makes himself into a spectacle daily, indeed, earns money by performing exotic animality, Gena might also be read as intentional camp (Sontag, 1964/1999). His personality, like all camp, challenges the notion of performance as a vertical structure in which a "real" person is presumed to dwell beneath the performed identity. In the case of the crocodile, a preconstructed "Gena" (a reptile who lives as a human among humans) animates the performed role of the Crocodile in the zoo. Hence, we see him reclining under a tree, surrounded by a wire fence, posing flamboyantly (not at all like a crocodile) for the spectators, reading a newspaper and smoking a pipe when the patrons are not around, and periodically glancing at his watch. When the workday ends, Gena puts on his shirt, tie, coat, and fedora and resumes his life in human society, waving goodbye to the zookeeper on his way out. The extravagance of the character "Gena" exceeds his crocodile role.

Literary theorist Jonathan Dollimore (1991) is particularly incisive about this aspect of camp, arguing that it

> undermines the depth model of identity from inside ... [it is] a kind of parody and mimicry which hollows out from within. ... Rather than the direct repudiation of depth, there is a performance of its excess: depth is undermined by being taken to and beyond its own limits.
>
> (pp. 310–311)

Camp style is associated with queer counterculture and especially drag because it utilizes over identification, exaggeration, the blurring of autobiography and public image, performance and audience, in order to denaturalize desire, gender roles, and the concept of authenticity itself. When newspaper-reading Gena, respectable in his neat working-class attire, steeped in *kul'turnost'* (cultivation) and attentive to etiquette and hygiene, camps it up, treats work as theater and working-class identity as a role, he strikes at the very foundations of socialist values.

~

If questions of identity, loneliness, and acceptance are salient in the Cheburashka series, queer time is its reigning preoccupation, textually embedded and poignantly expressed in the music, especially the two instantly classic songs from *Cheburashka* (1971) and *Shapokliak* (1974)—respectively, "Goluboi vagon" ("The Blue Train Car") and Gena's Birthday Song, or "Pust' begut neukliuzhe." The episode *Cheburashka* opens with the sound of rain and a sky-blue delivery truck bearing the words *"den' rozhdeniia"* (birthday). The truck and its lethargic driver putt-putt toward Gena, who sits on a bench playing an accordion and singing a sentimental birthday song:

> Let pedestrians clumsily
> Wade through the puddles
> As water streams down the street.
> Passersby just don't get why
> On this rainy day
> I am so happy.
> [Refrain:]
> I am playing my accordion
> Outside for all to see.
> What a pity that a birthday
> Comes but once a year.
> What if suddenly a magician arrived
> In a blue helicopter
> And showed a movie for free.
> He would wish me a happy birthday
> And maybe leave
> A present of 500 ice cream bars for me.
>   (Kachanov, 1971, 0:52)

One is immediately struck by the unmistakably doleful quality of what is supposed to be, if we believe the lines, a celebratory song. "Pust' begut neukliuzhe" is in melancholic C minor and played on an accordion, the loneliest of instruments, a one-man band with melody on the right hand and preset chords on the left. The solitary Gena, basically a street musician, performs for an audience of one, the delivery man. Indeed, the lyrics are belied by a gaping absence of people. There are no "clumsy pedestrians," just as there are no soaked passersby wondering about Gena's happiness. Not only the magician and ice cream, but also the entire song can be interpreted as a hallucination narrated to cover over various lacks: deficits of consumer goods, crop failures, and eroding sociability due to time spent in queues. In Brezhnev's era of space program achievements and food shortages, Gena's free movie and mountains of ice cream bars dropped from the sky are the perfect fantasy.

But perhaps the most wistful and famous line of the song, "what a pity that a birthday comes but once a year," is also the most explicitly about temporality. Gena expresses a wish for repetition, a disruption in the calendar, perhaps, a reorganization or manipulation of time. Such temporal pliability is signaled by the arrival of a blue, or *goluboi*, helicopter: Here again, the color blue is used to express queerness, a shift in temporal and spatial coordinates. The helicopter transports Gena to a magical space of amplitude and freedom.

"Goluboi vagon," the other meditation on time in minor key, is sung by Gena in the third episode as he sits, accordion in tow, on top of a sky-blue caboose with Cheburashka and their erstwhile adversary, Old Lady Shapokliak:

> Slowly the minutes flow past
> Don't expect to see them again.
> And even though we mourn the past a little bit
> All the best, of course, is still ahead.
> [Refrain:]
> Smoothly, effortlessly the long path spreads out
> And runs straight into the horizon.
> Everyone, everyone hopes for the best
> And our blue train car rolls forward.
> Perhaps we hurt someone needlessly
> The calendar will turn that page for us.
> Toward new adventures let's run my friends.
> Hey, driver, speed it up!
> The blue car races and shakes,
> The express train's picking up speed
> But why does this day have to come to an end
> I wish it would last the whole year.
> (Kachanov, 1974, 16:10)

In animation, as in the animal kingdom, depth and complexity are relative matters. Gena is clearly a simpleton if juxtaposed with a character from Leo Tolstoy or Fyodor Dostoevsky. But compared to his former self, say, in the first episode, he is a world-weary sage, thoroughly devoid of his former unselfconsciousness. In "Goluboi vagon," Gena is a veritable philosopher, the sort of protagonist who would go mad if forced to pose before spectators at a zoo. And, befitting an intellectual, he can even be abstruse: "perhaps we hurt someone needlessly"—what or whom is he talking about? One is tempted to say that Gena is wholly out of character here, acting as a Greek chorus or an internal object voice.

What is more, "Goluboi vagon" is both about time and against it, situated outside the time and space of the film's narrative and functioning vertically, as a reflective postscript and halt in the action. The lyrics of the song present us with an apparent contradiction as well. The emotionally weighted message at the start seems to be: *Turn the page.* Despite possible loss and difficulty, we must let go of past grievances, direct our attention toward the future, and seek new adventures. Do it now, accelerate, move along; the best is ahead! But almost instantly the impatient, forward-looking optimism is subverted. As the train chugs to a nostalgic minor tonality, Gena and the others sit at the rear of the caboose, looking not to their future, but backward, as it were. The unnecessary "of course" in "the best, of course, is still ahead" raises the sort of skepticism commonly elicited by overinsistence: Is it sarcasm or a defensive posture concealing contrary feelings? And in a final, dramatic reversal of sentiment, the lines after "the express train picks up speed" suggest time is passing too quickly: "Why does this day have to come to an end / I wish it would last the whole year." Even more overtly than in Gena's Birthday Song, "Goluboi vagon" articulates a desire for the postponement of the future, if not a foreclosure of futurity. It is a longing for an eternal moment of reparation and plentitude, a dilated present lived to the fullest.

~

If alternative temporality is at the heart of late Soviet children's culture, how do we account for its continued resonance? Why were songs about time consciousness especially popular in the 1970s, and why does their gentle plaintiveness pervade television airwaves and YouTube channels, seducing émigrés and Russian speakers even today (Katz, 2016, p. 121)? One might ask, too, why Gena wants birthdays more than once a year and a day without end given the gloominess suffusing the present in the two songs: Is he yearning for more nasty weather and prolonged infliction of petty miseries? The answer, of course, is *yes*, and the reason for Gena's wish for sorrowful rehearsal is also the reason for the attachment of post-Soviet adults to their favorite childhood fictional characters: Both are products of a melancholic position, a difficulty in mourning the halted socialist dream.

To complicate the matter still further: Is not the very idea of a sudden breach of temporality already represented in Brezhnev-era children's films and musicals? They seem simultaneously to acknowledge the 1977 Soviet Constitution's foreclosure of communist futurity and to anticipate the 1991 rupture, to give it voice avant la lettre. "The wheels of Time / Wore down from friction," croons Vladimir Vysotsky in *Alisa v strane chudes*, "And then Time was offended— / And the pendulum of time stood still."

~

Perestroika means, literally, reconstruction; it also implies systemic decline. Mikhail Gorbachev carefully chose this term, along with others like *uskorenie* (acceleration) and *glasnost'* (publicity, openness), to invent and undo what came before, *zastoi* (stagnation). In the late 1980s "stagnation" was a retrospective designation grafted onto an era previously unaware of itself as such, as economically and culturally stagnant. With this new periodization, Gorbachev aimed to distract from the regime's failures and to deny continuities with the past—the Chernobyl accident, poor living standards, food shortages, and other signs of destruction and decay—that is, to deny the prostheticity of both the Brezhnev years and his own policies. But stagnation as slogan and as the Before of perestroika functioned pro-leptically and retroactively. Its silences and unfinished sentences met their signi-fiers in Gorbachev's reforms.

Perestroika reconstructed *nothing*. The slogan was just that, a signifier veiling—and thereby marking—incompleteness, deferred meaning, a never-arrived com-munism. "Developed socialism" had prepared the path for Gorbachev, and he unwittingly delivered the final blow to the communist project, convulsively intro-ducing markets, inviting alternate viewpoints, emphasizing speed, and undermining its temporality. By distancing his person and reforms from the preceding, slacking decade, he pointed to a glitch in the progress toward utopia. Perestroika—a mask, a cover-up, a fetish—alerted Soviet citizens to the ways Gorbachev's errors had been prefigured in the 1970s, that which was *placed before*, a hole, antagonism, or impasse, *prosthesis*: the point of Communism's internal impossibility that would eventually become another Event, the dissolution of the Soviet Union.

~

Stagnation-era animators registered temporal fracture in their obsession with failed masculinity, depicted through the relationship between boyish protagonists and avuncular companions (Kliuchkin, 2008). In addition to Kachanov's Cheburashka and Gena, there were Vinni-Pukh and Piatachok (Winnie-the-Pooh and Piglet) in Fedor Khitruk's trilogy (1969–1972) and the duo I loved most in childhood: the Kid and Karlson in Boris Stepantsev's two animated shorts adapted from Astrid Lindgren's Karlsson-on-the-Roof books. It is not simply that the films spotlight older eccentric figures with little sidekicks but that they portray them queerly, in uneasy relation to gender, identity, social space, and time. Gena and Karlson are decidedly awkward and immature, inveterate bachelors ill-suited to their appar-ent mentoring roles. The queer nature of the older characters emanates from their ambiguous developmental stages, the non-filial register of their interaction with younger mates, and their association with other socially marginal or unreproductive characters: the trouble-making Old Lady Shapokliak in the Cheburashka series and the Kid's manifestly neglectful housekeeper, Freken Bok (Fröken Hildur Bock).

Gena's identity and connection to Cheburashka are murky, at best. The croco-dile's pipe smoking and dark timbre, provided by actor Vasilii Livanov, code him as an older male, as does the sonic distance between him and the reedy-voiced Cheburashka of Klara Rumianova. After Gena leaves his post at the zoo, we observe him beset by loneliness in a cluttered and untidy house, playing chess with an imaginary partner and composing a flyer seeking friendship. Gena's fatherly attitude can be detected in his concern for the welfare of the local children (who inspire him to build a playground) in the second episode and in his decision to send Cheburashka to school in the last installment of the series. The bond between Gena and Cheburashka seems, at least at some points, to carry the sort of intense emo-tional investment we attribute to parent–child relationships. When Cheburashka accidentally latches onto a launched toy helicopter and perilously whizzes through the air before landing safely, Gena is beside himself with worry, racing after his buddy and breathlessly inquiring about his physical well-being.

But at many other moments the generational difference between Gena and Cheburashka breaks down, along with their filial rapport. For example, in the second episode, it is Cheburashka who shyly gives Gena the toy helicopter for his birthday, and, later in the film, the two aspire to become Young Pioneers as if they are coevals. Gena describes himself as a "young crocodile" in tentative, childlike scrawl at the beginning of the series, but since youth is a relative concept and Gena is an animal, the matter of his age remains unresolved: Is he adolescent, unintelligent (hence "young") in some specifically reptilian way or, on the contrary, urbane, coy, self-promoting, and therefore ever youthful?

Weighing these multiple readings and tensions, one might surmise that Gena's infantile manner signals and rejoices in the stereotype of stunted queerness, tacitly referencing the notorious Freudian association of homosexuality with regression. Various aspects of Gena's character support such a view. He has no interest in female companionship or conjugal life, preferring to spend eternity with a toylike orphan. While Shapokliak's pranks might be viewed as disguised or disavowed declarations of love for Gena, the crocodile returns the Old Lady's modest overtures with a formal gentlemanly posture and an absolute indifference to heterosexual romance. And, as is plain from his two songs, Gena is not altogether innocent of pain and loss: By the third episode he is a psychological being, gripped by a desire for the impossible. Gena sings "The Blue Train Car" with the longing depressive's typical ambiguity of purpose, wishing for movement but toward no particular aim. We know that the train is en route to Moscow and that Gena's goal is friendship, but Gena himself does not experience his needs in such specific terms. He does not want, as children do; he yearns in the shadow of disappointment born of lived experience.

Like Gena, Karlson seems to have no significant attachments other than his young friend, and his relationship with the Kid has all the ingredients of a passionate love affair. Their romance is palpable from the moment the propellered trickster first lands on the Kid's windowsill. With Karlson's prompting, the two flirtatiously exchange information about age and personal proclivities with plenty of shoulder shrugs, giggles, and bashful head tilting. The Kid hesitatingly reveals that he is 7 years old, while Karlson, theatrically stroking his hair and waving his hand, declaims that he is "in the prime of his life" (Stepantsev, 1968, 5:06). Later, as the Kid weeps bitterly after his eighth birthday party because he mistakenly believes his parents neglected to buy him a puppy, Karlson asks, on his knees and in a stunned half-whisper, "A dog? But what about me? Kid, am I not better than a dog?" (Stepantsev, 1968, 17:30). And when the Kid's parents finally surprise him with a puppy, Karlson cannot bear the competition and disappears, leaving the boy bereft. In the episode's final frame, washed in a grayish blue, the Kid stands motionless with the dog under his arm, waiting and hoping for Karlson's return to the strains of a mournful tune.

But who, after all, is Karlson? And what about him communicates advanced age even as his small stature (he is shorter than the Kid), grandiosity, silly antics, and insatiable appetite for sweets signal prepubescence? Does he represent what Sedgwick called the "avunculate" (1993c, p. 63)? Is Karlson, in other words, a gay uncle type? He certainly is queerly embodied: Thick in the waist and carrot-topped, with a triangular head, he wears pants held up asymmetrically by one suspender. Though much of his dressed body is clownish and infantile in appearance, Karlson is readable as an adult principally because of his throaty baritone, furnished by actor Vasilii Livanov (also the voice of Gena). Livanov's is a masculine pitch that finds somewhat shaky corporeal support in his character's black bushy eyebrows and broad-palmed bravado.

It is precisely such vocal incongruence that seems partly responsible for the Brezhnev-era Karlson's enduring popularity. As literary scholar Maria Maiofis (2008) discusses at some length, the 2002 Russian release of a dubbed version of the Swedish animated film *Karlsson on the Roof* (Idsøe, 2002) elicited a flood of very critical reviews and, perhaps inevitably, many invidious comparisons between the familiar Soviet interpretation, deemed definitive, and the latest "foreign" iteration. Critics expressed dismay over most of the performances and yearned for the warm and loving Karlson of Livanov. Still, they were mildly impressed by the efforts of the well-known actor Sergei Bezrukov, who attempted to imitate Livanov's timbre and intonation (Maiofis, 2008, pp. 241–244).

The attachment of post-Soviet audiences to the 1968–1970 Karlson therefore appears to be rooted in a specific sonority, as well as a particular form of vocal drag: By locating Livanov's deep and weatherworn voice in a destructive but ultimately benevolent trickster, the animators at Soiuzmul'tfil'm performed and rejoiced in a failure—an excess or heterogeneity—showing that the vocal object cannot reliably be traced to a given body. They also attenuated and tamed the sound of a much less sympathetic adult Russian masculinity, associated after many years of war and Stalinist policies with arbitrary violence and carceral life.

~

Karlson-Livanov's queerness and attendant commitment to pleasure also contributes to the radical undermining of linear time. When Karlson arrives, the Kid's world immediately intensifies: Colors become saturated, and the grays of family routine vanish from the Kid's visual field—and ours. Daily rhythms are interrupted, and life is lived more vividly and urgently. Karlson swings from a chandelier that comes crashing down, takes the Kid flying over rooftops, and plays pranks on the newly hired Freken Bok. A steady supply of fruit preserves is brought out to keep Karlson content, and there is jazzy music and dancing. The imaginative flexibility necessary for such a queer mode of living is facilitated by Karlson's histrionic movements, retro aesthetics, and extravagant self-presentation. Operatic poses, splashy gesticulation, and costumes from the avant-garde early 1900s hint at artistic and sexual license.

The limits to this queer temporality are set by the comings and goings of sober intelligentsia parents whose entrance immediately curtails the expansive living and reinstalls clock time—at least until the second episode, when the division between normative adult and "Karlson time" is violated by the inclusion of the middle-aged Freken Bok. Or is it? The initially prim Freken Bok, it turns out, is quite labile and eccentric, as much an outsider as Karlson and in many ways allied with him. With her voluminous body, floral smock, and hair wrapped unfashionably in a bun, she is matronly but in no way maternal: When asked by the Kid's father if she likes children, she pauses for an uncomfortable length of time before proclaiming, "madly!" in an affected manner (Stepantsev, 1970, 21:10). Like Karlson, Faina Ranevskaia's Freken Bok is vain, juvenile, and dwells in the lower vocal range. Her magisterial contralto is larded with hyperbole and her pantomime is imbued with decadent fin de siècle emotionalism. Out of bounds sexually and temporally, unmarried and without children (and a bit too attached to her cat Matilda), the housekeeper joins Karlson in delimiting queer time and space.

Old Lady Shapokliak, Freken Bok's counterpart in the Cheburashka series, is also a woman without family and in gender trouble. Though she is utterly different from the housekeeper in embodiment and sonority—Shapokliak is ancient, wiry, and, in the first of the Cheburashka films, voiced by a male actor—her stance toward the world and place in the narrative evokes a similar politics. She is a meticulously attired androgyne clad in a turn-of-the-20th-century black dress with a white ruffle lace collar and, as her name signals, a 1940s *chapeau claque*. With both figures, as with Gena's fedora, stiff collar, and 1920s coat, Soviet animators used temporal drag—that is, sartorial and bodily references to all that is obsolete and outmoded—to disrupt straight, continuous maturation and its reproductive rationale (Freeman, 2010, pp. 59–65). Both Shapokliak and Freken Bok exhibit a denatured femininity permanently excluded from procreative life and traditional family units. Yet their work as foils and collaborators on the margins of the Karlson–Kid and Gena–Cheburashka relationships help constitute new forms of kinship.

~

While Disney innovators embraced cel and 2D animation in the 1970s, the new wavers at Soiuzmul'tfil'm revived stop-motion, a technique first employed in 1898 by Albert E. Smith and J. Stuart Blackton in the lost film *The Humpty Dumpty Circus* (Kornhaber, 2020, p. 82). Using puppets, cutouts, and clay figures, Soviet animators expressed something of stagnation, delay, a trace of deferred trauma. Cheburashka's movements are as twitchy as his gender, as if stuck in the wrong body, assembled from random shaggy parts, evidence that mistakes had been made. As with the Hedgehog and all stop-motion figures, his fluttering mouth and eyelids often lag behind his speech and speed ahead at random intervals.

"Life is movement," writes Jack Halberstam (2011): the "dynamic between motion and stillness is the dynamic between life and death that is nowhere more dramatically captured than in stop-motion animation, [making it perfect for portraying] toys transforming from wooden to animated, coming to life" (pp. 177–178). Introducing momentary pauses, stop-motion undermines the illusion of immediacy and presence and brings technology—one might say *prosthesis*—into visibility. "In stop-motion the themes of remote control, manipulation, entrapment, and imprisonment are everywhere" (Halberstam, 2011, pp. 178–179), as are the shifting borders among humans, animals, and machines.

Perhaps Soviet animators, primarily Jewish and queer, excluded from much of Brezhnev-era's culture industry (Katz, 2016), loved stop-motion for such evocations—and for its animation deformity, the capacity to disrupt one's rooted-ness in "real time," one's sense of coincidence between time and bodies in space. Stop-motion generates uncanny effects as Freud (1919/1955f) had explained them, whiffs of primal repression, the originary passage into life and the march toward death. Its animation deformity replays the loss incurred through separation from the mother, the Other, provoking morbid anxiety. "Stop-motion lends animation a spooky … quality," Halberstam notes (2011): "It conveys life where we expect stillness and stillness where we expect liveliness" (p. 178). The Hedgehog's stutter reminds me that the mechanical lurks beneath the willful, that I exist between two deaths, prenatal nonexistence and my impending mortality.

Like opera and psychoanalysis, stop-motion animation is extravagant, a notori-ously slow and laborious art:

> After each shot, a figure or puppet or prop is moved slightly; thus a stop-motion or claymation feature is made one frame at a time. Motion is *implied* by the rela-tion of one shot to another rather than *recorded* by a camera travelling alongside moving objects. … Unlike classical cinema, in which action attempts to appear seamless and suture consists in the erasure of all marks of editing and human presence, stop-motion animation is uncanny precisely because it depends on the manipulation of figures in front of the camera by those behind it. These relations of dependency, submission even, are precisely ones that we go to the cinema to forget. … The ghostly shifts that stop-motion animation records and incorporates, the shifts between action, direction, intention, and script, desire and constraint, force upon the viewer a darker reality about the human and about representation in general.
>
> (Halberstam, 2011, p. 178)

The ax falls again and again, *e pur si muove*. Stagnation was one such cut, a lull amid motion, the queer failure of socialism. Perestroika would be its recapitu-lation, the uncanny return; but in the 1970s there was no reconstruction yet, no perestroika, only socialist construction. Nonetheless, a parapraxis was registered, an animation deformity inaudibly etched, a scission that would later be named and rethought as stagnation, the harbinger of the death of the Soviet Union.

~

In his commentary on repetition in Seminar XI, Lacan posits the traumatic (missed) encounter with the Real, a recurrent stumbling on an unsymbolized kernel that establishes the subject as such. The Real of which Lacan (1964/1998a) speaks, however, ought not be viewed as purely external. The encounter is awaited, pre-pared by the real signifier, that which represents the outside for the subject *and resides within* (pp. 53–65). Lacan maintains that untouched reality is inaccessible to the speaking being, but this is not the entire story. Objective reality, the so-called phenomenal field, does not simply continue to exist elsewhere, undisturbed and whole (albeit beyond apprehension) once language is acquired. "External reality" is also ontologically incomplete—self-limiting—containing within itself the potentiality of subjectivity. "The hole in reality," moreover, "the inaccessibility of the transcendent In-itself, is a result of the inscription of the perceiving subject *into reality* [emphasis added]" (Sbriglia & Žižek, 2020, p. 10).

The subject is riven, containing in herself something more than herself (and less, the unconscious), something constitutive of subjectivity, object *a*. Reality, too, has its object *a*: the human. In this way the human is matter's prosthesis, its subjective excess, the gap that makes its every iteration inconsistent (Sbriglia & Žižek, 2020, p. 10). The human, Alenka Zupančič (2017) asserts, is the incomplete animal, the proof that there is no pure animality. The speaking being, in other words, is the impasse of the natural world: "Man [*sic*] is not an exception (constituting the whole of the rest of nature), but the point at which nature exists (only) through the inclusion of its own impossibility" (p. 93).

~

In "The 'Uncanny,'" Freud (1919/1955f) drew on his colleague Otto Rank's ideas to speculate that ancient peoples and young children invent the doppelgänger to compensate for their dire powerlessness: to protect the embryonic ego from castrating blows and to deny death. Spirits, ghosts, and imaginary friends do not vanish with scientific progress and the fading of primary narcissism, however. In modern times and later in life, the figure of the double returns as a sinister rival, eliciting uncanny terror, reminding the subject of his former helplessness, blending the strange and the intimate, the automaton and the human (Freud, 1919/1955f, pp. 247–248). Intersubjectivity, the *rapport sexuel*, is myth, implies Freud. Two subjects cannot share space: There is only the *I* and the object. When I am confronted by the other qua subject—like me, yet separate—the double becomes my mortal enemy.

Upon reading Freud's paper in graduate school, I wondered whether the double appears anymore in our secular, non-superstitious epoch, or whether it ever appeared except in literature and in Freud's poignant example of his unpleasant encounter with a strange old man—his reflection—in a train compartment mirror. These initial thoughts were revised under the pressure of my own specular clashes with a foreign self, the one-breasted woman, and by the uncanny effects of breast reconstruction, my repeated efforts at doubling.

The infant's mind and the traumatized person require mirroring for survival. But the mirror invariably cracks: Narcissistic illusion breaks down, and anxiety and shame emerge in the fracture. Psychoanalyst Carolyn Feigelson (1993) explores the connection between the plight of the survivor and the uncanny double through a very specific case, "the state of mind produced in the survivor-beholder, the healthy partner, of a head-injured person." She is eager to note that her "particularized" example might prove widely applicable, relevant to other circumstances "in which a unique event leaves an individual stranded with a psychological stranger" (p. 331).

Feigelson goes on to examine the disturbing experience of living with a close relation who is physically recognizable but otherwise profoundly changed, behaving bizarrely or mechanically, and always in the shadow of his former personality:

> In the situation of personality death, it is not the [brain] injured person but the witness who contends with a ghastly alter ego. First, the bifurcated object acts upon the observer in a real sense. Second, the damaged person attracts projected elements of frightening early representations of the parents. ... Third, this alter ego at the same time invites projected, unwanted self-representations of the witness. The injured person is a "double" of his former self, but he also stimulates projections and identifications of various kinds and intensities. Early repressed conflicts, old narcissistic deficits and sensitivity to empathy-withdrawal, and elements of fantasy-capacity ... may hook on to the impact of real trauma.
>
> (1993, p. 342)

Feigelson details the impact of the injured person's internal transformation on the beholder, the "healthy partner," who

> is required to shift back and forth between past and present images of the object, oscillating between the image in memory and the present moving creature: a situation in which the image of the past feels more real than its current, deformed counterpart.
>
> (1993, p. 334)

For the "survivor-beholder," the "deformed" partner eventually becomes a hated intimate whose "new and different personality is superimposed like a film, upon the original" (Feigelson, 1993, p. 331). The judgment and affect regulation of the noninjured are thrown into disarray. Everyday activities and dialogue become "unpredictable, ambiguous, presenting illusory sameness (the former person is still 'there,' in many respects) oscillating with strangeness, and involving antithetical images of 'death in life'" (Feigelson, 1993, p. 334). Witnesses are compelled into disavowed identification with the injured as "universal fears of inner deadness, devitalization, passivity, madness, stupidity, helplessness, and subjugation are stirred up" (Feigelson, 1993, p. 344) and an endless mourning follows (Feigelson, 1993, pp. 340, 343).

Feigelson (1993) writes mainly about the "survivor-beholder," "the witness," and the "observer" (p. 340) of the injured. The healthy partner, importantly, is one who *sees* the deformity in the other and suffers a rupture in the circuit of recognition, the one who experiences anxiety as well as the affect unmentioned but everywhere in evidence in Feigelson's account—shame. Shame—the urge to hide the otherness in oneself after it has become spectacle—is precisely what floods the subject when the brain-injured object, previously a good-enough reflecting surface, becomes a funhouse mirror. Scared of facing their "inner deadness, stupidity, helplessness, and subjugation"—their castration—children and partners of the injured wish to murder them or lock them up, perhaps to conceal forever the uncanny reminder in a tomb or an asylum.

Like the psychotic, the brain-injured person both witnesses and represents the alien part of the subject, the reality-threating *das Ding*, the animation deformity. Feigelson (1993) quotes Patient D, who "felt sex with his [injured] wife to be like a sacrifice because she made 'weird noises' and had 'a funny look on her face like a confused dog'" (p. 344). Are the only options for this patient endless mourning or wild denial? What would have to happen for him to accept the confused dog, the doubling of his incomplete animality, his own drives? The wife's partial defamiliarization would have to be completed so that the jouissance-soaked dog inside the patient could be handled. The doppelgänger would then transform into a stranger to be welcomed, afforded hospitality (Derrida & Dufourmantelle, 1997/2000).

Feigelson's case brings to mind acceptance of the reconstructed breast, of course, but the metaphor quickly fails. Maybe it is too much to ask a spouse or a child to grant hospitality to the loved one as foreigner, in all his radical alterity, the way one would a prosthesis. The injured relative might be removed, disowned, divorced, hidden. But the defamiliarized reconstructed breast and mastectomy scar must eventually be reabsorbed into the self-image. I cannot hide body parts from myself without irreparable damage to my sense of reality.

~

In Lacan's account of the mirror stage, the infant or toddler faces a mirror, and the mother (or primary caregiver) stands nearby looking on. She might nod in delight or point and say, "Look, that's you!" The child then turns to the mother and grasps, from the vantage point of her gaze, that he represents something for her—something enigmatic, not fully understood—that the mirror image is attributed to him through a nomination emanating from the Other, the primary caregiver as representative of language and Law. This moment introduces a dual alienation: from the image, and also from culture, or the symbolic order. When the infant pivots again to face the mirror, his image fundamentally changes because it is now mediated by the meaning of the Other's gesture. In the aftermath of the mirror stage, the child sees himself at a distance, through the Other's eyes, and seeks love and approval from others (Lacan, 1949/2006a; Vanier, 2012, p. 297). The infant recognizes himself and takes pleasure in his image, but at a cost, the part of his being obliterated by vision and metaphor, object *a*. As we know from the myth of Narcissus, who drowns in an attempt to reach his reflection, the mirror stage introduces both self-love and a mortal tension: If self-distance (and therefore time) narrows, so does the symbolic dimension. The lost object feels too close, the double appears, and the subject's existence is threatened.

The double for Lacan, then, is the mirror image in which the object of primordial loss, object *a*, is included. It is the specular moment when "the imaginary and real coincide, provoking a shattering anxiety," offers Mladen Dolar (1991) in an essay on the uncanny:

> The double is the same as me plus the object *a*, that invisible part of being added to my image. … For the mirror image to contain the object *a*, a wink or a nod is

enough. Lacan uses the gaze as the best presentation of that missing object; in the mirror, one can see one's eyes, but not the gaze which is the part that is lost. But imagine that one could see one's mirror image close its eyes: that would make the object as gaze appear in the mirror.

(p. 13)

Lacan names several quintessential manifestations of object *a*—the fantasmatic extimate—objects internalized, conjured, and shed since infancy: the gaze, the voice, feces, and the breast.

~

My reflection is uncanny because the reconstructed breast transforms into the double of its amputated predecessor. When I move, it ceases to be itself, to behave like a breast, to do what I expect: It contorts and collapses, displaying its animation deformity. The implant under my skin is and is not a breast; it returns to me a foreign image, revealing my *I* as the prosthesis of the world. In those moments I *am* a body.

The subject is not a body; it possesses one. When I am a subject, I forget my gaze, my framing position within the scene. There is a lack where I am, a hole, and this hole is hidden from me. The emergence of myself qua body part in the visual field produces annihilating horror, a lack of lack. The sight of my animation deformity—the uncanny me-not-me, the interstitial gap—renders visible the mediating gaze. I am reminded of my object status, I cannot maintain subjectivity, myself as *I*. What is my reality? How am I located in space and time?

Identifying with the *sinthome*, Lacan taught, is the singular process of coming to own the strangeness of one's body; it means knowing what to do with one's psychic deviations and deformities. This is the end of analysis, the taming and reduction of the uncanny. But how does this process begin post-mastectomy, after a violent alteration of the body's surface? For me, it did not begin with writing. As in infancy, it began with the mirror. It began, paradoxically, with the double: not with the uncanny double that returns but rather with the double that inaugurates, establishing mythical coherence and the body ego. Eventually, for my new reflection to be drained of its most terrifying aspects—for the process of integration to continue—my *I* needed ratification, inscription: a third to acknowledge the reflection as mine.

~

Frankenstein's creation, monstrosity of the Enlightenment, is utterly alone. He desperately longs for a double, a reflection of his mien, and of his secret longings, his most private self. Like Cheburashka and Karlson, Mary Shelley's creature is without "a genealogy, without anybody who would recognize or accept him (not even his creator)" (Dolar, 1991, p. 16). The creature seeks friends who might grant him culture, a stable identity and a place in the world. Most fundamentally, he wishes for a proper mirror stage. Dolar (1991) remarks:

[The monster's] narcissism is ... thwarted from the outset, and the main part of the plot ... springs from his demand for a partner, somebody like him, a wife, so that he could start a line, a new filiation. He is One and Unique, and as such he cannot even have a name: *he cannot be represented by a signifier*—(the absence of which is often "spontaneously" filled in by his "father's" name)—he cannot be a part of the symbolic.

(p. 16)

Dolar (1991) suggests that the story itself has become a "modern myth" in the Lévi-Straussian sense of a "'logical model to resolve a contradiction,' an insoluble task, the contradiction between nature and culture" (p. 16). Frankenstein's monster epitomizes the central concern of the Enlightenment: the discovery of a "zero degree" of subjectivity, the capture of the moment when nature becomes culture, "the point where the spiritual would directly spring from the material." Enlightenment discourses, from John Locke's tabula rasa to Jean-Jacques Rousseau's *Émile*,

> aim at a subject ... singularly deprived of a mirror stage, a ... subject from which the imaginary support in the world has to be taken away ... in order to reconstruct it, in its true significance, from this "zero" point.
>
> (Dolar, 1991, p. 17)

The predicament of Frankenstein's monster—the quintessential missing link produced by science, the subject produced out of nothing—is that, unlike Cheburashka, who finds structural support for his project of subjectivization, he must "create the whole complexity of the spiritual world *ex nihilo*," to live an excruciating and deadly irony:

> As the embodiment of the natural zero state, he is counter to nature, a monster, excluded from nature and culture alike. Through his tragedy, culture only gets back its own message: his monstrosity is the monstrosity of culture. The noble savage, the self-educated man, turns bad only because ... culture turns him down. By not accepting him society shows its corruption, its inability to integrate him, to include its own missing link. Culture judges by nature (that is, by his looks), not by culture (that is, by his good heart and sensitivity). The creature as the Unique only wants a social contract, but being refused one he wants to destroy the contract that excludes him and so to vindicate himself.
>
> (Dolar, 1991, p. 18)

The monster fails in his attempt to found a social contract with "his like," to be recognized as family, and so he kills the family of his creator, his one potential connection to culture. The paradox of Frankenstein's creature, finally, Dolar (1991) claims, is that as the missing link created to restore "the great chain of being," to make the universe continuous and full, he becomes its double, "the horror of an unsplit world" (p. 18), the uncanny anxiety brought on by overproximity, the lack of lack—the reflection in the mirror that blinks when you do not, that does not mimic your movements in absolute synchronicity. The double is where object *a*, the gaze, is included, and it must be eradicated to ensure the ego's survival:

This embodiment of the subject of the Enlightenment directly disrupts its universe and produces its limit. ... Frankenstein brings to humanity, like Prometheus, the spark of life, but also much more. There is a promise to provide it with its origin, to heal the wound of castration, to make it whole again. But filling the lack is catastrophic: the Enlightenment reaches its limit by realizing it, just as the appearance of the double produce[s] the lack of lack.

(Dolar, 1991, p. 18)

~

The reconstructed breast is not a functional prosthesis. Unlike other prostheses, say, artificial limbs or jaws, it cannot be loved for its function. Arguably, it helps during sex, if only in a passive, aesthetic sense, to the degree that it is recognizable as a breast. The reconstructed breast must therefore be loved for its superficiality, for its appearance, and via a complicated dialectical procedure of defamiliarization and refamiliarization, again and again, through retroaction. The acceptance of prosthesis requires a sinthomatic act: the binding of the Real of the body with its specular image and its signifiers in a knot around a "true hole"—an unknowable part to which one surrenders—that holds fast against spectral reminders (Lacan, 1975–1976/2016). I am forced under great duress to choose mastectomy, prosthesis, a mangled body—and I choose it, nonetheless. I claim the strangeness of my deformed breast. I do not adopt an identity of martyr, cancer patient, survivor. I am one who survives.

The specular is crucial for identificatory processes. The mirror might take the form of a mother's face, a caregiver who looks on lovingly, and of the voice, through which exquisite warmth and acceptance are expressed. But for an *other* to function as *the Other*, the other's bodily presence is necessary, since it is the human body in its three dimensions (and not merely as an image) that exudes the silence of the drive, the medium of subjectivity. The body of the maternal other in its ineffable materiality—as biological entity and carrier of signification—supports subjectivizing operations. The analyst, too, performs this function: the analyst as incarnation of object *a*, the excluded part, the unconscious.

~

My mother does not wish to replay the mirror stage, to ratify my reconstructed breast, to nod or point and say, "That's you! You're still *you*! A somewhat different you, to be sure, and yet continuous with the previous one, yes, *yes*!" *I see you; you are beautiful and you are yourself.* She hopes, rather, that I will inter the monstrous prosthesis, stuff it in a bra and veil it with baggy blouses and patterned scarves draped on my neck and chest. She wants me to put it away; she cannot bear the uncanniness, the anxiety. I am the injured double, I am offspring yet strange to her, now.

Instead, perhaps my analyst will recognize me, offer his gaze, a gesture of structural support. How will he do it? Not by looking at my bare breasts or scars, surely, nor with interpretation: for what I need concerns the very limit of interpretation. In this latest rite of passage, as in all the previous mythic ones, being comes to occupy the place where interpretation stops: being as the gaze, the voice shorn of speech, the body as *das Ding*, as biological substance. My analyst acts as the Other and as object *a* by receiving my vocal narration of corporeal events, by reading this text—and through his being-there—in a shared space with me. The analytic act requires the analyst as an embodied presence, as prosthesis: the Real of his body, the hollow of his ears, his gaze receiving the voice as pure sonority, receiving me with the analyst's voice, with silence. In the end, I do this for myself, by myself. I internalize the prosthesis; I become my own analyst: the one who listens, the one who survives, and continues surviving.

The writing of the *sinthome*—one's prostheticity—never ceases.

References

Derrida, J. (1995). Archive fever: A Freudian impression (E. Prenowitz, Trans.). *Diacritics, 25*(2), 9–63.

Derrida, J., & Dufourmantelle, A. (2000). *Of hospitality* (R. Bowlby, Trans.). Stanford University Press. (Original work published 1997)

Dolar, M. (1991). "I shall be with you on your wedding-night": Lacan and the uncanny. *October, 58*, 5–23.

Dollimore, J. (1991). *Sexual dissidence: Augustine to Wilde, Freud to Foucault*. Oxford University Press.

Feigelson, C. (1993). Personality death, object loss, and the uncanny. *International Journal of Psychoanalysis, 74*, 331–345.

Freeman, E. (2010). *Time binds: Queer temporalities, queer histories*. Duke University Press.

Freud, S. (1955f). The "uncanny." In J. Strachey et al. (Eds. & Trans.), *The standard edition of the complete psychological works of Sigmund Freud* (Vol. 17, pp. 217–256). Hogarth Press. (Original work published 1919)

Freud, S. (1961a). Civilization and its discontents. In J. Strachey et al. (Eds. & Trans.), *The standard edition of the complete psychological works of Sigmund Freud* (Vol. 21, pp. 57–146). Hogarth Press. (Original work published 1930)

Freud, S. (1961b). The ego and the id. In J. Strachey et al. (Eds. & Trans.), *The standard edition of the complete psychological works of Sigmund Freud* (Vol. 19, pp. 1–66). Hogarth Press. (Original work published 1923)

Halberstam, J. (2011). *The queer art of failure*. Duke University Press.

Idsøe, V. (Director). (2002). *Karlsson på taket* [Karlsson on the roof] [Film]. AB Svensk Filmindustrie.

Kachanov, R. (Director). (1969). *Krokodil Gena* [Crocodile Gena] [Animated short]. Soiuzmul'tfil'm. Retrieved August 21, 2024, from https://www.dailymotion.com/video/xkb9ys

Kachanov, R. (Director). (1971). *Cheburashka* [Animated short]. Soiuzmul'tfil'm. Retrieved August 21, 2024, from https://www.dailymotion.com/video/x3ayizu

Kachanov, R. (Director). (1974). *Shapokliak* [Animated short]. Soiuzmul'tfil'm. YouTube. Retrieved August 21, 2024, from https://www.youtube.com/watch?v=ZPoFhdDeJqo

Kachanov, R. (Director). (1983). *Cheburashka idet v shkolu* [Cheburashka goes to school] [Animated short]. Soiuzmul'tfil'm. YouTube. Retrieved October 5, 2024, from https://www.youtube.com/watch?v=Fk3rvl6VfV0

Katz, M. B. (2016). *Drawing the iron curtain: Jews and the golden age of Soviet animation.* Rutgers University Press.

Kliuchkin, K. (2008). Zavetnyi mul'tfil'm: Prichiny populiarnosti "Cheburashki" [A cherished cartoon: Reasons for the popularity of "Cheburashka"]. In I. Kukulin, M. Lipovetskii, & M. Maiofis (Eds.), *Veselye chelovechki: Kul'turnye geroi sovetskogo detstva* [Merry little fellows: Cultural heroes of Soviet childhood] (pp. 360–377). Novoe literaturnoe obozrenie.

Kornhaber, D. (2020). *Silent film: A very short introduction.* Oxford University Press.

Lacan, J. (1998a). *The seminar of Jacques Lacan: Book XI. The four fundamental concepts of psychoanalysis* (J.-A. Miller, Ed.; A. Sheridan, Trans.). W. W. Norton & Company. (Original lectures presented 1964)

Lacan, J. (2006a). The mirror stage as formative of the *I* function as revealed in psychoanalytic experience (B. Fink, Trans.). In *Écrits: The first complete edition in English* (B. Fink, Trans.; pp. 75–82). W. W. Norton & Company. (Original work published 1949)

Lacan, J. (2016). *The seminar of Jacques Lacan: Book XXIII. The sinthome* (J.-A. Miller, Ed.; A. R. Price, Trans.). Polity. (Original lectures presented 1975–1976)

Lin, L. (2017). *Freud's jaw and other lost objects: Fractured subjectivity in the face of cancer.* Fordham University Press.

Maiofis, M. (2008). Milyi, milyi trikster: Karlson i sovetskaia utopiia o "nastoiashchem detstve" [Sweet, sweet trickster: Karlson and the Soviet utopia of "real childhood"]. In I. Kukulin, M. Lipovetskii, & M. Maiofis (Eds.), *Veselye chelovechki: Kul'turnye geroi sovetskogo detstva* [Merry little fellows: Cultural heroes of Soviet childhood] (pp. 241–286). Novoe literaturnoe obozrenie.

Matviyenko, S., & Roof, J. (2018). Introduction. In S. Matviyenko & J. Roof (Eds.), *Lacan and the posthuman* (pp. 9–21). Palgrave Macmillan.

Santanelli di Pompeo, F., Paolini, G., Firmani, G., & Sorotos, M. (2022). History of breast implants: Back to the future. *JPRAS Open: An International Open Access Journal of Surgical Reconstruction, 32,* 166–177. https://doi.org/10.1016/j.jpra.2022.02.004

Sbriglia, R., & Žižek, S. (2020). *Subject lessons: Hegel, Lacan, and the future of materialism.* Northwestern University Press.

Sedgwick, E. K. (1993b). Privilege of unknowing: Diderot's *The nun.* In E. K. Sedgwick (Ed.), *Tendencies* (pp. 23–51). Duke University Press. (Original work published 1988)

Sedgwick, E. K. (1993c). Tales of the avunculate: Queer tutelage in *The importance of being earnest.* In E. K. Sedgwick (Ed.), *Tendencies* (pp. 52–72). Duke University Press.

Smith, M., & Morra, J. (2007). Introduction. In M. Smith & J. Morra (Eds.), *The prosthetic impulse: From a posthuman present to a biocultural future* (pp. 1–14). MIT Press.

Sontag, S. (1999). Notes on camp. In F. Cleto (Ed.), *Camp: Queer aesthetics and the performing subject; A reader* (pp. 51–65). University of Michigan Press. (Original work published 1964)

Stepantsev, B. (Director). (1968). *Malysh i Karlson* [The Kid and Karlson] [Animated short]. Soiuzmul'tfil'm. Retrieved August 21, 2024, from https://www.dailymotion.com/video/x41pyqe

Stepantsev, B. (Director). (1970). *Karlson vernulsia* [Karlson returns] [Animated short]. Soiuzmul'tfil'm. Retrieved August 21, 2024, from https://www.dailymotion.com/video/x41pyqe

Sterne, J. (2003). *The audible past: Cultural origins of sound reproduction.* Duke University Press.

Stiegler, B. (1998a). *Technics and time: Vol. 1. The fault of Epimetheus* (R. Beardsworth & G. Collins, Trans.). Stanford University Press. (Original work published 1994)

Stiegler, B. (1998b). *Technics and time: Vol. 2. Disorientation* (S. Barker, Trans.). Stanford University Press. (Original work published 1996)

Vanier, A. (2012). Winnicott and Lacan: A missed encounter? (K. Valendinova, Trans.). *Psychoanalytic Quarterly, 81*(2), 279–303.

Wills, D. (2007). Technology or the discourse of speed. In M. Smith & J. Morra (Eds.), *The prosthetic impulse: From a posthuman present to a biocultural future* (pp. 237–264). MIT Press.

Wills, D. (2021). *Prosthesis.* Stanford University Press. (Original work published 1995)

Zupančič, A. (2017). *What is sex?* MIT Press.

10

Perestroika

My second reconstructive surgery, 7 months after the initial cut, had a triple purpose, a three-in-one job. It consisted of mastopexy of the left breast; nipple "reconstruction" on the mastectomy side using loose skin gathered and twisted into a knot; and lipofilling, the transfer of fat tissue from the belly area to the right breast for a fuller cleavage. On the left breast, Dr. Forceps employed a technique commonly called the "anchor lift": The incision is made around the areola and then straight down the center and around the crease under the breast. The nipple is thereby raised, along with the nerve tree attached to it, giving the breast (if all goes well) a high-sitting, Barbie-doll look. After such a lift, the areola is no longer a true areola, irregularly shaped, but a bull's-eye, with the postsurgical scar acting as its new, perfectly circular border. If the original areola is very pale, its reconstructed version has an especially artificial appearance. Most nipple reconstructions fail, that is to say, flatten, or lose "projection" over time. I was only told this at my post-op appointment.

Sprawled on my couch in an abdominal compression garment and surgical bra almost a week after the surgery, I noticed that my left breast was not healing properly. Some bruises had evolved from fluorescent yellow to blackish purple and then faded. But fresh purpuric geographies and inflammation had surfaced on large areas of the breast, and the vertical incision site had transformed into a raw, umber fault. I sent pictures to the plastics team through the FHC portal and received a prompt reply. The wound dehiscence was undesirable, certainly unattractive, though "common." It meant more scarring, but the incision would heal on its own. The extreme swelling and new bruising were indicative of a hematoma and potentially more serious. I was told by the nurse to come in for a closer look.

Dr. F's waiting area was uncharacteristically empty. I was quickly fetched and escorted to the examination room, where I sat, jaw clenched, nervously contemplating my impending flight to Los Angeles. In several days I was expected at a workshop organized as part of a 2-year research grant on Soviet-era hippies. A friend and colleague had invited me to be a researcher on the project, which helped financially support my psychoanalytic training.

I was to spend 3 days in Venice Beach with my fellow researchers mining the archive of the recently deceased hippie poet Azazello and attending the opening

DOI: 10.4324/9781003498582-11

of an exhibit on Soviet hippies at the Wende Museum. Though in considerable discomfort and worried about the healing process, I was determined to show up in LA to prove my gratitude and commitment.

As the nurse practitioner examined me, I scanned for blanching and other signs of horror or concern. Her eyes were holograms.

"It's not the worst I've seen … not enough for a return to the OR, I don't think. With large hematomas we sometimes have to go back in and drain. As you can probably tell, certain areas are already healing … You should be fine to fly."

She was unconvincing.

"Might I see Dr. Forceps?"

"Yes, a doctor will look at it and confirm … It will have to be Dr. Scissors. Dr. Forceps is on vacation this week."

A man of spellbinding beauty soon entered the room. Dr. Scissors could have been a runway model or a Verdi baritone capable of the highest tessitura in his *fach*. I imagined him in full-throated, tremolo-free song as he hovered over my supine wounded body, "Non morire, mio tesoro, pietade! Mia colomba, lasciarmi non dêi!" Embarrassment and titillation pummeled my mind into confusion.

He palpated every centimeter of my throbbing chest and concluded wanly, "You can fly to California. Take ibuprofen, and if the breast swells to three times its normal size, go to the emergency room."

~

In Venice I sat cross-legged and fully dressed on the beach watching my colleagues change into their swimsuits and jump into the ocean. Back at the Airbnb, redolent with salt water and interdisciplinary chatter, I made frequent trips to the bathroom while the others pored over and discussed Azazello's personal papers. Transfixed by the vanity mirror, I lifted my dress again and again, as if persistent staring would lessen the pain and make the bruises disappear. Though I went to great lengths to conceal my swollen, asymmetrical body from my collaborators, I did not attempt to cover up the pain management. Tylenol every 4 hours; Advil every 5. I popped pills surrounded by hippie portrayals of drug use: drawings of severed body parts in dog-eared notebooks, poems on scraps of rusted paper, ancient Soviet-era photographs.

~

The archive of Azazello, writer, artist, opiate addict, and boyfriend of the nomenklatura hippie muse Ofelia, consists of 36 notebooks crammed with sketches, original poetry, barely legible scrawl, contact details, and song lyrics produced and reproduced between 1972 and 1993. It is a rich source of hippie sensibilities and material life and a fitting backdrop for a body in pain. Together with a collection of loose papers of original poems, the notebooks outline a coherent aesthetic and worldview at the center of which are an ethic of play and a temporality that privileges childlike ruthlessness, make-believe, authenticity, and spontaneity. Azazello probably would have denied that hippiedom was a worldview. For him, the hippie was anti-ideological, an affect or phenomenon of the psyche rather than conscious thought: "Hippie is not fashion and not a philosophical current, and it is not a sociological phenomenon. Hippie is a psychic condition of a human being. It cannot be otherwise" (Azazello Collection, 2015.075.012, p. 43).

The papers resound with a yearning to seize the object of primordial loss, to witness and capture the evanescent in-betweenness of things: one's own birth, the materiality of speech, the gaze that supports visual memories, the real of a childhood created retrospectively. "Immense is the number of words / lost because of significance / inherent in them," Azazello muses in his 1992 poem "On Childhood":

> The best years are remembered / the way one thinks of summer / in springtime. / a tribute to sentimentality— / childhood. / after my birth— / for I was born, that much is certain— / eternity retreated into the realm of legends, / myths and fairy tales became my signposts.

Further in the poem, another reference to erasure, a fleeting gesture, that which is forfeited to memory or repression: "mental memos taken as mementos / abandoned or deleted in a hurry, / or burned upon departure" (Azazello Collection, 2015.075.403). In another, untitled, poem Azazello expresses an excruciating, impossible wish to recover the pieces of a shattered self, and for transcendence:

> I am approaching the critical mass, / my own 'EGO.' / I am approaching the start / of the final countdown. / I am approaching the borders of memory, / the regions where it becomes fictionalized. / I am not able to forget everything, / and it's killing me.
>
> (Azazello Collection, 2015.075.389)[1]

Azazello depicts the hippie as a destructive child, a figure that, for him, was not incompatible with drug use. Drugs enable a departure from linear time and actualize a space and time of ecstatic play. The notebooks feature drawings of broken clocks, trips to the moon, fairy-tale knights, and *Alice in Wonderland* characters that signal the stoppage of linear time. Because time is disorganized, gender and sexuality are as well. Bodies are fragmented—often presented as part objects—most commonly as eyeballs pierced with needles and dripping syringes. Human figures appear androgynous, naked and emaciated, and without genitalia (Azazello Collection, 2015.075.003, pp. 19–20). "When kingdoms collapse, you walk and sing," writes Azazello (Azazello Collection, 2015.075.012, pp. 12–13). Destruction is part of the creative process of becoming, where the future is so open, so vague and ever-growing, as to be unrepresentable. The fluidity of time is rendered as aesthetic pastiche. The blending of "adult" and children's themes conveys an oceanic temporality: cats, poppies, castles, and multicolored kingdoms cover page after page. Princesses, syringes, and Pierrots repeatedly illustrate a dark innocence (Azazello Collection, 2015.075.012, pp. 4–43).

~

I apprehended as never before Jacques Lacan's dictum: The subject's desire is the desire of the Other. What had I attempted with this surgery? To reconstruct a symmetry that I imagined I'd once possessed. To reunite with the breast, regain a prosthetic maternity. I longed to undo the separation from my mother. I fantasized being in my analyst's belly and birthing myself by myself, using him as a temporary vessel. A second sarcophagus, a reabsorption into the omnipotent maternal body. The operation fell short. Aching and bruised, I was caught in the specular. The sites of the Other's gaze: a hippie archive, the Soviet past, a bathroom mirror in Venice Beach.

~

Stagnation-era hippies adopted Friedrich Nietzsche's critique of metaphysics and embraced his elevation of *play* and *becoming* in defiance of Soviet official ideology, with its emphasis on a higher purpose and rationality. Azazello, nicknamed after the demonic character from Mikhail Bulgakov's *Master and Margarita* (1967), communicated this Nietzschean perspective, including its queer temporality and glorification of lethal innocence. Like other hippies of the Soviet 1960s and 1970s, Azazello was a frequent inpatient of psychiatric hospitals and paid mightily for "dropping out of socialism" (Fürst, 2018; Fürst & McLellan, 2017). Despite attacks on his mind and on his person, he continued to make art and poetry, take solace in music, and seek freedom and sublimation in opiates and psychedelics. The hippies of Azazello's circle probably did not read D. W. Winnicott, but that did not preclude their Winnicottian theorizing, the extolment of play and adaptation of the figure and temporality of the child for therapeutic and creative ends. Their childlike fantasies and playfulness maintained a space of spontaneity and unrestraint amid the violence of everyday socialism.

Winnicott viewed the psychotherapeutic clinic as a domain in which an experience of life as play could be taken up, elaborated upon, and renewed. In his oft-cited words: "Psychotherapy takes place in the overlap of two areas of playing, that of the patient and that of the therapist. Psychotherapy has to do with two people playing together." Winnicott quotes the poet Rabindranath Tagore in his classic *Playing and Reality* (1971/2005): "On the seashore of endless worlds, children play" (p. 128). Tagore's lines are appropriated from the Presocratic philosopher Heraclitus (also central to Nietzsche's Übermensch), who described existence as "a child building sandcastles on a shore, eagerly awaiting the next wave to wash away his creation so as to begin creating again" (as cited in Russell, 2017, p. 100). Soviet hippie aesthetics utilized the paradoxical language of childlike playing to experiment in the protected space between chimerical fancy and the physical world. Through the systematic use of drugs, music, poetry, and art, hippies considered possible trials and rehearsed various endings. Their perspective, moreover, was not confined to the small and rarefied milieu of privileged youth. Hippie aesthetics and sensibility were made palatable to broad audiences by Soiuzmul'tfil'm in two of the most beloved animated films of the stagnation era: Inessa Kovalevskaia's *Bremenskie muzykanty* (*Bremen Town* Musicians; 1969) and Vasilii Livanov's *Po sledam bremenskikh muzykantov* (*On the Trail of the Bremen Town Musicians*; 1973). The films' popularity testifies to the influential reach of hippie culture and situates it at the very heart of late Soviet life—and my early childhood.

In the film *Bremenskie muzykanty*, the heroes enter on a donkey-drawn modish plaid suitcase-as-wagon to a rock and roll drumbeat and rhythm guitar. The Donkey, wearing a matching plaid mantle of saturated blue and red, provides an occasional accompaniment of "la-la-la, yeah, yeah-yeah, yeah-yeah" as the other band members—a teenaged Troubadour, Cat, Rooster, and Dog on bass and electric guitars—sing their theme song:

> There's nothing better in this life,
> Than to roam the world with friends!
> In friendship struggles aren't daunting.
> We take every path!
> We will not forget our calling—
> To bring laughter and joy to others!
> For palaces' seductive domes
> We'll never trade our freedom!
> Our floors are fields of flowers.
> Our walls are giant pines.
> Our roof—the clear blue sky.
> Our good fortune—to live this fate!
> (Kovalevskaia, 1969, 0:09)

The lush voice of actor and pop singer Oleg Anofriev belts out the tune as his character, the Troubadour, lies on his back atop the hurtling wagon, effortlessly strumming a guitar and swinging his leg to its rhythm. Blinding yellow curls caress his neck, and a bright orange Baja jacket and matching embroidered bell bottoms hug his strapping physique: The young man is carefree, happy, and chic. His animal friends, too, are decked out in the latest Western fashions. The white and black striped cap perched on the Donkey's long blonde mane contrasts nicely with his plaid attire; the Rooster's large cherry-red comb, oversized belt buckle, and thick-rimmed blue glasses are decidedly rockabilly revival; the Cat's colorful bow tie suggests psychedelic; and the floppy-eared Dog's gold medallion and black and red upright electric bass epitomize cool.

Before most Soviet children and adults had seen or heard of hippies, they learned to recognize them by watching and listening to *Bremenskie muzykanty* on screen and records. Though Soiuzmul'tfil'm's Bremen musicians perform circus acts for a vaguely 17th-century kingdom in the early part of the cartoon, they communicate sartorially and musically that they are a rock band, one that manages to evoke both home and abroad by moving seamlessly among musical styles: from psychedelic rock to nostalgic doo-wop, so-called gypsy art songs and 1960s *estrada*, Beatles-style melodies and funk. In their generic eclecticism the *Brementsy* truly resemble the first generation of Moscow hippies, who adapted flower children's costume, musical taste, and gentle politics of peace and personal freedom to hard-boiled Soviet conditions (Fürst, 2014).

By popularizing hippie culture, *Bremenskie muzykanty* gave expression to a nonteleological, queer time and space of playing and becoming. Both the original film and its sequel, *Po sledam bremenskikh muzykantov*, distilled and presented to the Soviet public the hippie worldview by linking the presentist and free-flowing worlds of children, traveling musicians, and animals in variously intricate and flamboyant ways. The temporality instantiated by the animators and composer Gennadii Gladkov through such linkages did not stand in diametrical opposition to the Soviet way of life. Nor did the films' values pose an overt challenge to socialist ideals. Like actual Moscow hippies, they offered utopian depictions of friendship, love, egalitarianism, creativity, and spontaneous collaboration. What they failed to portray was movement—or, rather, linear movement. Instead of proffering a happy cadence of progress and the approach of a tangible and radiant future, the Bremen musicals enticed audiences with sudden eruptions of emotional intensity, a road going nowhere, genre mixing, and the overcoming of generational logic through sincere, childlike outlooks and postures.

~

Brezhnev-era hippies may not have been aware of Winnicott, but they were passionately engaged with the work of Nietzsche, another influential theorist of play. Azazello's friend and housemate in the 1970s, Il'ia Kestner, recalls that hippies

> definitely read [Nietzsche] although it was difficult [to obtain] such literature. We frequently read books aloud, and group readings were popular. Authors varied ... we read lots of banned American literature, [as well as] poetry and philosophy. ... Books were copied and passed around, not always in their entirety. Often there were articles where authors [like Nietzsche] were cited, and people read fragments [of their work]. Most knew *Thus Spoke Zarathustra*—some had prerevolutionary editions.
>
> (Kestner to Irina Gordeeva, personal communication,
> May 19, 2018; see also Gordeeva, 2017, pp. 503–504)

Following the philosophical tradition of Heraclitus, Nietzsche challenged metaphysical thinking by putting forward *becoming* as the innocent play of the world. For Nietzsche, the becoming of play operates as the main category of ontology,

> displacing the privilege of atemporal, substantial Being: metaphysics as the attempt at an impossible reversal of time—a source of bad conscience, nihilism, and *ressentiment*—is overcome in a gesture that inaugurates new opportunities for action and new horizons of life.
>
> (Russell, 2017, p. 99)

Nietzsche (1873/1962) explains:

> In the world only play, play as artists and children engage in it, exhibits coming-to-be and passing away, structuring and destroying without any moral additive, in forever equal innocence. And as children and artists play, so plays the ever-living fire. It constructs and destroys, all in innocence.
>
> (p. 62)

In Nietzsche's early writings, the child and the artist are symbols of the "pursuit of ideals without ideality," modeling

> a future that has not been absolutely determined and programmed in advance by a subject. … The child and the artist do not submit themselves to the play of becoming knowing *what* they are going to create, only *that* they are going to create.
>
> (Russell, 2017, p. 99)

This sort of creative capacity was equated by Nietzsche with his much vaunted "innocence," the generative innocence he sought and held to be the consummate testament to the life of "will to power" (Nietzsche, 1884/1961, pp. 160–162).

In *Thus Spoke Zarathustra*, the figure that Nietzsche utilizes to convey that which elevates itself—that which overcomes—is the Übermensch-as-child:

> The child is innocence and forgetfulness, a new beginning, a sport, a self-propelling wheel, a first motion, a sacred Yes.
>
> Yes, a sacred Yes is needed, my brothers, for the sport of creation: The spirit now wills *its own* will, the spirit sundered from the world now wins *its own* world.
>
> (1884/1961, p. 55)

Close readers of Nietzsche emphasize that his symbolic child, while placed at the pinnacle of the process of self-overcoming, should not be understood as a model of subjectivity superior to all those preceding it. The Übermensch as Heraclitean child, in other words, is not meant

> to explain human life in terms of some ultimate goal, either as history or of the individual, but on the contrary to indicate that such processes have no goal—are properly liberated or affirmed to the extent that they are recognized, joyfully, as open and indeterminate. The identification of self and becoming that erases the opposition between self and action is what Nietzsche calls "life."
>
> (Russell, 2017, p. 100)

Soviet hippies' version of Nietzschean becoming found its fullest expression in the notion of *kaif*, a feeling of elation—even transcendence—a high achieved through drugs, music listening, haptic pleasures, and other ephemera (Fürst, 2021, pp. 229–289). *Kaif*—its ethos, its ability to open areas of experience and enable dreaming—can be grasped on nearly every page of Azazello's notebooks. Sketches, song lyrics, and original poetry that span almost 2 decades conjure an ecstatic temporality, celebrating willful abandon and guileless destructiveness.

Azazello, self-styled Übermensch, intrepid child-hero of poetry and art, was also an unwitting Winnicottian analyst. Within the transitional space of his notebooks, between fantasy and reality, he played with genre and poetic verse in order to heal himself—to write himself back into existence after a deadening 3 years of incarceration in a psychiatric hospital in the latter 1980s. From the harsh reality of the *psikhushka*, where post-Stalinist political dissidents were commonly confined for their nonconformist "delusions," he mapped a path of fantastical, lyrical rebirth, mixing the vocabularies and sensations of children's fairy tales and legends with the songs of Jim Morrison and the Rolling Stones.

Azazello undertook his own cure in a world where psychiatry was coopted by the carceral state for the purpose of social control. As the infant uses its transitional object, he fashioned common notebooks into a material basis for the sacred spatiotemporal dimension of *kaif*. Like therapy sessions, the notebooks framed a locus of play and illusion, a way of asserting subjectivity in an ever-encroaching Soviet environment.

~

After the drain had been removed post-mastectomy, I decided to ditch the hospital's pink surgical bras, gather courage, and get fitted for something reminiscent of the lacey pushup numbers I used to wear. The obvious place to visit was the Breast Center Boutique, which I had spied on the second floor between appointments. The store has a fairly sizable selection of surgical, compression, and pocketed bras. It offers variously shaped breast prosthetics and accessories, as well as head scarves, wigs, swimwear, caftans, and the ultimate oxymoron: cancer gifts. To the uninitiated, it is the least sexy lingerie shop imaginable; to breast cancer survivors, it is the promise of normality and a wellspring of desire.

Stupefied, I slouched at the counter next to a tall glassy-eyed woman as we waited patiently for the clerk's attention. From behind a giant curtain, we overheard the fitter explain to another customer that the ideal, really the *only*, option for women in the initial phase of breast reconstruction is a stretchy sports bra with internal pockets for cotton puffs that are reduced in size after each expansion and eventually plucked out of existence. The woman beside me bleated her agony: "I just had two drains removed, and I'd been wearing those compression bras … I had a double mastectomy … I'm very swollen." She and I were now members of the same breast cancer sorority, a club of women who love and hate one another fiercely, in equal measure. Oh, the lacerating irony of a lingerie shop in the breast pavilion of a cancer hospital! "Where, o where have you gone, / Golden days of my youth?" sings, andante, Petr Tchaikovsky's naive poet Lensky, slain in a duel by his friend Onegin and by insufficient irony toward Romantic clichés (Boym, 1994,

p. 176). Homesickness brought me to the Breast Center Boutique, where a maternal figure would make me two-breasted again.

~

Bremenskie muzykanty appealed to spectators of all ages, but one nevertheless wonders why librettist Entin, Gladkov, and Soiuzmul'tfil'm chose to evoke hippiedom in an adaptation of a Grimm folktale ostensibly aimed at children. The Bremen town musicians of the 1973 sequel are markedly more hippie than their 1969 predecessors: The V neckline of the Troubadour's shirt plunges further to reveal a larger portion of suntanned chest framed by an oversized pointed collar. He and his girlfriend, the Princess, don crowns of flowers. She prances barefoot across meadows in a red skin-clinging micromini dress, as their animal friends fish and dance around a campfire. In the penultimate scene, the animal musicians perform psychedelic tunes for the kingdom while impersonating "foreign singers" in Jim Morrison wigs, pointed-toe high-heeled shoes, tie-dyed shirts, giant sunglasses, and the inevitable patched bell-bottomed jeans.

A likely reason for the felicitous incorporation of hippie aesthetics and themes into these late socialist animated films was the already established link between hippiedom and childhood, both in the popular imagination in the West and, as Azazello's archive demonstrates, in Soviet hippies' self-stylization and politics. Juliane Fürst's oral history of the relatively small but vibrant stagnation-era hippie scene informs us that Soviet audiences were first introduced to the new subculture by a 1967 youth magazine article, "Children With Flowers and Without Color." While the piece excoriated hippiedom as a capitalist diversion of youth from truly leftist activism, it also pointed to the affinity between childlike and hippie behaviors, describing in detail the predilections and attitudes of young Hyde Park hippies, "barefoot and clad in colorful … attire, in search of a life without money and materialism" (as cited in Fürst, 2012, pp. 7–8, 2016, p. 126). The Moscow hippies affirmed their identification with children in 1971 by adopting the Day of the Defense of the Child as a special hippie holiday and insisting that they too were children, "the true subjects of the celebration." The same year, Fürst notes, Moscow hippies "planned a demonstration in defense of Vietnamese children and against the Vietnam war in front of the American embassy" (Fürst, 2012, pp. 13–14, 2014, p. 571).

Nietzsche was not the only source for countercultural appropriations of the child. Children were especially apt symbols of generational rebellion against both capitalism and the socialist state because childhood, as delimited in the 20th century, signifies a queer temporality, a period of delay, and a world apart from adult concerns. Children allow adults to imagine a space of not-yet and, as Kathryn Bond Stockton (2009) suggests, sometime grow sideways rather than up, forming horizontal alliances that eschew parental, domestic, or future-oriented temporality. In their supposed flower-picking innocence and through play with siblings, friends, and animals, real and figural children offer adults the possibility of a life and pleasure outside the normative family and law-enforcing state (Sedgwick, 1993c).

In the stalled time of childhood hippies found a subversive potential because, in Stockton's words, delay always betrays: "How can children be gradually led by degrees toward domains they must never enter at all as children?" Paradoxically, children-as-innocents represent danger: the danger of managing their own delay and of agency in their own pleasure (Stockton, 2009, p. 62).

Many paradoxes also structured the lives of Brezhnev-era flower children. Although their modes of identification and beliefs ran parallel to those of family and the state, hippies, initially in Moscow and then gradually throughout the major cities of the Soviet Union, forged lines of filiation, meeting places, and rituals in the very heart of educational, ideological, and cultural institutions: at Moscow State University, the Komsomol, and the Bol'shoi Theater. Hippies called themselves a system, *sistema*, suggesting rigid structures and explicit rules, but, really, the *sistema* was a loose and informal social network. Soviet hippie culture took shape at specific public sites, friends' apartments, and in imitation of mainstream Western youth culture (not always actual hippie aesthetics in the West). Yet, it advocated aimlessness, a peripatetic life, and outsider status. Initially, the *sistema* consisted of children from the Soviet ruling bureaucratic class, but eventually the network grew more inclusive, and by the mid-1970s its members faced arrest, caroused with queer youth, and shared spaces with gay cruising grounds (Fürst, 2012, p. 416, 2014, p. 586). Like actual children who engage in fantastical and strange play enabled by the benign neglect of nearby but preoccupied adults, flower children initially met and played rebelliously *beside* but in full view of their law-creating, privileged Communist Party parents, managing to fashion rich emotional and aesthetic worlds. When the long-haired *Bremenskie muzykanty* wandered onto Soviet screens, parts of these colorful, obscure hippie subcultures were made known and vivid to the wider public.

~

The original folktale "Bremen Town Musicians" is not a story about humans. Its animal heroes talk, think, and act in solidarity in order to rebel against their ruthless owners and establish a just and happy life. In the Grimm brothers' version, Donkey, Dog, Cat, and Rooster, all of advanced age and no longer fit for labor, run away from their respective farms, where they are targeted for slaughter. The Donkey sets off first, and the others join one by one on the road to Bremen, a place of freedom and hope—a town where the fast friends plan to become musicians. Toward evening, on the way to Bremen, they see light coming from a cottage, peer inside, and discover robbers enjoying drink and food. The hungry animals devise a plan to scare away the robbers and take their provisions. The Donkey stands upright and grabs the windowsill with his forefeet. The Dog climbs on the Donkey's back, the Cat jumps on the Dog, and the Rooster flies onto the Cat's head. Perched securely atop one another, they begin to make "music" in unison: the Donkey brays, the Dog barks, the Cat meows, and the Rooster crows. They then shatter the window, burst into the room, and startle and spook the robbers with their cries. The terrified robbers, convinced a ghost has invaded the cottage, flee into the forest. The animals proceed to occupy the cottage, enjoy a fine supper, and fall asleep. Later that night, the robbers return and order a member of their crew to go inside and investigate. A series of ambushes rapidly follow, and the robbers abandon the cottage forever. The four animals enjoy the place so much that they forgo Bremen and live there happily for the remainder of their days (Grimm et al., 1987/2003, pp. 96–98).

Bremenskie muzykanty is also about collective heroism and friendship—minstrels banding together, employing their musical skills and smarts to create unshackled, fulfilling lives. The hippie comrades, too, encounter and outwit a group of "robbers" (in the film they resemble gypsy singers and perform a tuneful number), and more than once stand on each other's shoulders to score a victory. But here the similarities, important though they are, end. Human characters abound in the world of *Bremenskie muzykanty*, and the motive for action in the film is not ageist oppression but romantic love.

In the Soviet version, the animal musicians from the start travel with a human troubadour who acts as a bandleader. They arrive draped in psychedelic sartorial splendor in a place belonging to a remote time, a sort of campy Middle Ages with Baroque elements. The hippie friends find there a 17th-century monarch, judging by dress and court etiquette, in a Versailles-like palace, incongruously surrounded by medieval fortifications and cavalry, infantrymen, and loyal subjects. The musicians entertain the denizens of the superannuated town with a series of circus and variety theater acts.

Against the background of the high-tempo rhythms and raucous proceedings of their performance emerges a moment of exquisite refinement and transcendence. It conjures a realm of experience completely cut off from the time-soaked beat of everyday life. As in the Grimm tale, but for a different end, the *Brementsy* mount one another's shoulders. The acrobatics here are meant to entertain rather than frighten, of course, and instead of the Rooster, the Troubadour acts as the crowning figure of the precariously vertical stack of bodies. He leaps, to a suspense-building drum roll, onto the Cat's pate and lands upside down. Standing on his head, he bows his guitar, holding it like a violin. The Troubadour then spots the Princess on a balcony. As their faces meet (his upside down, hers right side up), and they look into each other's eyes, blushing, the sweetly stringed euphoniousness produced by the Troubadour provides the perfect accompaniment to him and the Princess falling suddenly and hopelessly in love. But then, "falling in love" misrepresents what really takes place, since the phrase suggests a process, even if meteoric. The love that envelops the two teenagers is instantaneous and intrinsically timeless. The onlookers recede into oblivion, and the moment hovers in oscillating suspension, removed from all things diachronic and ordinary. A solo violin punctuates it with a lilting, sentimental tune, motion within an everlasting now. But as instantly as it was created, this interlude of timelessness is shattered: The assemblage of animals on which the Troubadour's head has been comfortably resting begins to teeter, and he manages a far-fetched airborne somersault straight into the Princess's chamber, prompting the outraged King to throw him and the other musicians out of his castle.

All this probably sounds very familiar, and it is. There is nothing especially radical or queer about the Romantic connection between young love and a sense of timelessness, nor the 20th-century notion that young adulthood is an italicized and intensified stage mediated by a zeal for freedom from parental control. But *Bremenskie muzykanty* offers its viewers much more than typical fairy-tale romance. Once their timeless interval dissolves, the lovers do not reenter, as most fairy-tale and late 19th-century fictional couples do, the thoroughly timebound reproductive family. The pair does not ride off into the sunset of nuptial blessedness.

The Bremen musicians plot to bring the Princess and Troubadour together. They dress up as bandits, abduct the cowardly King, and then stage a rescue by the Troubadour. In gratitude, the King allows the lovesick young man to marry his daughter and invites him into the palace. The happiness of the bride and groom is disturbed, however, by the absence of their animal friends, who have been excluded from wedding. The couple quits the scene as the guests continue dancing, unaware, and abandon the patriarchal family and the royal bloodline, too, to join the Donkey, Dog, Cat, and Rooster on the road to Bremen—or nowhere in particular. The Princess, having discarded her crown and royal robes for tall modish boots and an A-line mini, now stands atop the wagon with the Troubadour as all six friends, reunited and free, recapitulate their theme song.

Timelessness is queer in *Bremenskie muzykanty* because its evocation does not ultimately endorse or result in traditional gender roles, normative family arrangements, and dyadic heterosexual union. The Princess's tale is not a Cinderella story leading her from a perverse fatherless stepfamily to a natural, nuclear one. Indeed, the human couple's love has no meaning, and happiness remains elusive, outside the extended kinship structure of animals and its emancipatory magic. The Princess substitutes a five-piece band for the harpsichord, and an exceptional state of temporal deviance becomes a permanent mode of being.

~

"Animal/child affectionate bondings," writes Stockton (2009), "offer opportunities … for children's motions inside their delay"—their pause on the threshold of adulthood—by "making delay a sideways growth the child in part controls for herself, in ways confounding her parents and her future" (p. 90). Stockton suggests, with Gilles Deleuze and Félix Guattari, that the family dog can function not simply as a sentimental domestic relation but "rather as a loving, growing metaphor for the child itself … and for the child's own propensities to stray." The dog, in Stockton's view,

> is a vehicle for the child's strangeness … [and] her companion in queerness. As a recipient of the child's attentions … and a living screen for the child's self-projections, the dog is a figure for the child beside itself, engaged in a growing quite aside from growing up.
>
> (Stockton, 2009, p. 90)

Stockton's sideways growth closely resembles Deleuze and Guattari's concept of plateau, a "state of intensity leading to irreducible dynamisms … and implying other forms of expression." One such plateau, *becoming animal*, is an alliance between human and animal that "traverses human beings and sweeps them away." This alliance is anti-oedipal because it is not filial, and "a question not of development or differentiation," but of increase in magnitude, degree, and quantity: movement and transport. Deleuze and Guattari claim, and Stockton echoes, that "children are particularly 'moved' by animals in this way and 'continually undergo becomings of this kind.'" Animals are parts of the many "assemblages a child can mount in order to solve a problem from which all exits are barred to him" (as cited in Stockton, 2009, p. 94).

As we have seen, animal assemblages are mounted quite literally in *Bremenskie muzykanty*. The musicians, in a layered stack, like a metaphor that pauses time, a moving suspension that swells meanings, enable the Troubadour and Princess to meet and to fall in love (Stockton, 2009, p. 92). The animals' formidable bodies, on which the Troubadour stands, act as bridge and transport between the radically different aesthetic and temporal worlds of the two young lovers, allowing a timeless interval, merger, and enlargement. One can easily imagine that if not for the aid of the Donkey, Cat, Dog, and Rooster, the hippie Troubadour and medieval Princess would remain in their separate temporalities without hope of convergence.

~

"Time is *out* but this is the moment to live and love and sing loud" enigmatically serves as a banner atop Azazello's drawings of clocks, a hippie swinging from a pendulum, harlequins, and maniacal children (Azazello Collection, 2015.075.012, p. 29). Ink bleeds and oozes over once crisply sketched portraits, giving some of the notebooks a palimpsestic quality. Reproductions of album covers are sprinkled among transcribed song lyrics from the Beatles and Pink Floyd. An atomic cloud hovers over flower children dancing and playing music (Azazello Collection, 2015.075.020, p. 28). Drug-induced *kaif* is held up as the ultimate experience. The hippie-as-child is a Spirit, a destructive force that invents a new world and transmits novelty itself among flower children and, also, adults. Azazello's hippie manifesto proclaims:

> We, the hippies, are the makers and creators of the New Spirit, which we pass on through pictures and drawings, poems and prose, through music, through song and dance, through outfits and ornaments, through relationships among ourselves as well as with the social world of Adults.
>
> We want to see ourselves united by a creative force whose aim is the creation of a Luminous Space that will overtake our Mind and Soul.
>
> We want our relationships with each other to be pure, without deception. ... Sincerity is the fulcrum of our friendships.
>
> Each one of us carries the fire. For some, it is brighter, for others less so; still others don't even know about the fire, but they have it nonetheless, even if only a spark.
>
> Just as before, we reject violence and intolerance, conformism, hypocrisy, dishonesty, and other muck that the Adults use in attempts to raise others to be like them. These are not for us.

(Azazello Collection, 2015.075.444)

In a similar philosophical statement, Azazello declares:

We force the smoke to crawl through our lips / into our lungs in quick eruptions, / we splash around our long hair / intertwined with the grass in the sun, / we've soared over the earth and are flying through the sky like the waning fire of the rainbows.

(Azazello Collection, 2015.075.450)[2]

Hippies are as pure as the elements, attuned to all that is experiential and sensorial. Their creative productions carry messages across ever-expanding time and space.

Azazello often endeavored to compose from the perspective of a child rather than an adult looking back on childhood. Like a child at play, he lived in a malleable present—the immediacy and pulsation of the moment—and often denied generational time. Juxtaposing references as diverse as A. A. Milne, Kornei Chukovskii, and Jimi Hendrix, Azazello made art in an external yet close relation to late Soviet culture (Azazello Collection, 2015.075.012, pp. 7–8).

~

The notebooks and poetry functioned for Azazello as a therapeutic project of self-expression and healing and, more radically and urgently, a sinthomatic inscription that ensured his subjective consistency while partaking of the drives. Writing and drawing allowed him to play with time and identity while remaining securely anchored in the Symbolic. In the role of the Übermensch-child who creates and destroys innocently, Azazello etched for himself a space of freedom and fantasizing that transferred the past into the present and amplified both, instantiating a reverberant temporality: Jack Halberstam's queer time, José Muñoz's dual notions of ecstatic time and queer potentiality (Halberstam, 2005; Muñoz, 2009/2019).

Azazello's personal papers produce spatiotemporal effects similar to those of the psychoanalytic session. Every notebook, precisely because of its attention to chronology (for example, constant mention of seasons and engagement with the latest albums and songs), is a space of temporal plasticity and dynamism: Some artistic productions are forms of temporal drag, drawing from the past, while others crisscross historical periods, genres, and generations, undermining doxa and remapping knowledges. Such temporal and symbolic fluidity is not especially nostalgic; it aims forward, toward future audiences who wish to understand hippie community and values. The notebooks, then, were not only used as instruments of self-care; they also were conceived from the outset as an archive.

Azazello's archiving impulse illuminates something essential about hippies and the Soviet culture they tried to escape from within, as it were. *Kaif* was an instance of ecstatic time, a hole in late socialism, a dizzying potentiality. The materiality of the notebooks helped Azazello to stretch the ephemeral zone of *kaif* long enough to capture its traces. The notebook pages reek of cigarettes and are textured by irreverent wear and tear: a blood stain, a phone number scrawled over meticulously drawn art, water and ink spilled on a hastily sketched pattern for a blouse or blue jeans. Each stroke of the pen that repeatedly drew faces, eyeballs, and sinewy hair and muscles, each ink blot that bled over English song lyrics meticulously copied, held onto and documented the ephemera of a pulsating, nonchronological temporality. Azazello's notebooks, like every "unofficial" or queer archive conceived as such, preserved in partial and faint form an extraordinary and expansive subject, and the promise of associative leaps into futures yet unthought.

~

Ecstatic time was evoked by Azazello through references to fairy tales and childhood, animals and castles. He and his lover, the "princess" Ofelia, appeared on horses and among knights and kings in a place intimate yet temporally far away. Like a child, he engaged in repetitive play, rendering similar images over and over, as if chasing and failing to grasp *kaif*. In the notebooks, animals and medieval fortresses flow from twisting 1970s bodies, making them capacious vessels of mythical events and personages. Azazello and his fellow hippies (whose sketches and scribble pepper the journals) thereby acquired bigger selves and a wider impact (Azazello Collection, 2015.075.012, pp. 13, 40, 2015.075.013, pp. 8–9).

What can be made of Azazello's repeated efforts to make visible his own gaze, to recover the lost object, to get to other side of the looking glass? Is his artistic activity a childlike fascination with repetition, or darkness and nihilism—a destructive idée fixe? He writes:

> when i finally die, and i won't die anytime soon,
> although i will certainly die young,
> i want to behold my eyes as a child
> in the broken mirror
> that the wind knocked down and shattered.
> or could it be that i shattered myself,
> that i trampled and crushed my own self?
> that i mixed myself with my own blood,
> having drowned in my black blood
> my grownup eyes
> reflected in the mirror shards.
> (Azazello Collection, 2015.075.488)[3]

Against the tenets of Nietzschean overcoming, and in conflict with playing, Azazello here longs to turn back the clock and reacquire his childhood eyes, darkened and broken through adult living. In a similar vein, in the notebooks he frequently draws the eye separated from the body. Sometimes it appears pierced by a syringe, sometimes marked by a line, arrow, or conical shape, a representation of the gaze (Azazello Collection, 2015.075.013, p. 22, 2015.075.003, pp. 36–37). Recurring part-objects such as eyeballs and needles articulate, paradoxically, Azazello's larger theme: the return to wholeness through drug use and intoxication. In chronicling his efforts at integration and transcendence, Azazello tries recursively to seize the ephemeral encounter with the drive and the cause of his desire: rapturous *kaif*. It "drowns him in his own blood," overwhelming him with simultaneous pleasure and pain. The archive therefore can be viewed as a compulsion to repeat, the testament and result not of sublimation or play but, rather, of a masochistic, futile, and ultimately self-destructive project. The attempt to seize the object that makes possible the visual field *through its very exclusion* was destined to end, as it did for Narcissus, in death.

Ofelia's body was found in the River Setun in 1991. She died, like many Soviet hippies, from an overdose of *vint*, a synthetic heroin circulating in Moscow in those days. Her relationship with Azazello, marked by addiction and violence, had ended around 1982. The Princess of *Bremenskie muzykanty* represents a different trajectory. While under her father's aegis, she inhabits a realm not of a specific generation, but representative of generational time itself. It is pastiche, a pastel mixture of bygone times and towns ruled by a dithering King who perpetually carries between two pink fingers an egg in a holder, a singular soft-boiled egg that he sometimes slurps with a spoon. Neither the egg, clearly symbolic of feminine brittleness and reproduction, nor the kingdom proves appealing to the Princess. In trying to soothe his daughter and after briefly abducting her in the 1973 sequel, the King proposes rather pathetic salutary measures: "Your condition is hysterical, try this dietary egg, my dear girl … or maybe we'll send for the doctor" (Livanov, 1973, 10:17). The Princess rejects the King's offer, and with it the bondage of oedipal striving, the feminine gamete, and growing up (or old). Thanks to the prompt rescue efforts of her dear animal friends, she soon escapes once again to the temporal domain of the hippie Troubadour—to all that is present, free, and eternally novel—and to the queer time of infinite delay, hippie exuberance, colorful desires, and planning-free, animal existence.

~

I balk at lingering on Ofelia's ugly death, the image of a decomposed corpse in a river in Moscow. Instead, I contemplate a Tchaikovsky heroine's operatic demise, her suicidal dive into a Petersburg canal. A memory of the 1999 Metropolitan Opera production of *The Queen of Spades* (1890). It is scene 2 of act 3. Liza waits for her lover Gherman on the banks of the Winter Canal, a picturesque spot for her final hour. Midnight strikes, Gherman is late, and Liza fears the worst, that he has betrayed her. Even before Liza utters a sound there is an orchestral fate motif, a funereal march. Roland Barthes (1977/2001) would later echo Tchaikovsky's musical statement, "The lover's fatal identity is precisely: *I am the one who waits*" (p. 40).

Maestro Valery Gergiev is in the pit, his hands feverishly quivering in attempts to tame the death drive's rhythmic spams. The baton gyrates as fate courses through his rapturous grip. Gergiev's face tells of harsh Russian winter nights when distressed damsels wait for men who arrive late, or not at all. This particular man, Plácido Domingo–Gherman, arrives late enough for Liza's soaring account of her anguish and disappointment. Gherman might be a cad, perhaps worse: a murderer. The voice of dramatic soprano Galina Gorchakova is in top form: "It is close to midnight already, but still no sign of Gherman—no sign! I know that he will come and quell my suspicion … I am weary and worn out with suffering! … Night and day I think only of him." A fortress tower clock strikes in the distance. "O time, wait but a moment and he will be here!" Then despair: "It is true, then! I have … given my soul to a murderer and a monster, for eternity! My life and my honor lie in his wicked hands!" (Tchaikovsky & Tchaikovsky, 1890/1993).

Liza waits and waits for what turns out to be mere minutes. When Gherman appears, all is forgiven: "You have come, you have come, and you are not a criminal! You are here. My agonies are over, and once again I am yours! No more tears, worries, and doubts!" (Tchaikovsky & Tchaikovsky, 1890/1993). Liza collapses into Gherman's embrace. He is hers again, albeit briefly, for those who wait are always alone in their love. Gherman wants knowledge more than he wants Liza, knowledge in the form of a secret, the secret of the magic winning three cards that the heroine's grandmother took to her grave. Gherman cannot love. He is obsessed with gambling, the mother, zombielike repetition. Liza looks at Gherman, but he looks maniacally elsewhere, toward the card table. Gherman runs off. His disappearance into the wings extinguishes all remnants of hope. The fate motif returns, insists, and with the capping assistance of the bass clarinet and bassoon it swells into a unified orchestral verdict. Liza dives into the dark, frigid canal. Gorchakova falls off the stage, quite literally, in a *passage à l'acte*. The scene ends.

~

When Lacan introduces the *passage à l'acte*, or "passage to the act," he immediately distinguishes it from "acting out." Acting out can be an isolated or recurrent action, within or outside the consulting room. Often it is a misrecognition of the analytic transference and therefore carries traces of the repressed. Acting out is, above all, a repetition of a fantasmatic scenario, an unconscious address. The analysand acts out unwittingly to reach the analyst, to show and rebel against the analyst's (mis)interpretation or the failure to interpret. Whether in or outside of an analytic context, acting out gives expression to a scene that cannot be thought or said. It is irruptive, external to the subject's time-bound personality. Acting out is an extravagant staging, a desperate love letter to the Other. Whereas acting out is the enactment of unconscious fantasy (or *fantasme*), the *passage à l'acte* is the *fantasme*'s disappearance: The curtain closes on the unconscious scene in which the subject maintains a desirable and desiring position for the Other, that is to say, in the world.

Lacan elaborates the difference between acting out and the *passage à l'acte* in his discussion of Sigmund Freud's "The Psychogenesis of a Case of Homosexuality in a Woman" (1920) in Seminar X. Later, in Seminars XIV (1966–1967, pp. 147–155) and XV (1967–1968), he draws a further contrast between the *passage à l'acte* and the psychoanalytic "act." While the *passage à l'acte* is a quitting of the *fantasme*—a definitive crossing of the threshold of the Law—the act proper entails a resignification and therefore reinauguration of the subject. The former is suicide, the latter a rebirth.

~

Sidonie Csillag,[4] Freud's Young Homosexual Woman, was an attractive and intelligent 18-year-old from a distinguished family, sent to treatment by her father after a suicide attempt. The trouble began for Sidonie when she fell in love with an older woman, a "lady" of dubious reputation, a "cocotte," as Freud puts it, taking a cue from the patient's parents. Public opinion and family opposition did not deter the infatuated young woman. On the contrary, she devoted all her energy to courting the lady while neglecting herself, her friendships, and her previous interests. Sex appears to have been of little importance to Sidonie. In the manner of a virile courtly lover, she required only the presence and minimal attention of her beloved. One day while walking with her lady friend through the "most frequented streets" of Vienna, Sidonie ran into her father, who shot an angry, ominous glance in the couple's direction as he walked by (Freud, 1920/1955e, pp. 147–148, 161). Upon discovering the identity of the disapproving man, the lady ended the affair, and Sidonie promptly jumped, à la Anna Karenina, over a wall and onto the tracks of the local railway line.

Freud believes that Sidonie's homosexuality is a response, in part, to an oedipal trauma (1920/1955e, p. 159). A few years before the commencement of her chivalric romance, Sidonie suffered a great blow to her feminine self-regard, just as she was "experiencing the revival of her infantile Oedipus complex" and unconsciously desiring her father's male child:

> It was not she who bore the child, but her unconsciously hated rival, her mother. Furiously resentful and embittered, she turned away from her father and from men altogether. After this first great reverse she forswore her womanhood and sought another goal for her libido.
>
> (Freud, 1920/1955e, p. 157)

Sidonie became homosexual, according to Freud, because her heterosexual desire, aimed at her father, was frustrated. The patriarch clearly preferred his youthful and still-attractive wife, who was able to give him a son. Sidonie's homosexuality, moreover, was fueled by her father's exasperation over her relationship with the lady, transforming it into a vehicle of revenge. Freud implies that Sidonie deliberately (consciously?) strolled with the lady by her father's place of work, hoping to meet him and provoke the very reaction she ultimately received. Why, then, would an irate stare from her father immediately send Sidonie over the edge? Freud ventures that the suicide attempt was self-punishment for the unconscious wish to "fall" pregnant. And there was an additional oedipal motive: Homosexuality and its fallout were for the young woman a means of evading rivalry with her mother.

Having provided an oedipal explanation for Sidonie's homosexuality and masochistic infatuation, Freud remains unsatisfied. After all, not every girl reacts to the birth of a male sibling by throwing herself at the feet of an older woman and onto railway tracks. He introduces another line of argument to account for Sidonie's same-sex object choice: a predisposition to homosexuality of "an internal nature," that is, an original bisexuality of all human beings (Freud, 1920/1955e, pp. 168, 171). Intended to shore up the oedipal psychogenetic theory, Freud's second, hereditary causality undermines the first and casts doubt on the entire construction.

The Oedipus complex was conceptualized by Freud mainly within the narrow confines of the study of obsessional neurosis but soon became for him an essential and universal element of subjectivity. But as the Oedipus complex transformed into an intricate web of familial identifications and wishes enabling sexual identity and access to culture, it never completely shed its obsessional neurotic, masculine cast, and arguably proved inadequate in elaborating hysteria, the feminine, and homosexuality (Van Haute & Geyskens, 2012). For decades Lacan wrestled with the Freudian Oedipus in an attempt to disentangle it from its developmental, normative, and biological foundations. In the 1950s and early 1960s, under the influence of Claude Lévi-Strauss, Lacan formulated the Oedipus complex as a historically contingent interpretation of a kinship structure requiring exogamy. Hysterics are individuals (women or feminine identified) who are reluctant to assume the role of exchange objects within such a kinship structure and its phallic economy. Lacan also saw hysteria in this period as an exaggerated dramatization of the universal problematic of desire. Hysterics systematize and testify to the impossibility of filling the constitutive lack (primordial loss) in the subject, the irreducible gap between demand and desire. Every proffered object fails to satisfy desire, reproducing the lack from which desire springs once more.

Lacan reinterprets Freud's study of the Young Homosexual Woman several times. In Seminar X, he proposes that Sidonie's episode with her lady is an exquisite example of an acting out, followed by a *passage à l'acte*. The whole situation—which involves flowers, hand kissing, ostentatious promenading, and so on—is staged for the father's gaze. It is an attempt to demonstrate to him what true love is all about, precisely the sort of love refused to Sidonie. It is no accident that Sidonie's object choice is worshipped, on the one hand, and of questionable morality, on the other—an object that requires saving; also unsurprising, the relationship with the older, unmarried, and childless woman is platonic. Sidonie is sending a message to her father by way of this idealizing, hopeless infatuation: One can love someone for what she does not have. Love exceeds every gift, every concrete object (for example, a son) through which it may be expressed. The lady cannot give Sidonie what she unconsciously wants, a child to compensate for the missing phallus (by which Lacan means the signifier of lack). Sidonie asks her father to consider that his wife's ability to offer him something that the girl cannot is no justification for his preferring the mother to the daughter. Sidonie gives her phallus (a minus) to the lady despite her being both out of reach and unworthy, in other words, despite a lack of fulfillment (Lacan, 1962–1963/2014, pp. 109–113, 122–128).

In acting out her wish to be loved for something in herself that is more than her person—in staging the very structure of love—Sidonie remains unconscious of her addressee, the audience as the support and impetus for the play. She therefore has a certain metonymic distance from the motor of her desire. In the moment her father looks at her with bitter disapproval, Sidonie identifies with his gaze, the object-cause of her productions. When Sidonie's unconsciously projected gaze is returned to her in a hateful guise, it pierces and obliterates her subjective position.

As Lacan would have it, she "passes to the act." The distance between Sidonie and her scene shrinks until she falls off the stage.

Lacan's apparent structural explanation of the suicide attempt presents a problem, however: It only makes sense within the very Freudian oedipal scheme that he tries to neutralize. In Lacanian terms, Sidonie has not gone beyond the Oedipus complex due to an overidentification with her father's (actual) gaze. And while there are ample references to the phallus-as-*signifier* and lack-as-*symbolic* castration, the young woman's fixation and homosexual object choice are here, as in Freud's paper, subtended by a normative developmental psychology and sexist view of anatomy: The girl's interest in the lady is attributed to her unconscious wish to have her father's baby in order to remedy the absence of a penis.

In the late 1960s and 1970s Lacan gradually abandons the Oedipus complex, calling it "Freud's dream," a symptom that must be interpreted. Like all symptoms, the Oedipus complex is a compromise formation that both reveals and obscures the fundamental truth of desire. It thematizes not the father's murder but, rather, the master's castration as an effect of language, showing that even the wisest among us can never know and say all, that something of reality always slips away in speech, and truth and knowledge never completely coincide. Hysterical subjects in particular *unconsciously* stage this impossibility (Lacan, 1969–1970/2007, pp. 87–132).

Lacan claims in Seminar XVII that Freud's leitmotif of the murder of the father—the invocation of his own father's death and various dead father dreams in *The Interpretation of Dreams* (1900/1953b), the origin myth in *Totem and Taboo* (1912/1953g), and the Oedipus story—constitutes an attempt to obscure the father's castration, his real limitations, failures, and mortality. So long as we unconsciously think that the father's death is the consequence of murder, we hold fast to the belief that his death, and perhaps death generally, *can only be due to* murder. In other words, if we believe that collective patricide terminated the primal father's jouissance (his enjoyment of all the women), we also misrecognize the structural character of castration, that is, the impossibility of limitless jouissance external to the Law. Lacan's assertion is that *Totem and Taboo as myth* testifies to the fact that jouissance is only possible when the father is a dead father: When an unlimited enjoyment can be posited *outside* the social order (the sons can only realize sexuality after they murder the primal father). This does not mean that there existed an actual, historical primal father who enjoyed all the women (as Freud seems rather naively to accept!) but that we depend on such a figure—unrealizable, external to the human realm—to safeguard our own enjoyment (Lacan, 1969–1970/2007).

Given the latent content of the myth of the primal father, the true importance of Oedipus for Lacan is that he replaces the (murdered) father as well as figures the "castrated master": He represents both the desire and the inability to know fully. Oedipus solves the riddle of the Sphinx in an effort to help his community—to save it through knowledge—but when the plague ravages Thebes, he is confronted with the impossible truth that he is to blame. Through the act of gouging out his own eyes, Oedipus enacts and embodies the truth of the master, the truth of his symbolic castration. Neurotics do not assimilate the castrated master and instead conjure in their fantasies the father of the primal horde—the omnipotent father who holds the answers to pressing questions, like: *What does a woman want? Am I a man or am I a woman?*

It is this perspective that Lacan applies to Sidonie Csillag and the operations of hysteria more broadly. He reinterprets the hysteric's discourse as the incarnation of "the truth of the master," the master's deficiency or castration. Hysterics seek to become enigmatic objects that stoke curiosity in the Other by inviting others' desires to know, to solve mysteries at the level of being (*What is a woman? Who am I?*). But hysterics also resist becoming phallic objects and purposely choose masters who are inaccessible (and supposedly beyond desire), like teachers, analysts, clergy, or self-absorbed and morally compromised figures. If such figures show themselves as desiring subjects by striving to meet hystericized demands, they lose their appeal, becoming incapable of satisfying hysterics' unconscious desire for unfulfilled desire. The illusion of these masters' omniscience is shattered, and they are abandoned (Lacan, 1960–1961/2015, p. 366, 1969–1970/2007, p. 129).

~

The 2015 documentary *The Babushkas of Chernobyl* chronicles the daily lives of several of about 100 elderly women who returned to the villages around Chernobyl shortly after the accident. They crossed into the Exclusion Zone illegally, digging tunnels and crawling under barbed-wire fences. Brooking no substitute, the women reconstituted their former lives in decaying huts and houses. They are shown drinking vodka together and singing songs, making do with mushrooms, herbs, and berries. They produce jam with obscene quantities of sugar. Some keep radiated chickens. Good-humored Ukrainian scientists periodically check in on the babushkas. The casually dressed men from Kyiv exchange greetings and accept moonshine from the natives while collecting soil samples, eggs, and produce for transport to a lab and the monitoring of radiation levels. Sometimes the scientists take the aging grandmas into town so that they may receive the barest medical care. A local post office employee, herself a babushka, delivers to the Exclusion Zone denizens their monthly pensions (Bogart & Morris, 2015).

The babushkas tell the filmmakers that all the men have died. Some disclose that they have buried young children without mentioning causes of death. When the babushkas are asked why they returned to Chernobyl, they reply simply, frankly, "this is my motherland" (Bogart & Morris, 2015, 17:10, 58:51). Unlike Kupny and his fellow adventurers who risked their lives to penetrate the sarcophagus, these women did not go to the Zone seeking knowledge. They did not return for symbolic import or documentation. They came back to be with the earth, their place of birth. One woman describes falling to the ground and putting clumps of soil into her mouth upon reentering her village (Bogart & Morris, 2015, 9:52). Theirs is not a comeback in the name of reconstruction, for the sake of historical truth. It is a restoration that aims at denying change and the passage of time. A reversal of chronology. A negation of temporality.

~

In his late paper "Constructions in Analysis," Freud (1937/1964) throws into question the difference between construction and reconstruction:

We all know that the person who is being analysed has to be induced to remember something that has been experienced by him and repressed. ... The analyst has neither experienced nor repressed any of the material under consideration; his task cannot be to remember anything. What then *is* his task? His task is to make out what has been forgotten from the traces which it has left behind or, more correctly, to *construct* it. The time and manner in which he conveys his constructions to the person who is being analysed, as well as the explanations with which he accompanies them, constitute the link between the two portions of the work of analysis, between his own part and that of the patient. His *work of construction, or, if it is preferred, of reconstruction* [emphasis added], resembles ... an archaeologist's excavation of some dwelling-place that has been destroyed and buried or of some ancient edifice.

(pp. 257–258)

Though "reconstruction" and "construction" for Freud are virtually synonymous, the tricky aspect is that their connotations can be quite different: The former may refer to the linking of facts and artifacts in narrative, while the latter might be a made-up story; one is historically accurate and "objective," while the other is a fabrication (Benvenuto, 2020, p. 105).

When Freud put psychoanalysis on the side of construction, he placed fantasy together with reality. For analytic interpretation is neither strictly a decoding of memories nor is it merely the construction of a new life narrative: At its most daring, it rejects positivistic outcomes, uncorrupted objectivity. Every construction is a reconstruction, a return, a refinding. But that which is refound was never possessed in the first place, obviating the distinction. The temporality of the psychoanalytic session is queer, *nachträglich*. Originary violence, childhood traumas, are brought to light, indeed, *invented, après-coup*. Analytic reconstruction is not restoration or a search for historical truth. It is the creation of a novel, subjective truth. This is what Lacan calls the act.

~

Psychoanalysis, *my* psychoanalysis, pursues the terribly obscure, utopian. A comeback with nothing to prove. A retroactive revision. Is the analytic act a restructuring, a perestroika? It asks the analysand to do the impossible, to cross the border of her psychic reality, to step outside the Law—everything she holds dear and true—and then reconstitute knowledge and sense, to push against silence and live with freshly acquired know-how.

An overly strong attachment to the object threatens de-subjectivization, suicidal merger. But what of attachment to objects, to *things*—is it salutary or disastrous? Like many Soviet refugees, Harvard literature professor Svetlana Boym left Leningrad in 1979 with two suitcases and a 90-dollar allowance (Boym, 2001, p. 332). She died from cancer at age 56, having spent much of her career returning to Russia in order to recapture a personal truth and, more ambitiously, nostalgically, to reconstruct the faded truth of the last Soviet generation.

Mikhail Gorbachev, too, staged a return so as to reconstruct socialism, to renew a Soviet project that would eventually crash from the weight of internal contradictions. But socialism was always and only about construction: It was forward facing, linear, and could not bear the signifier *perestroika*.

~

Psychoanalysis had an auspicious beginning in the Russian Empire, but Joseph Stalin extinguished its societies and journals and ultimately the analysts themselves. Psychoanalyst Sabina Spielrein, author of the death drive, pediatrician, colleague of Freud and Carl Jung, analyst of Jean Piaget, teacher of Lev Vygotsky, returned from Geneva to postrevolutionary Moscow in the early 1920s, and then to her hometown, Rostov-on-Don, where she worked as a paedologist at a school. Was her comeback an acting out? A *passage à l'acte*? She chose a place without psychoanalysis, a place more dangerous than the method she once practiced.

The most gruesome of many impossible returns: After briefly occupying Rostov in 1941, the Nazis came back the following year and murdered 27,000 people, including Spielrein, and with her two daughters.

Notes

1 Azazello's poems translated by Margarit Ordukhanyan and reproduced here with permission.
2 Azazello's above philosophical statements translated by Margarit Ordukhanyan and reproduced here with permission.
3 Translated by Margarit Ordukhanyan and reproduced here with permission.
4 The pseudonym of Margarethe (Gretl) Trautenegg, née Csonka.

References

Azazello (Anatolyi Kalabin) Collection, 2015.075 (1972–1993). Wende Museum.
Barthes, R. (2001). *A lover's discourse: Fragments* (R. Howard, Trans.). Hill and Wang. (Original work published 1977)
Benvenuto, S. (2020). *Conversations with Lacan: Seven lectures for understanding Lacan.* Routledge.
Bogart, A., & Morris, H. (Directors). (2015). *The Babushkas of Chernobyl* [Film]. Chicken & Egg Pictures; Fork Films; PowderKeg Studios. YouTube. Retrieved August 18, 2024, from https://www.youtube.com/watch?v=q-WWiOUQeSY
Boym, S. (1994). *Common places: Mythologies of everyday life in Russia.* Harvard University Press.
Boym, S. (2001). *The future of nostalgia.* Basic Books.
Freud, S. (1953b). The interpretation of dreams. In J. Strachey et al. (Eds. & Trans.), *The standard edition of the complete psychological works of Sigmund Freud* (Vols. 4–5, pp. 1–625). Hogarth Press. (Original work published 1900)
Freud, S. (1953g). Totem and taboo. In J. Strachey et al. (Eds. & Trans.), *The standard edition of the complete psychological works of Sigmund Freud* (Vol. 13, pp. 1–255). Hogarth Press. (Original work published 1912)
Freud, S. (1955e). The psychogenesis of a case of homosexuality in a woman. In J. Strachey et al. (Eds. & Trans.), *The standard edition of the complete psychological works of Sigmund Freud* (Vol. 18, pp. 145–172). Hogarth Press. (Original work published 1920)

Freud, S. (1964). Constructions in analysis. In J. Strachey et al. (Eds. & Trans.), *The standard edition of the complete psychological works of Sigmund Freud* (Vol. 23, pp. 255–270). Hogarth Press. (Original work published 1937)

Fürst, J. (2012, March 31). *"When you come to Moscow, make sure that you have flowers in your hair (and a bottle of portwine in your pocket)": The life and world of the Soviet hippies under Brezhnev* [Conference presentation]. Reconsidering Stagnation International Workshop. Amsterdam, Netherlands.

Fürst, J. (2014). Love, peace and rock, 'n' roll on Gorky Street: The "emotional style" of the Soviet hippie community. *Contemporary European History*, *23*(4), 565–587.

Fürst, J. (2016). If you're going to Moscow, be sure to have some flowers in your hair (and bring a bottle of port wine in your pocket). In D. Fainberg & A. Kalinovsky (Eds.), *Reconsidering stagnation in the Brezhnev era: Ideology and exchange* (pp. 123–146). Lexington Books.

Fürst, J. (2018). Liberating madness, punishing insanity. *Journal of Contemporary History*, *53*(4), 832–860.

Fürst, J. (2021). *Flowers through concrete: Explorations in Soviet hippieland*. Oxford University Press.

Fürst, J., & McLellan, J. (Eds.). (2017). *Dropping out of socialism: The creation of alternative spheres in the Soviet bloc*. Lexington Books.

Gordeeva, I. (2017). Tolstoyism in the late-socialist cultural underground: Soviet youth in search of religion, individual autonomy and nonviolence in the 1970s–1980s. *Open Theology*, *3*(1), 494–515.

Grimm, J., Grimm, W., & Zipes, J. (2003). *The complete fairy tales of the brothers Grimm: All-new third edition* (J. Zipes, Trans.). Bantam Books. (Original work published 1987)

Halberstam, J. (2005). *In a queer time and place: Transgender bodies, subcultural lives*. New York University Press.

Kovalevskaia, I. (Director). (1969). *Bremenskie muzykanty* [Bremen town musicians] [Animated short]. Soiuzmul'tfil'm. YouTube. Retrieved August 21, 2024, from https://www.youtube.com/watch?v=d7NpFhucGbg

Lacan, J. (1966–1967). *The seminar of Jacques Lacan: Book XIV* (C. Gallagher, Trans.). Unpublished manuscript. Retrieved October 5, 2024, from http://www.lacaninireland.com/web/wp-content/uploads/2010/06/14-Logic-of-Phantasy-Complete.pdf

Lacan, J. (1967–1968). *The seminar of Jacques Lacan: Book XV* (C. Gallagher, Trans.). Unpublished manuscript. Retrieved October 5, 2024, from http://www.lacaninireland.com/web/wp-content/uploads/2010/06/Book-15-The-Psychoanalytical-Act.pdf

Lacan, J. (2007). *The seminar of Jacques Lacan: Book XVII. The other side of psychoanalysis* (J.-A. Miller, Ed.; R. Grigg, Trans.). W. W. Norton & Company. (Original lectures presented 1969–1970)

Lacan, J. (2014). *The seminar of Jacques Lacan: Book XX. Anxiety* (J.-A. Miller, Ed.; A. R. Price, Trans.). Polity. (Original lectures presented 1962–1963)

Lacan, J. (2015). *The seminar of Jacques Lacan: Book VIII. Transference* (J.-A. Miller, Ed.; B. Fink, Trans.). Polity. (Original lectures presented 1960–1961)

Livanov, V. (Director). (1973). *Po sledam bremenskikh muzykantov* [On the trail of the Bremen town musicians] [Animated short]. Soiuzmul'tfil'm. YouTube. Retrieved August 26, 2024, from https://www.youtube.com/watch?v=X3xNJSpOgWk

Muñoz, J. E. (2019). *Cruising utopia: The then and there of queer futurity* (10th anniversary ed.). New York University Press. (Original work published 2009)

Nietzsche, F. W. (1961). *Thus spoke Zarathustra* (R. J. Hollingdale, Trans). Penguin Publishing Group. (Original work published 1884)

Nietzsche, F. W. (1962). *Philosophy in the age of the Greeks* (M. Cowan, Trans.). Regnery Publishing. (Original work published 1873)

Russell, J. (2017). *Nietzsche and the clinic: Psychoanalysis, philosophy, metaphysics.* Karnac.

Sedgwick, E. K. (1993c). Tales of the avunculate: Queer tutelage in *The importance of being earnest.* In E. K. Sedgwick (Ed.), *Tendencies* (pp. 52–72). Duke University Press.

Stockton, K. B. (2009). *The queer child, or growing sideways in the twentieth century.* Duke University Press.

Tchaikovsky, P., & Tchaikovsky, M. (1993). *Pique dame* [Album recorded with the Kirov Opera and Orchestra, St. Petersburg, Valery Gergiev, conductor]. Philips. (Original work published 1890)

Van Haute, P., & Geyskens, T. (2012). *A non-oedipal psychoanalysis? A clinical anthropology of hysteria in the works of Freud and Lacan.* Leuven University Press.

Winnicott, D. W. (2005). *Playing and reality.* Routledge Classics. (Original work published 1971)

11

Anniversary

Having and surviving cancer are an exercise in waiting. Waiting for imaging and biopsy results, waiting for pathology reports, waiting for doctors to return your calls; waiting rooms, surgical theaters, dens of uncertainty; waiting in hospital gowns, in degrees of undress and distress; waiting with mind-serrating fear for the unwanted guest, Recurrence.

Waiting will never be the same again, liberated from associations to misfortune, medical settings, disease. I am declared cancer free, but yearly scans bring explosive anxiety. Will cancer return? When and where will it arrive? And in what guise?

In "Waiting," Roland Barthes concludes, "wherever there is waiting there is transference" (1977/2001, p. 40). What is the meaning of the ultrasound technician's sigh? Why did she linger on a given area of my breast, applying extra pressure with the wand? The radiologist is not emerging from his office, or he has come back too quickly—*with a death sentence?* The nurse approaches me with a subtle rubato, holding a sheet of paper, the verdict. Uncertainty and anxiety are merged in waiting: I am not sure what the mammographer, the doctor, the Other will do to me, but I know that my fate is in their hands. They might spare me, love me, or mortally wound me, take everything from me, condemn me to death.

Even 19th-century operas offer respite from melodrama; not every aria is superlative, not every note is forte. There are filler ensembles, extended mezza voce passages. Similarly, as Barthes notes, "the anxiety of waiting is not continuously violent; it has its matte moments" (1977/2001, p. 38). An acquaintance unexpectedly turns up on the mammography floor of the Breast Center—*Why are you here?* A family history of breast cancer: "I have to come here for checkups every 6 months." *How ... fortuitous?* A woman enters the Famous Cancer Hospital's waiting room at the height of the COVID-19 pandemic with her mask pulled down and chats up another patient at the coffee machine. Indignation temporarily organizes your frayed psyche. The young person a few chairs away receives bad news, and pity pulls you out of a narcissistic fog.

The checkup is over, the wait is over. You resume a subjective position; you reenter your singular body. Until the next anniversary, the next appointment, the next recurrence scare.

~

DOI: 10.4324/9781003498582-12

Desperate situations call for desperate somatic measures. The anniversary of the diagnosis: September 11. The anniversary of the mastectomy: October 5. The body knows, and the body reacts; it replays moments I have repressed. My body keeps a complete record and irrupts periodically in spectacular hypochondriacal displays.

I notice that psychosomatic ailments flare up in August, and I can't tell if it is because of the impending cancer anniversaries and oncological checkups or the humid weather or my vacationing analyst's absence: skin reactions, pointillist rashes, the coming to the surface. The psychosomatic symptom is a deconstruction, the stripping away of hard-won defenses. How far will the regression go? Will my body fragment, along with my reality, until I am a constellation of dots? Will I be reduced to dotted calcifications, ductal carcinoma in situ? I lose control over my body ego. The biological, indeterminate lamella-body threatens to attack and subsume coherent self-representation. A long-held belief system feels to be unraveling, a structure that once fastened in place corporeal limits, body language, the internalized mirror image. But maybe that's not really it.

Maybe the allergy storm, the persistent itch, the red dots blanketing my arms are an urgent call to my mother, via my analyst, an acting out, a question, a pleading cry: *Where are you? Can you see me? I am an amputee! Defend me! Restore my confidence, my sense of safety in the world!*

~

Hypochondria vexed Sigmund Freud. He did not believe it could be analyzed and classified it as a stubborn "actual neurosis" rather than a treatable "psychoneurosis." In Freud's differential diagnostic scheme, psychoneuroses were psychic articulations: They involved repression, transference, symbolization, and distortion through defensive operations. Psychoneuroses were linked to "signal anxiety" alerting subjects to imminent dangers derived from the past: For hysterics and obsessional neurotics, infantile sexual conflicts produced symptoms that could be interpreted. But hypochondria, neurasthenia, and other actual-neurotic pathology were caused by the dumb pain of present-day or "automatic" anxiety and said nothing. They were not meaningful; they did not signify. Actual neuroses were manifestations of somatic events (headaches, irritability, dyspepsia) coupled with supposed sexual dysfunction such as abstinence, excessive masturbation, and coitus interruptus (Freud, 1894/1953c, 1898/1953e, 1914/1955d, 1926/1961c).

From its earliest mention, psychoanalytically conceived hypochondria was a miscarried attempt at binding excitation, an inability to relieve endogenous "pressure," a tension arising internally that Freud eventually would call the drive. As Freud continued to conceptualize drive and anxiety—at the frontier of soma and psyche—the etiology of hypochondria became clearer and its emergence more ominous: It could slide into paranoia—it involved projection of badness onto organs or perhaps the perception of the body itself as a persecutor. The failure of modulating the drive—corralling somatic arousal into the realm of ego, into language—was, moreover, a failure of fantasy and maturation, a malfunction of identity (Freud, 1914/1955d).

Freud's wayward disciple Sándor Ferenczi surmised that hypochondria is a response to trauma in early childhood. He described it as an "auto-narcissistic splitting": the division of the psyche-soma into a healthy part and a sick part. The dichotomization enables self-observation and protection of the once-endangered self—its representative could be the mind, for example—from the afflicted portion of the body, which might stand for an abusive parent (Stathopoulos, 2017, pp. 362–363). Melanie Klein and her object-relations followers built on Ferenczi's ideas, attributing hypochondria to the primitive mechanisms of projection and introjection: Persecutory internal objects attack good ones, or else the ego fights against itself (Klein, 1935/1984, pp. 156–159; Meltzer, 1978/2018).

I conceive breast cancer as an enemy intruder, yet it is intimate, internal, ravaging the first and quintessential source of nurturance and infantile sexuality, the consummate representative of maternal care. Mastectomy is therefore always a double sacrifice, a reprise, an *après-coup* reminder and revision of ineffable primordial loss: It reeks of weaning, separation. It is the cut of a cut, the falling of an object already at the edge of corporeality and psyche. Is, then, my hypervigilance—my pressing concern about recurrence or a new cancer—actual-neurotic pathology or, rather, depressive paranoia, a healthy suspicion of the fantasied division between neighbor and foreigner?

~

Freud placed hypochondria into the actual neurosis category because for him it derived from the darker, psychotic reaches of the mind. Though it might accompany organic disease, hypochondria is primarily a narcissistic difficulty, excessive preoccupation with bodily phenomena, a pulling away of libido from external objects and toward the self—a self, moreover, prone to fragmentation. Hypochondriacs distort reality, break down, retreat from relationships. Is transference or cure even possible with such subjects?

Recent currents within psychoanalysis offer more sanguine prognoses for somaticizing patients, drawing on a congruity between hypochondria and dreams delineated by Freud in one of his less cited papers: "In dreams, incipient physical disease is often detected earlier and more clearly than in waking life, and all the current bodily sensations assume gigantic proportions. This magnification is hypochondriacal in character" (1917/1955c, p. 223). In a review of psychoanalytic approaches to hypochondria, Georgios Stathopoulos (2017) observes that

the parallelism … relating hypochondria and dreams prompts the question of the diagnostic capacity of an overinvestment of bodily sensations, and hence the question of the *minimal hypochondriacal investment of the body that would be protective* [emphasis added] for the timely diagnosis of physical diseases.

(p. 362)

Passionate attention to the tinglings of the body might be an "infantile theory of the somatic" (Stathopoulos, 2017, p. 362). Or *perhaps I am protecting myself from future incurable disease!* I was caught off guard, ambushed: A routine mammogram yielded a cancer diagnosis. There are no more routine mammograms. Hypochondria is a signal, a warning. *This time I will be prepared.* Anxiety attaches to a sensation or bodily manifestation: an itch, a freckle, a chest pain. I attack myself before a new cancer attacks me.

~

Psychoanalyst Paul Verhaeghe (2015) tells us that if we remove Freud's sexual etiology from actual-neurotic pathology (its connection to excessive masturbation and so forth), we see that it emanates primarily from a faulty relationship to the Other. He elaborates hypochondria and other actual neuroses by grafting Lacanian theory onto Freud's aforementioned types of anxiety, hierarchically organized: automatic anxiety, separation anxiety, and signal anxiety. Each of the three types is connected to a developmental stage marking the subject's capacity for regulating the drive, that is, internal tension, the bodily demand upon the mind for work; and to the quality of the subject's interactions with caregivers (their words and ministrations), namely, all those figures who come to represent the Other for the subject.

In earliest infancy, hunger and thirst are experienced as unbearable anguish; the boundary between internal and external, self and other, is blurred. Bodily tension cannot be managed due to the newborn's physical and psychical immaturity and manifests as automatic anxiety, the overwhelming feeling of coming apart. Months later, the Other is recognized as such: as a separate object, a signifying mirror, a presence or absence. The caregivers that constitute the Other are expected to remedy excruciating drive arousal, and their inevitable failures to provide adequate comfort induce separation anxiety. Finally, in late toddlerhood, or by the end of the oedipal period, anxiety might arrive in the form of a signal, a warning of impending internal or external danger—perhaps the return of the original anxiety or a potential loss. Such signal anxiety, it bears repeating, is defensive, psychically elaborated and interpretable, at some distance from the flooding, automatic variety. Signal anxiety becomes possible due to the subject's internalization of, and ultimate identification with, the Other's words and gestures. Verhaeghe (2015) notes that while separation anxiety is often dominant in early development, it diminishes in intensity and frequency with the acquisition of identity and object permanence: When "the Other is internalized, her actual presence is no longer needed" (p. 75). Identity development and drive regulation (with the aid of signal anxiety) therefore arise in tandem, both taking as their basis the representations proffered by the Other.

The hypochondriac, in this framework, has stalled at the level of automatic or separation anxiety. Her means of self-expression and drive regulation are underdeveloped, and the intersubjective dimension is disturbed. "Excitation begins from the body and ends in the body; it is discharged in it, without mental mediation, due to the deficit or failure of psychic defenses and the malfunction of the preconscious system" (Stathopoulos, 2017, pp. 370–371). The hypochondriac is compelled to seek help from the Other in a regressed manner: "words are not enough; word representations are not easily formed and are ultimately replaced … with an 'organ-speech' … or a thought that concentrates only on the literal, missing the symbolic foundations with which language is usually formed" (Stathopoulos, 2017, p. 371).

Verhaeghe and analysts of various French schools maintain that where there is regression, *progression is also possible!* With the help of an analyst's presence and the mirroring therapeutic relation, the Other might be more securely internalized, enabling bodily events to be symbolized, that is, deadened via discourse.

~

Mourning is a paradoxical and highly repetitive *signifying* process. You invent substitutes, metaphors for departed objects; perhaps the metaphors are accompanied by musical memories, vocal intermezzi again and again tethering the object to the ego. Marrying music and language, mediated by the grain of the voice, you tolerate the umbra of absence and eventually forget. This is *introjection* at its truest and most rigorous: a taking-in enabling a letting-go, ingestion of the object for the purpose of its integration and ultimate release. Introjection is diachronous and hence might be distinguished from sudden and gluttonous *incorporation*: Introjection is not an immediate swallowing whole—the encryption and denial of a loss—but, rather, a slow and deliberate recognition of the *difference* between you and the lost other (Abraham & Torok, 1972/1994). In mourning, as in introjection, you identify with this gap or differential, transforming it into prosthesis, into part of your psyche. Assuming responsibility for the loss, you find words and more words, skeins of words set to melodies bridging you and your most precious object. You put yourself, enlarged by the lost other, in the other's vacated place. The first such activity is taken up in weaning, in separating from the maternal breast, actual and metaphorical, from the caregiver's touch and smell, and many, many times over a lifespan: goodbyes to lovers, countries, analysts, friends, ideologies, ideals.

When disfiguring illness strikes, a mourning of the former body is required. Where does one begin and end such a process? Mourning a breast can feel like an insurmountable task. Aging is gradual, prosthetic: Over time, hopefully, you increasingly accept and adjust to its devastation. Mourning is waiting. So how does one mourn a swift and violent amputation?

Perhaps the cancer survivor's hypochondria is an instance of impossible mourning—or the avoidance of mourning altogether (Aisenstein & Gibeault, 1991), an expression of a melancholic attachment to the extracted organ. Psychoanalyst Marie-Claire Célérier suggests that "in hypochondria, neurotic or delusional, the object that suffers in the body (the hypochondriacal organ) takes the place of an object whose loss cannot be psychically elaborated by the subject" (as cited in Stathopoulos, 2017, p. 366). The breast cancer survivor's hypochondria, then, might be the remaining breast's dirge for its dead counterpart or the phantasmatic missing breast's lament, displaced onto surviving organs.

~

To Freud's tripartite classification of anxiety, the cancer survivor contributes a fourth: scanxiety. The portmanteau was invented to convey the specific predicament of the cancer patient: the terror of waiting for imaging scans and their results. With its attendant aches and pains, scanxiety is a blend of the automatic, separation, and signal varieties. It is the breaking of what Freud called "the stimulus barrier," the intrusion of the Real glimpsed in a traumatic moment, an acute reaction to imminent and external danger: the "suspicious finding." And it is an address to the Other, a performative gesture that may be misrecognized or refused. Scans show the body's caverns, revealing extimate regions, as does my hypochondriacal dermatitis: imaged cancer as separation anxiety, the blazon of shame, cancer as the me-not-me destined to be discovered or missed by doctors and loved ones. *Aren't you ashamed? The tumor had been growing silently for years.*

For the cancer patient in remission, scanxiety is also a signal—less a deafening alarm than a defensive, pessimistic assessment of a potential outcome—a message hearkening to past traumatic experience. *The worst has already happened ... but has it?* I brace myself for another bad scan.

~

The hypochondriac lives in terror of the organismic body—convulsive, menacing mortal flesh—and this terror is not without masochistic enjoyment. Perseverative excursions over phantom aches and corporeal deteriorations drip with libido and epistemophilia. Indeed, "before having anything to do with the body," writes Lacanian Leon Brenner (2017),

> *hypochondria* is an affliction which revolves around *the desire for knowledge.* It is an obsessive attempt to know what our body hides from us, what goes on inside of it, and how it affects us. Some might even call it an academic endeavor, attempting to articulate something of the inarticulability of our inevitable death.

After my fourth surgery I became obsessed with documentaries about people with terminal disease. Several times I watched *Cristina* (2016), a 39-minute documentary about a 37-year-old film script supervisor diagnosed with metastatic breast cancer. Director Michèle Ohayon began filming soon after Cristina's recurrence with the intention of making a full-length feature, but only managed 20 minutes of footage. Though Cristina was told by oncologists she had 5, maybe even 10 years left, she died a mere 5 months after the second diagnosis. Every treatment failed.

My preoccupation with recurrence deepened as memory of the mastectomy dimmed. I kept track of colleagues and acquaintances whose breast cancer had metastasized. What would the dying teach me about death? Was it less enigmatic and terrifying at its edge?

Death is rarely fully out of awareness for the hypochondriacal cancer survivor. Her brush with mortality is transformed into fascination, repeated efforts to study, know, and understand death:

> [The] *hypochondriac's* ... pains [ought to be viewed] as pieces of knowledge provided in the hopes that somebody could make sense out of them—like a doctor for instance. Through the interaction between "bodily-knowledge" (pain) and the knowledge of practitioners, the *hypochondriac* hopes to learn something of ... the body which can only be mastered in actual death.
>
> (Brenner, 2017)

~

The cancer survivor's hypochondria presents a cornucopia of etiologies, diagnoses, and prognoses. It is the imperfect binding of anxiety related to the loss of the object, to loss of love; it is the dressing of narcissistic wounds, efforts at healing and reinvention. Hypochondria post-mastectomy is a drastic defense against the ego's undoing: I am preoccupied with a given organ in order to avoid assimilating that another is gone—to ignore the fact that the body is riven.

Hypochondria is a failure of introjection, the return to the body of messages meant for the Other: *undeliverable*. The skin's eruptions are attempts to reach the gaze of the Other—the other as bearer of sociality, of language and sense—*I am in pain, in search of a shiny new ego ideal. I do not recognize my body; a cracked mirror that needs mending, a necessary regression; put me back together, throw me a line ("that's you!") after the catastrophe.* Except none of these sentences are strung together or pronounced. The utterance, instead, is registered as pain, numbness, a tugging ache: the physical body as the only channel of communication, a substitute for the returned letter. Insofar as the cancer survivor's hypochondria expresses that which cannot be symbolized, it is like other actual-neurotic pathology: a partial collapse of the symbolic dimension, a call for narcissistic and symbolic restoration, the suture of the body and its image via signifiers.

The breast cancer survivor post-mastectomy, and especially following reconstruction, is dealt an impoverished vocabulary, a dearth of representation for the missing breast. To remedy such a situation, she requires what Jacques Lacan would call a *sinthomatic solution*: a creative act of sublimation, a process of inscription, the relinking of the body as observable and felt surface to its intrinsic, raw materiality.

What would a cure look like? Words would have to be discovered, new metaphors for the amputated body part, and not just any body part, but the maternal phallus, the archetype of separation, of the interstitial, object *a*, the drive.

~

Wolfgang Mozart's *Idomeneo* (1781) has a gallery of fathers and no mothers. The looming paternal feels apt in an opera focused on love, identity, and personal autonomy. With *Idomeneo* Mozart salutes and bids farewell to opera seria—to its omnipotent gods wielding absolute control over the fates of humans—and introduces instead an Enlightenment universe of subjects defying patriarchs in pursuit of love and their own moral principles. In the first scene, a dead father, the defeated Trojan king Priam, is invoked in an aria by his bereaved daughter Ilia ("Padre, germani, addio!") whose pledge of vengeance is fully consonant with amorous daydreaming about the Cretan enemy prince ("Ill-fated life, o sweet death! ... But does Idamante love me?"). The primal father is the god Neptune, slain by Idamante in effigy—in the guise of a ferocious sea monster prone to screaming piccolo threats. Finally, the castrated master is the eponymous ruler of Crete who is allowed by Neptune to save his son from sacrifice on the condition that he yield the throne to Idamante and his beloved.

With such a collection of father figures, the mothers, perhaps long-buried and mourned, are less relevant. For at stake in the Mozartian model of subjectivity is the possibility of a "gesture of mercy on the part of the Other"—a reprieve granted to those ready to risk everything in an act of "defiant renunciation" (Žižek, 1993, p. 168). The savage freedom on the part of the subject—the blasphemous *No!*—is made possible and reciprocated by the father's symbolic castration.

The feared and loved fathers must be killed, if only metaphorically, so that the Cretan line may continue. Sexuality blooms and society functions when patriarchs soften, hesitate, grow compassionate and open to influence. The purpose of *Idomeneo*'s fathers, ultimately, is to fail nobly, ceding their authority to the next, gender-troubling generation. Paternal foibles and weaknesses result in the recognition and ascendance of a new couple: Ilia and her paramour Idamante, a figural father with an asterisk, a role written originally for castrato, then tenor, often sung by a mezzo-soprano.

~

Lacan, famously preoccupied with fathers, gave mothers short shrift. But, explains Joan Copjec (2002), Lacan's neglect of mothers in the family romance is not an oversight; rather, it is his conceptualization of the mother "as a void, a hollow." The mother in psychoanalytic and literary works is commonly depicted as the "fully supplied container," a "beyond or elsewhere … of pleasure," an Eden "from which the subject has been banished and to which he or she endeavors to return." Lacan's near erasure of the figural mother is the deliberate elimination of this "metadimension," of the "outside of history" (p. 100).

While Lacan's mothers might be hollowed out, his fathers are rarely biological or fatherly in any quotidian sense. In the late 1930s Lacan writes about the decline of the paternal imago; by the 1950s references to living, flesh-and-blood fathers all but vanish. Lacan instead lays emphasis on the *symbolic function* of the father, the father as Law, the incest taboo; the "father" as signifier, as name and metaphor (Lacan, 1938, pp. 44–46, 1956–1957/2020, 1957–1958/2017). The mirror stage produces the *ideal ego*, which gives the uncoordinated infant a false sense of mastery over its own and the other's body. The ideal ego, therefore, is an *imaginary identification*—a dual and fixed *relation* based on likeness—in which both ego and the mirroring gaze of the other are held in mind and aggrandized. The imaginary identification develops alongside a symbolic relation, the *ego ideal*, the structuring outcome of nomination: kinship obligations, the initiation into language and the social sphere. If the mother's role in the subject's emergence is to generate desire by establishing her "lack"—a hole in being that cannot be filled by the child—then the father's role is to give shape to this desire through signification, to symbolically individuate it through the *paternal metaphor*.

In the paternal metaphor, as in all metaphors, one signifier is substituted for another, which is repressed, destined to live on silently: The Name-of-the-Father, the signifier of the symbolic order, is substituted for maternal desire. The consequence of this substitution is the incest prohibition, the tearing of mother–infant duality, in short, triangulation. This is the structure of symbolization, the enabling of metaphorical substitutions, signifiers for other signifiers that represent parents, objects, and images stored in consciousness.

The subject is born! The infant gives up trying to become the maternal object's lack, what Lacan called the *phallus*, and pursues desire instead via the many associative pathways mapped by his unconscious. The phallus, in other words, is repressed and becomes a generalized signifier of the desire of the Other. Through displacement and condensation, the phallus qua object of desire transforms into the *object-cause of desire*, prefiguring object *a* of Lacan's later writings. Abstract thinking is possible, bodily coherence without constant mirroring is now possible; longing for an object that cannot be reduced to concrete *things*, that slips and slides out of the subject's reach, remaining beyond the perceptual field, shrouded in many veils: *All this becomes possible!* Having acquired the capacity to symbolize, secured by the Name-of-the-Father, the child ceases being the sole object of parental desire, identified in an imaginary manner with their desire, and becomes a desiring subject in their absence (Lacan, 1957–1958/2017, pp. 145–196).

Since the Name-of the-Father is a function (sustained by various statements invoking judgment, authority, and prohibition) not to be conflated with the family name, it is pluralizable. Eventually Lacan introduces various *Names of the Father*: Woman, God, James Joyce—whatever works, whatever establishes a place in the world for the subject—whatever might supply a bar, a prohibitive "No!" perched over the mother's desire. Every symbolic identification is an identification with an empty signifier because it stands for the unknown—it is the signifier for the very lack of imaginary identification—the signifier without a signified. The Name-of-the-Father, therefore, is "virtual," as Slavoj Žižek (1993) puts it, "the paternal metaphor is an 'X' in the sense that it opens up the space of virtual meaning; it stands for all possible future meanings" (p. 79).

Lacan's extraction of the empirical father (and even his actual name) from the paternal function allows for the development of radical, nonbiological, and gender-neutral concepts like the Real, object *a*, and the *sinthome*. The genesis of the subject becomes not only feasible but also expected, perhaps even necessary, in new family configurations: single mothers without fathers, same-sex parents, adoptive nonbinary uncles, may, according to Lacanian theory, rear high-functioning, garden-variety neurotics.

Lacan does reference an originary split outside of time and outside of language: the interstitial spark of metaphorical substitution, the inaccessible Thing from which spring both symbolically structured reality and the void of the Real, the index of the Thing forever lost, the mythical object whose imagined possession would yield full satisfaction of the drive. In the 1960s Lacan elaborates his object *a*, the subjective vanishing point creating a subject's reality. But, importantly, nothing can be known by the subject about this structuring, vanishing point—the hollow of the gaze, the voice qua silence—just as nothing can be known about one's own death (Lacan, 1962–1963/2014, 1964/1998a).

By the mid-1970s Lacan delves obsessively into topology, and the Name-of-the-Father ceases to be symbolic. To the three rings of the Borromean knot—which formalize the relation among the Real, the Symbolic, and Imaginary—Lacan adds a fourth, the *sinthome* (an archaic spelling of "symptom" and a play on *saint-homme*, sublime trash, a no-thing, ex-sistence). The *sinthome* is alien to the other three registers, yet paradoxically it links them via the human being's insertion *of himself* into language in a singular manner, through invention rather than substitution (Lacan, 1975–1976/2016). If the Name-of-the-Father fails or isn't provided, no matter! You can create one for yourself! A prosthetic paternity.

The *sinthome* adheres to and molds the subjective Real. What does this mean? At the place of the lack in the Other, Lacan invites you to come up with a unique, nonsensical way of organizing sense, and of managing and enjoying your body. For women without breasts, for breast cancer survivors, Lacanian psychoanalysis offers a compensatory structure, a way of giving up and mourning the "maternal"—the Other's desire to look like the idealized mother, that is, two-breasted. And it posits something even more radical: the possibility of making the "reconstructed" breast into true prosthesis, turning reconstruction into your own construction, tying your body qua Thing—pure materiality—with signifiers like "breast" and with novel identity and self-possession.

I know my body maintains coherence without having to look at the mirror repeatedly; I can hold the image in place without beseeching another to say "that's you!" over and over. I separate from the imaginary without hypochondriacal breaking or dissolution. I can stitch the symbolic, imaginary, and real elements together with an act of ineffable inscription, through a kind of writing.

References

Abraham, N., & Torok, M. (1994). Mourning or melancholia: Introjection versus incorporation (N. T. Rand, Trans.). In N. Abraham, M. Torok, & N. T. Rand, *The shell and the kernel: Renewals of psychoanalysis* (Vol. 1, pp. 125–138). University of Chicago Press. (Original work published 1972)

Aisenstein, M., & Gibeault, A. (1991). The work of hypochondria: A contribution to the study of the specificity of hypochondria, in particular in relation to hysterical conversion and organic disease. *International Journal of Psycho-Analysis*, *72*(4), 669–681.

Barthes, R. (2001). *A lover's discourse: Fragments* (R. Howard, Trans.). Hill and Wang. (Original work published 1977)

Brenner, L. (2017, September 5). Hypochondria. Retrieved August 28, 2024, from https://leonbrenner.com/2017/09/05/hypochondria/

Copjec, J. (2002). *Imagine there's no woman: Ethics and sublimation*. MIT Press.

Freud, S. (1953c). The neuro-psychoses of defence. In J. Strachey et al. (Eds. & Trans.), *The standard edition of the complete psychological works of Sigmund Freud* (Vol. 3, pp. 41–61). Hogarth Press. (Original work published 1894)

Freud, S. (1953e). Sexuality in the aetiology of the neuroses. In J. Strachey et al. (Eds. & Trans.), *The standard edition of the complete psychological works of Sigmund Freud* (Vol. 3, pp. 259–285). Hogarth Press. (Original work published 1898)

Freud, S. (1955c). A metapsychological supplement to the theory of dreams. In J. Strachey et al. (Eds. & Trans.), *The standard edition of the complete psychological works of Sigmund Freud* (Vol. 14, pp. 217–235). Hogarth Press. (Original work published 1917)

Freud, S. (1955d). On narcissism: An introduction. In J. Strachey et al. (Eds. & Trans.), *The standard edition of the complete psychological works of Sigmund Freud* (Vol. 14, pp. 67–102). Hogarth Press. (Original work published 1914)

Freud, S. (1961c). Inhibitions, symptoms and anxiety. In J. Strachey et al. (Eds. & Trans.), *The standard edition of the complete psychological works of Sigmund Freud* (Vol. 20, pp. 75–176). Hogarth Press. (Original work published 1926)

Klein, M. (1984). A contribution to the psychogenesis of manic-depressive states. In R. Money-Kyrle (Ed.), *Love, guilt and reparation and other works, 1921–1945* (pp. 262–289). Free Press. (Original work published 1935)

Lacan, J. (1938). Family complexes in the formation of the individual (C. Gallagher, Trans.). Unpublished manuscript. Retrieved August 28, 2024, from http://www.lacaninireland.com/web/wp-content/uploads/2010/06/FAMILY-COMPLEXES-IN-THE-FORMATION-OF-THE-INDIVIDUAL2.pdf

Lacan, J. (1998a). *The seminar of Jacques Lacan: Book XI. The four fundamental concepts of psychoanalysis* (J.-A. Miller, Ed.; A. Sheridan, Trans.). W. W. Norton & Company. (Original lectures presented 1964)

Lacan, J. (2014). *The seminar of Jacques Lacan: Book XX. Anxiety* (J.-A. Miller, Ed.; A. R. Price, Trans.). Polity. (Original lectures presented 1962–1963)

Lacan, J. (2016). *The seminar of Jacques Lacan: Book XXIII. The sinthome* (J.-A. Miller, Ed.; A. R. Price, Trans.). Polity. (Original lectures presented 1975–1976)

Lacan, J. (2017). *The seminar of Jacques Lacan: Book V. Formations of the unconscious* (J.-A. Miller, Ed.; R. Grigg, Trans.). Polity. (Original lectures presented 1957–1958)

Lacan, J. (2020). *The seminar of Jacques Lacan: Book IV. The object relation* (J.-A. Miller, Ed.; A. R. Price, Trans.). Polity. (Original lectures presented 1956–1957)

Meltzer, D. (2018). *The Kleinian development part 2: Richard week-by-week*. The Harris Meltzer Trust. (Original work published 1978)

Ohayon, M. (Director). (2016). *Cristina* [Film]. Kavana Entertainment.

Stathopoulos, G. (2017). Hypochondria: A review of its place in psychoanalytic theory. *Psychoanalytic Quarterly, 86*(2), 359–381.

Verhaeghe, P. (2015). Today's madness does not make sense. In P. Gherovici & M. Steinkoler (Eds.), *Lacan on madness: Madness yes you can't* (pp. 68–80). Routledge.

Žižek, S. (1993). *Tarrying with the negative: Kant, Hegel, and the critique of ideology*. Duke University Press.

12

The Voice

To take tamoxifen or not to take tamoxifen? One of several forced choices faced by the breast cancer survivor. Until the postsurgical pathology report I had not been given much of a choice: *Your money or your life? Your breast or your longevity?* At the mastectomy follow-up visit, without a gun to my head, the choice was less clear: *Your money or your ... savings*? A one in eight chance of developing estrogen-receptor positive cancer in the contralateral breast (as for a woman without a personal history of breast cancer) and a 1% chance of DCIS recurrence on the mastectomy side; or, with tamoxifen, a 30%–50% reduced risk of developing cancer in the remaining breast and potentially debilitating side effects for the treatment's 5-year duration (Jayasekera et al., 2023, para. 2), including vaginal dryness, leg swelling, weight gain, rashes, fatigue, headaches, and loss of sex drive, as well as the much rarer and infinitely more serious deep venous thrombosis, pulmonary emboli, cataracts, stroke, uterine cancer, bone loss ... *loss of the object, loss of love, loss of pleasure, loss of the will to live.*

~

After months of agonizing procrastination and with no time to spare, I looked forward to my appointment with the medical oncologist recently assigned by Famous Cancer Hospital (FCH). As the dreaded cancer anniversary approached, Dr. Confusing would grant clarity: She would help me decide whether to take tamoxifen. Firm and caring, she would arm me with knowledge, transform the forced choice into *my* choice, one I wouldn't regret years later. At the annual checkup, my surgeon, Dr. G, had advised refusal. Reluctantly, she'd confessed: "It's the medical oncologist's area but, personally, if I'd had a mastectomy for DCIS, I wouldn't take it. It's about quality of life, and the risk reduction isn't sufficient." Would a healthy woman take tamoxifen to lower her breast cancer risk from 8% to 4%?

Dr. Confusing did not possess the placid charm of some of the other FCH doctors. Anxious, unblinking, disturbingly gaunt, and a little peaked, she insisted that I would be jeopardizing my life by forgoing tamoxifen, that I'd be faulted for my own illness and dying, that, in fact, I was at greater risk of developing a tumor than a woman without a history of breast cancer. When I cited contradicting research and my surgical oncologist, Dr. Confusing became exasperated: "No!

DOI: 10.4324/9781003498582-13

That's plainly wrong. I *just* examined a patient with a recurrence of DCIS—she is in the next room—she also refused to take tamoxifen! It *does* happen. You *are* more likely to get a new cancer."

Dr. Confusing offered several other muddled impressions and threatening anecdotal evidence. At this point, as with Echo and Narcissus, the interrogative and the imperative became almost indistinguishable:

"I read that tamoxifen increases risk of endometrial cancers?"

"... Endometrial cancers."

"My aunt died in your hospital of endometrial cancer ..."

"... Endometrial cancer? ... Well, then we'll just take it out!"

Now I was Echo, she Narcissus, "Take it out?!—You mean, *my uterus?*"

The appointment became increasingly contentious and ended with Dr. Confusing rushing to another, more pliable patient. The following day I called my surgeon's office and demanded to be paired with a different medical oncologist. "I want someone who will be more patient-focused," I muttered, not knowing what that meant. "I want someone more flexible, nicer, who will not speak about my organs as if they were easily expendable." *I want someone to agree with me and love me!*

Several months passed without a referral to a new oncologist. At last, an "FCH patient advocate" called me to explain. It was not so easy to find another medical oncologist specializing in breast cancer. At FCH they all worked together, as part of a team, and supported one another's opinions. What, precisely, was wrong with the first one? Could I say more? I felt like I had done something wrong, like I was on trial. "Look," I explained, "I will not be pressured into endocrine therapy. I will not be sold tamoxifen as if it's snake oil or some street drug. I know it's not snake oil, but I also don't want to be told that I'll die without it. I want an oncologist who will present it as an option and not a necessity. I will not be bullied. I will go elsewhere for a consultation if FCH doesn't offer a gentler, more reasonable alternative." A few weeks later I received another phone call. The patient advocate had found someone, with a man's name: Dr. T. L. Irishman.

~

The visit with medical oncologist no. 1 had been in late September, and the appointment with medical oncologist no. 2 was scheduled for early January. In the meantime, I thought about tinkering with the shape and volume of the reconstructed breast. The perfectionist in me saw room for improvement, more belly liposuction and chest lipofilling for enhancing softness and a rounder appearance. I requested another "revision" surgery, knowing full well that most of the fat injected into the chest area would be reabsorbed by the body over time. A temporary solution at best.

The final reconstructive surgery would happen about a week after the appointment with Dr. Irishman. With my decision not to decide, and by opting to have yet another surgery, I prolonged the queer time in-between. Why would anyone choose more surgery, more hospitals, more anesthesia? Because of cosmetic considerations? A flimsy and partial rationalization. I was not ready to let go of my breast, my FCH caregivers, all those holding me tight. The fourth surgery was a deferral of reentry into sexuality and chronology, a postponement of life on the clock.

~

Opera fandom and a Soviet early childhood taught me to see the queue as an instance of queer temporality, akin to the analytic hour: a liminal arena enabling the separation of voices from bodies, the mingling of genders and identities, acousmatic flight, promiscuity of thought, the emergence of uncanny silences, distilled instances of the drive. In the 1990s, when AIDS and the closet were not yet relics, Wayne Koestenbaum (1993) brought queer delight and a keen poetic ear to the ticket line and standing room at the old Metropolitan Opera House, "spaces of mobility, cruising, maximum attentiveness; spaces where one broadcasts commitment, desperation, patience; spaces where one meets other fanatics; spaces of rumor, dish, cabal" (p. 44). At the new Met, I have not witnessed the salacious acts reported by Koestenbaum, but I do recall relationships contrived on camping stools and lawn chairs, "the friendships and enmities of the queue," the cheapness of my time (Koestenbaum, 1993, p. 44), lacerating arguments about the latest productions and rising stars.

~

Waiting in queue is perhaps the most emblematic experience of late socialism. Goods deficits and long lines were common throughout East European history, but in the 1970s they became exceedingly inconvenient and frustrating. Or, more likely, the queue grew strange and intolerable only retroactively, in the wake of perestroika. Since the end of the Soviet Union, the queue with its dilated temporality has continued to serve as a metaphor for the entire Brezhnev era, indeed, as its central organizing principle. In fictional and scholarly accounts, it both incarnates and comments on social relations, the second economy, and the logic of scarcity (Baranskaya, 1969/1990, pp. 1–62; Humphrey, 2002, pp. 40–64).

One particularly illustrative example of such scholarly focus is anthropologist Katherine Verdery's classic article "The 'Etatization' of Time in Ceaușescu's Romania." The queue is invoked as Verdery (1992/1996) explores the late socialist state's use of temporal politics to exercise power over its inhabitants. She argues that the regime's policies aimed to "seize time" from individuals by making exorbitant demands on the human body, "the site of many possible uses of time" (p. 40). Bodies often were appropriated and compelled into activities (or inaction) beneficial to the state. Since socialist regimes sought to accumulate means of production above all, and inputs counted more than outputs, the center constantly attempted to enhance its pool of resources by denying other, peripheral actors the ability to do so. This strategy caused an economy of scarcity that, in turn, resulted in an immobilization of bodies. Food shortages, for example, meant long stints in queues, while deficits of fuel rendered complicated and tiring such basic activities as getting to and from work. The binding of the labor force in queues was not seen as a cost to the socialist state because it accrued supplies and not profit (Verdery, 1992/1996, pp. 39–58).

Verdery views the involvement of bodies in idle time as a mechanism of subjugation because people were made unproductive and time was "flattened" (1992/1996, pp. 46, 57). Queues diverted energy away from undertakings that might have alleviated shortages, such as lower-level initiative and planning. Temporal organization, furthermore, is crucial to identity formation and sociability, and, implicitly, to the sustained relationships necessary for collective grassroots action. According to Verdery, as well as theorists from Pierre Bourdieu to Judith Butler, national-historical time plays a significant role in defining the self and forming alliances (Verdery, 1992/1996, pp. 53–56; see also Freeman, 2010, pp. 3–4, 18–19). Disturbance of temporality courts disturbance of subjectivity. But did accepting "queue time" mean accepting the abyss (Koestenbaum, 1993, p. 218)?

The line debuted as the central protagonist in Vladimir Sorokin's stagnation-era novel *The Queue* (1983). Its characters are divorced from an established time and place, taking shape largely through dialogue and without a narrative linking utterances to a particular setting. Through such stylistic choices the novel communicates the phenomenology of the queue: a cacophony of voices, statements without addressees—life as a series of disembodied sounds, truncated exchanges, and overheard snippets of conversation. On the one hand, *The Queue* explores the idea that ruptures in linear time result in depletion of the subjective and the relational. The novel's structure gives an impression of ephemeral and ultimately unproductive social bodies. On the other hand, since the queue exists in protracted time and is without purpose (no one knows what is being sold, and value is invested in the very act of lining up), the characters are free from material ties and have many opportunities for accidental loyalties and situational attachments. Those waiting in an unending line for an unspecified product or result embody and instantiate desire without object—or demonstrate an unrestrained desire that alights on random objects, such as strangers, adventures, and conversations. Sorokin's novel therefore conveys not only the despair of the queue but also its creative potential. Through renderings of episodic socialities and casual sex, it offers a fantasy of limitless possibilities and nonlinear temporality due, paradoxically, to interminable lines. Sorokin's characters find themselves in a swirling movement that, while seemingly without direction or aim, leads to entrancing discoveries and meaning making (Sorokin 1983/2008).

~

I am a child of the stagnation era and therefore ghostly to myself, in exile, the interstitial time and space of emigration. I am in the littoral, at the shoreline, a perpetual refugee. I wrote academic articles about stagnation's most quintessential cultural artifacts—its queue, its innovative animation—because they raise the ghost of the late socialist queer child, a child who did not grow up. The Soviet youngster's failure to become what she latently was brings to light the strange temporality haunting all children. Childhood, after all, is the retrospective work of adults. But if the figure of the child is always a memorial to the death of a former (fictional) self, then the Brezhnev-era child, fallen out of history, arrested in development, is not readily available to its adult subject for integrating infantile affects, desires, and fantasies.

Not properly assimilated, mourned, and let go, the late socialist way of living—and of being in time—is repeatedly staged by the Soviet diaspora.

Even more than Sorokin's queue, Russian American novelist Olga Grushin's line twists time, blurring historical periods and generational distinctions. In her 2010 novel, *The Line*, interior and exterior, domestic and foreign are rendered mutually constitutive and fantasmatic, produced and reproduced within the minds of its protagonists. Time pulsates and opens on the line, and past and present become interchangeable. The line is experienced as an ever-widening now.

Those queued wait to purchase tickets for a concert by the (fictional) composer Igor Selinsky, rumored to be returning to Russia to conduct his latest symphony on an unknown date. The line never budges, and the tickets are never sold. And yet we see how the line irrevocably transforms the material and inner lives of a family: Anna, husband Sergei, son Sasha, and Anna's uncommunicative mother. At the beginning of the novel their relationships are devoid of love, eroticism, and movement. An unbridgeable gulf separates the protagonists even though they live virtually on top of one another in a tiny apartment. Indeed, their proximity impedes rather than fosters affection, the clock on the kitchen wall a hovering witness to the hours spent in routine actions and sickening familiarity. The line breaks the stifling closeness of the family members, and each learns—through loss, surprise, and fleeting intimacies—how to love and how to want, eventually rediscovering one another as well (Grushin, 2010).

Connections forged on the line are not typically romantic or heterosexual: The middle-aged Anna grows fond of a 10-year-old boy, the teenaged Sasha spends time with the much older, debauched Nikolai and his gang of hooligans, and Sergei has an unconsummated emotional entanglement with a purge victim's pallid wife. Through these new queer relationships as well as their contact with the line-as-organism (the line is often described by Grushin as a unified, embodied entity that grunts, undulates, feels, and changes shape), the protagonists become their dreamed better selves (Grushin, 2010). In metaphysically exceptional states like lines, identity loses its certainty and reality cedes its hold.

The queerness or exceptionality of the line is conveyed, too, by its association with Selinsky/Stravinsky and, by extension, the fin de siècle world of Sergei Diaghilev, Vaslav Nijinsky, and the Ballets Russes—a world of modernist sexual dissidence and aesthetic practices linking the novel's characters to forgotten pleasures and experimentation. As in Sorokin's *The Queue*, we are shown in Grushin's novel that it is precisely the stagnant and initially enigmatic quality of the line that incites change and desire. As they wait, Anna and others in queue begin to fantasize about what might be sold, enjoying not knowing and awaiting surprise. The socialist state only issues concrete demands, but the queue poses open-ended questions and entices, awakening the libido.

~

Latvian-born David Bezmozgis's *The Free World: A Novel* (2011), like Grushin's *The Line*, is set in a time and place in-between. It narrates the experiences of the

Krasnansky family and fellow Soviet refugees in Rome and Ladispoli as they await entry visas to "Over There," that is, Canada, Australia, Israel, and the United States. Italy in Bezmozgis's novel is a metaphor that suspends time and expands the present, placing memories and identifications into synchronous arrangements and allowing characters to examine themselves and others from new vantage points. Those who can forgo yesterday, and to some degree tomorrow, thrive in this queer temporality. Others collapse under the burden of the present and cannot abide the hauntings of an unfinished Soviet past. The patriarch Samuil, war hero and Communist Party loyalist, does not live but merely "exists" in Italy as if between two deaths (symbolic and physical) and expires at the end of the novel, while his friend, fellow World War II veteran and amateur musician Josef Roidman, composes an opera and socializes, making the most of the moment.

The once successful and virile Samuil is marked by Stalinist antecedents—its masculine ego ideal, linear view of history, and promise of plentitude—and finds his current circumstances unendurable. But Roidman, having lost a leg in the war, welcomes the contingency of Ladispoli time, a temporality stripped of history and generational inheritance. Already queerly embodied, he embraces the disappearance of Soviet chrononormativity, the bound time that steered male bodies into labor productivity and ideological compliance. Roidman confides to Samuil that he "would continue to wait until one of two things happened: either Canada accepted him or he finished his opera about Fanny Kaplan," the terrorist Socialist Revolutionary famous for shooting Vladimir Lenin. Roidman

> found Ladispoli to be conducive to musical composition. There was the seashore, the mild climate, stimulating company, and few practical obligations. This was how he always imagined … creative people worked in their exclusive rest homes and union retreats. … What a charmed life [artists] led! What they did could not be considered work—it was such a pleasure. When he sat down to compose, the music poured out of him.
>
> (Bezmozgis, 2011, pp. 289–290)

Disfigured by the war, Roidman, unlike Samuil, admits that he is lacking, that he is castrated. When confronted with overt emasculation during the immigration, he is able to accept, even revel in, loss, which he finds emancipatory and affirming. A temporality where yesterday and tomorrow hold fast while the present moment is stretched and mined for potentiality—precisely for incompleteness—is encapsulated in Roidman's opera forever in progress. He has reached and is savoring, Roidman tells Samuil,

> the most stirring and hopeful part of the story. Fanny Kaplan has just recovered from blindness due to an accident caused by an exploding bomb meant for the tsar. A clinic in Kharkov has restored her eyesight. She is now fit to instruct the masses and foment revolution once again. In the spring of 1917, Lenin had not yet become *Lenin*. There is no reason to shoot him yet. … The spring of 1917

was as far as Roidman had progressed. He had arrived at the enchanted moment when, as in a fairy tale, the clouds part and the golden light streams in. In a fairy tale, this is where the story ends. Not so in life. But that doesn't detract from the enchanted moment. The moment remains the moment. And that which comes later, comes later.

(Bezmozgis, 2011, p. 291)

~

Internationally renowned opera diva Natalie Dessay lost and recovered her voice several times, enduring four vocal cord surgeries. French television recorded one such episode while following her daily activities for the 2005 documentary, *Natalie Dessay: La Voix*. A dress rehearsal at the Bastille Opera ends in despair: Dessay refuses to sing the role of Zerbinetta and withdraws from all performances of Richard Strauss's *Ariadne auf Naxos*. A voiceover by the one-named filmmaker Esti informs without ceremony: "Natalie cannot bear the vagaries of her voice any longer. She can't live with a voice that no longer responds" (Esti, 2005a, 1:33).

Dessay consults her doctor, a "speech pathologist" who has "examined her between 50 and 100 times." The doctor places a laryngoscope into Natalie's mouth, summoning her vocal cords. "Today we can see it clearly, it is not a dream": imaging reveals that her glottis isn't straight (Esti, 2005a, 2:25). The acousmatic Esti cannot make it out, the anomaly is too subtle, but Natalie insists, it's there in black and white: the queer glottis, two lips, one errant. Can an operation straighten Natalie's vocal cords, cure her of queerness? Temporarily, perhaps, but one senses the endeavor is ultimately futile, the impossible complementarity of two vocal cords, perfection that never was, an irreducible gap. At the filmmaker's prompting, Dessay contemplates the risks of another operation, her second. If it fails, she "will not sing anymore. Never again. Ever" (Esti, 2005a, 5:15).

In the next scene, the diva meets with her surgeon and again is asked to weigh the potential dangers and benefits of vocal cord surgery, especially for a barely visible flaw. The discussion is mostly phatic, for Dessay does not view the operation as a choice:

I cannot go on living like this! I'm even ready to switch careers if it doesn't work. If I'm unable to recover the means that I—and I alone—find acceptable, I'll do something else. I'll be 40 next year. Life can change at 40. It's not the end of the world. It's sad, but it's not a tragedy. Life goes on.

(Esti, 2005a, 9:56)

Just minutes before surgery, Dessay is shown on a gurney in a polypropylene bouffant cap and skimpy hospital gown. She confesses to stage fright. Why is she even having this surgery, risking everything? "It's dumb to be put under. I'm not sick. I feel good!" (Esti, 2005b, 3:30). She exercises her soprano, a preternatural vocalise, possibly her last, and disappears into the operating theater.

We learn post-surgery that something was in fact *there*, Natalie had not imagined it: a distended mucus membrane, a tiny polyp, now removed. Success! Nobody mentions that small polyps and nodules are a common occurrence, that perhaps the polyp would have healed on its own, with sufficient vocal rest, and that surgery might have been too radical and unnecessary. It hardly matters to Dessay, for after a week of mandatory muteness on the Normandy coast and a lengthy rehabilitation, she is again capable of a crystalline F above C. In January 2005 she wins Best Singer of the Year at the Victoire Music Awards. "The less often I sing, the more Victoires I receive," she quips (Esti, 2005c, 5:30).

In the penultimate scene, Dessay avows to her vocal coach that she does not want to be cured, that she is attached to illness. She wants to be left alone, to perform less, to have more time with her family, to be sick again, to be a better mother. We believe none of it. In the documentary's final sequence, Dessay performs a concert version of Lucia di Lammermoor's Mad Scene at the Theâtre des Champs-Elysées. When breaks from singing are stretched, comebacks are all the more anticipated. Dessay would leave and return to opera for another 15 years.

~

What would it mean to lose the lost object, to lose one's voice? What if it were damaged or stolen? To what lengths would one go to regain it, to traverse the breach? To catch up, to fuse with one's own voice as it escapes the throat, invites madness, or worse. Some marriages are deadly.

In 2011 I heard Natalie Dessay at the Met in Gaetano Donizetti's *Lucia di Lammermoor* (1835). Her voice sounded lighter, more fragile than I'd remembered. She was not the Natalie of my dreams but nonetheless managed all the roulades, trills, and mordents—the acrobatics and raptures of coloratura—sweeping me away. Natalie was back; she had made yet another comeback.

Like Dessay, Lucia has difficulty mourning. She loves Edgardo but is tricked by her brother into a more politically advantageous marriage to Arturo. On her wedding night, devastated Lucia murders the groom in their nuptial bed. Wild-eyed and disheveled, bridal gown splattered with blood, she descends an enormous staircase and performs a 20-minute "mad scene" cabaletta, hallucinating Edgardo's voice in suicidal ecstasy before a chorus of petrified guests. Lucia chases and chases Edgardo, represented by an echoing flute, until they finally merge, and their merger can only mean death. This is it. Lucia's falling in love with a family rival wasn't it; her brother's betrayal wasn't it; murdering her husband wasn't it; the blood-stained wedding dress also was not it. When Echo is extinguished, there is no longer any gap, no residue, no sexual difference. So long as there is an echo, so long as there is pursuit and repetition, there is life. But when Lucia and the flute sing in unison, we fall with her into the abyss. Now Dessay can emit the high F and expire, plunging from above the staff.

~

The throat is at the center of psychoanalytic practice, the aphonic reverse of the voice, the vanishing mediator of desire, a germinating navel of subjectivity. Koestenbaum (1993) notes that the glottis is "spookily genderless," a place where sexual difference disappears, and yet the voice box "has been clothed with a feminine aura" because it is "hidden from view," like the vagina, "a horizontal cleft, terminated by two lips" (p. 161). The feminine throat is a metaphor for all things internal and invisible—the psyche, the unconscious, the Real—that which cannot be glimpsed without a doctor, a laryngoscope, interpretation, the mouth held open.

In "Irma's injection," Sigmund Freud's paradigmatic dream of wish fulfillment in *The Interpretation of Dreams* (1900), the father of psychoanalysis pries open and peers into a woman's mouth and vanishes, falling into its deep mystery, a leuko-plakia presaging his own cancer. Freud extricates himself from the fleshy horror of Irma's throat by lending it symbolic support, by inventing psychoanalysis (Freud, 1900/1953b; Lacan, 1954–1955/1991, pp. 161–171).

Freud's famous patient Dora's symptoms originated in the throat—a cough, irri-tations, mucus, aphonia—cast and recast retroactively from an "imaginary mold," a childhood memory (the somatic prerequisite!) of sucking her left thumb while tugging with her other hand at her brother's earlobe (Freud, 1905/1953a; Lacan, 1952/2006b, p. 180). In Dora's throat Jacques Lacan finds the etiology of hyste-ria: not her repressed wish for fellatio or Herr K, as Freud thought, but rather the failure to "assume" her own body. Everything associated with femininity for Dora is folded into the oral drive, including a masculine identification through thumb sucking. Dora stitched together her identity by the only means available to her, via a male figure. This was her earliest imago, Lacan (1952/2006b) explains, and it constitutes "that primordial identification through which the subject recognizes herself as *I*" (p. 181). Dora's enjoyment of her body can only happen through her brother's body; hence her *I* is susceptible to "functional fragmentation and con-version symptoms" (Lacan, 1952/2006b, p. 181). The hysteric's ability to grapple with the feminine and to experience genital pleasure hinges on symbolization and analytic mirroring. Without verbalization and dialectization of Dora's identifica-tions and "transferences," various men will continue to organize her self-image, enabling her to open her mouth, to suck and speak, to experience and enjoy her own body (Lacan, 1952/2006b, pp. 181, 183–184).

The receptivity of the glottis keeps a person alive. Its hole must never cease producing itself, for it is the material guardian of the unconscious, the gatekeeper of humanity. Dessay's surgeon gives a less speculative rendering:

> The vocal cords shut off access to the trachea and the lungs when they close and let air through when they open. They control the swallowing mechanism, [enable you] to avoid drowning in saliva while you sleep. Or, in water, if you're napping by a river and fall in … your vocal cords will keep you from drowning. It's a vital reflex … that resists [all but the strongest anesthetics].
>
> (Esti, 2005a, 7:13)

Reading tattered voice manuals from the 18th and 19th centuries, Koestenbaum (1993) observes a striking similitude between voice culture and psychoanalysis:

> Both systems believe in expressing hidden material, confessing secrets. And both discourses take castration seriously: voice culture wants to recapture the castrato's scandalous vocal plenitude, while psychoanalysis imagines castration

as identity's foundation-star player in the psyche's interminable opera. Opera culture has always fantasized about a lost golden age of singing; accordingly, a central ambition of the voice manual is to preserve cantabile style against degeneration and newfangled vices.

(p. 159)

In opera as in an analytic session, the voice is the carrier of queerness. It meanders, it cracks, strains, exceeds its own limits. Operatic singing has no relationship to the speaking voice. It trespasses the sexed body and violates grammar; it becomes unmoored from gendered self-expression. Lacan drew attention to the materiality of the voice and the promiscuity of speech in analysis. He dubbed it *lalangue*: inexplicable events in the mouth and on the couch, the jouissance of uttering sounds, the playfulness and pleasures of orality, dangling phonemes and parapraxes of utterance (Lacan, 1972–1973/1998b, pp. 138–139, 141–142). The analyst receives and repeats back to the analysand her babble and its cleaving libido.

The object-voice—the silent, enjoying voice carried by speech—doesn't stop being generated. It is the sensual dimension of utterance, the registering of the place where meaning abuts affect. The voice as pure materiality may be viewed as the subject's inability to understand all, to close the gap in self-knowledge. It interrupts perfectionistic automatism, cuts ceaseless attempts at making the original look like the copy. The "natural" breast must achieve symmetry with the manufactured one, just as the early recording artist was encouraged to sing in a manner that suited the technology and boosted "fidelity." In Enrico Caruso's 1906 recording of Giuseppe Verdi's *La Forza del Destino* (1862), Victor "shifted the frequency range of the reproducing equipment upward to favor the higher registers, reinforcing the [tenor's] 'ringing tones.'" One Victor ad then proclaimed that "the sound [is] … 'so natural that it seems to be Caruso himself singing instead of the machine'" (Siefert, 1995, p. 439). Producers eventually learned that human warmth emerged not by technology vanquishing itself but in the incidental noises and blemishes of recordings. Audiophiles sought and continue to seek the gentle hiss of needle touching vinyl.

~

Reassuring and empathic Dr. Irishman helped me say *No!* to tamoxifen and *No!* to more surgery. At my presurgical appointment in January 2019, I asked the dashing red-headed doctor whether he would consider me crazy if I declined endocrine therapy, and he replied, "I would not think you were crazy." My efforts at prelapsarian return and immaculate symmetry were reaching a terminus: The fourth "revision" surgery would be my last. I expressed my gratitude to Dr. Irishman. I was very lucky to have found him—someone with whom I would have an enduring relationship—a trusted authority to guide me going forward. He chuckled and patted me warmly on the back: "I hope you never have to see me again!"

With a gentle push from Dr. Irishman, my ginger-haired twin, I stepped into myself. The voice emerges in the interstitial, in the impossibility of self-identity.

Assuming one's voice entails giving up the narcissistic project, embracing echo, and eventually, becoming Echo for oneself, one's own analyst.

~

In late fall of 2020 I received a letter via USPS from FCH informing me that Dr. T. L. Irishman had died suddenly and that I had already been assigned a new medical oncologist. An internet search revealed that Dr. Irishman "passed away unexpectedly" at FCH "while on duty" at age 38. He was predeceased by his brother, who died young from cancer. His partner's name was David; he was deeply loved.

References

Baranskaya, N. (1990). A week like any other (P. Monks, Trans.). In *A week like any other: Novellas and stories* (pp. 1–62). Seal Press. (Original work published 1969)

Bezmozgis, D. (2011). *The free world* (1st ed.). Farrar, Straus and Giroux.

Esti. (Director). (2005a). *Natalie Dessay, la voix* [Natalie Dessay, the voice] [TV documentary, part 1]. France. YouTube. Retrieved August 19, 2024, from https://www.youtube.com/watch?v=JOCcaveUSzI&list=PL2m6FD0rcM3Evg6A93yktYdwT2ZbAoBAX&index=1

Esti. (Director). (2005b). *Natalie Dessay, la voix* [Natalie Dessay, the voice] [TV documentary, part 2]. France. YouTube. Retrieved August 19, 2024, from https://www.youtube.com/watch?v=V8QdaR90MPg

Esti. (Director). (2005c). *Natalie Dessay, la voix* [Natalie Dessay, the voice] [TV documentary, part 5]. France. YouTube. Retrieved August 19, 2024, from https://www.youtube.com/watch?v=HTFjxTGNn5c

Freeman, E. (2010). *Time binds: Queer temporalities, queer histories.* Duke University Press.

Freud, S. (1953a). Fragment of an analysis of a case of hysteria. In J. Strachey et al. (Eds. & Trans.), *The standard edition of the complete psychological works of Sigmund Freud* (Vol. 7, pp. 1–122). Hogarth Press. (Original work published 1905)

Freud, S. (1953b). The interpretation of dreams. In J. Strachey et al. (Eds. & Trans.), *The standard edition of the complete psychological works of Sigmund Freud* (Vols. 4–5, pp. 1–625). Hogarth Press. (Original work published 1900)

Grushin, O. (2010). *The line.* G. P. Putnam's Sons.

Humphrey, C. (2002). *The unmaking of Soviet life: Everyday economies after socialism.* Cornell University Press.

Jayasekera, J., Zhao, A., Schechter, C., et al. (2023). Reassessing the benefits and harms of risk-reducing medication considering the persistent risk of breast cancer mortality in estrogen receptor–positive breast cancer. *Journal of Clinical Oncology, 41*(4), 859–870. https://doi.org/10.1200/JCO.22.01342

Koestenbaum, W. (1993). *The queen's throat: Opera, homosexuality, and the mystery of desire* (1st ed.). Vintage Books.

Lacan, J. (1991). *The seminar of Jacques Lacan: Book II. The ego in Freud's theory and in the technique of psychoanalysis, 1954–1955* (J.-A. Miller, Ed.; S. Tomaselli, Trans.). W. W. Norton & Company. (Original lectures presented 1954–1955)

Lacan, J. (1998b). *The seminar of Jacques Lacan: Book XX. On feminine sexuality: The limits of love and knowledge, 1972–1973* (J.-A. Miller, Ed.; B. Fink, Trans.). W. W. Norton & Company. (Original lectures presented 1972–1973)

Lacan, J. (2006b). Presentation on transference. In *Écrits: The first complete edition in English* (B. Fink, Trans.; pp. 176–185). W. W. Norton & Company. (Original work published 1952)

Siefert, M. (1995). Aesthetics, technology, and the capitalization of culture: How the talking machine became a musical instrument. *Science in Context, 8*(2), 417–449.

Sorokin, V. (2008). *The queue* (S. Laird, Trans.). New York Review Books Classics. (Original work published 1983)

Verdery, K. (1996). The "etatization" of time in Ceaușescu's Romania. In K. Verdery (Ed.), *What was socialism, and what comes next?* (pp. 39–58). Princeton University Press. (Original work published 1992)

13

Tattoo

Little Vinnie's Tattoos in Finksburg, Maryland, became a popular destination for breast cancer survivors in 2001, when its eccentric owner Vincent Myers decided to cease creating artistic tattoos and focus exclusively on what turned out to be a much more lucrative business: "3D" nipple and areola tattooing. Women from far and wide book months in advance to get their "Vinnies" (Bracken & Jensen, 2014, 1:16). Myers completes breast reconstruction post-mastectomy by helping women sinthomatize their prostheses, transforming nippleless domes into forms resembling breasts, draining mirror images of uncanny elements and symbolizing them through inscription of the skin that can be felt in the Real. Mastectomy leaves the chest area numbed, but the painful process of tattooing might still be felt and experienced, reanimating deadened flesh. With Myers' help, the extimate breast implant is subjectified and libidinized.

Vinnie Myers, accidental writer of the *sinthome. The New York Times* and *The Today Show* feature him tattooing nipples onto mastectomy scars, enabling "women to feel whole again" (Today Show, 2015, 1:56; see also Bracken & Jensen, 2014). *Whole again?* In one respect, maybe: He helps amputees tame unruly parts of their body egos, drive irruptions disturbing their visual and affective fields. Myers offers something else, too, a service far more radical and important. The act of tattooing invites women with reconstructed breasts to feel (the) *hole* again. Myers's work is sinthomatic because it makes Jacques Lacan's "true hole" from within a fracture in the ideal image-object, from the place at which the imaginary breaks its own unity and penetrates the Real (Lacan, 1975–1976/2016, pp. 15–16, 125, 155). Where there was a stain in the specular image and a sensory blank, comes to be a flat likeness of a body part, *the semblance* of a three-dimensional nipple–areola complex.

The act of tattooing transforms the subtracted corporeal into a locus of creative openness, a structural void in being. Mimicking the signifier, it burrows a hole in the biological substance of the body. The tattoo itself then operates as a null set within the imaginary, a representation of the beyond of representation: nothingness rather than absence. The 3D nipple–areola tattoo, remarkably, represents both finitude and its failure, the incompleteness of the visual and symbolic components of reality. It functions, in other words, not by deception and fantasy—through repression (it does not, in Lacanian terms, create a "false hole")—but by registering

DOI: 10.4324/9781003498582-14

emptiness, *das Ding*, the no-thing itself (Lacan, 1975–1976/2016, pp. 15–16, 155). The two-dimensional figure, therefore, is used in a symbolic way. Women are not stupid; they do not actually feel whole again; they do not repress the amputation. On the contrary, in getting their Vinnies, women identify with a structural impossibility, with their *not-all*.

~

In manner, gesture, and style, Vinnie Myers is what one might call a dandy. He shows up to work every day in a tilted porkpie, dress shirt, and vest. In a *New York Times* video interview, he sits ankle on knee with Wildean sangfroid, flashing polka-dotted socks and two-toned wingtips. Publicity photos show him smiling sardonically as he adjusts his bow tie for the camera. Vinnie's cool, his pale blue eyes complementing the neutral hue of his unstructured suit. Sartorial flair lends middle-class respectability to an otherwise plain-spoken tattoo artist, a feminizing veneer to a figure whose surroundings and humor suggest seedier, more masculine pursuits.

Vinnie is well suited to "putting the finishing touches" on women's breast reconstructions and making them (w)hole (Kreuz, 2013/2015, para. 2). He exhibits excess, drag, effeminacy. The wingtip shoes are a tad overly polished, the varied patterns on shirt, vest, and socks perhaps too meticulously chosen. Cool fastidiousness is the paradoxical raison d'être of the dandy, the flaneur, the homosexual, and the phallic woman. There is something in ostentatious masculinity—put-on virility, the raiment of symbolic power—that slides into the decorative, into the feminine.

Lacan named that "something" in the putting-on that signals femininity, castration, and more fundamentally, the dizzying gap in being: the phallus, the signifier of signification and its failure, the irreducible discomfort of the mortal, acculturated subject. Masculine and feminine positions are two ways of accommodating— of dealing *indirectly*—with this anxiety-inducing condition. The abyss born of the signifier can only be handled through what Lacan termed the phallic function, the veil and trace of primordial loss (for how could we look directly at death)? Put another way: We all fall short of fully occupying our own bodies. Occasionally we might become aware of our egos as sets of masks, as masquerade. *What if underneath my social roles, gestures, and identities—my symbolic support—I am nothing?* Unalloyed subjectivity is this ontological negativity, and the anxiety it induces must be warded off. The phallus (the signifier of lack, the cause of desire) can only be experienced—assume shape and be seen—when veiled.

What do sexed beings, then, *do* with the phallus? Lacan follows psychoanalyst Joan Riviere in positing that masculine subjects play at *having* the phallus through imposture, by keeping their lack concealed. Feminine subjects flaunt *not having* it through masquerade and, in doing so, paradoxically make the phallus visible (Lacan, 1958/2006c; Riviere, 1929). There is nothing extra or stagey about masculinity or masculine power; it is made to appear natural, effortless. Femininity is, by definition, excess: It is all extra, it is adornment itself. Scholar Todd McGowan (2018) felicitously describes Lacan's distinction between masculinity as imposture and femininity as masquerade:

> Imposture involves feigning as if one has something that one doesn't have, while masquerade involves acting like what one is not. The imposter hides what he has because he doesn't have the secret power that he pretends to have, whereas the masquerading woman puts a secret on display so that she will be loved for it even though it has nothing to do with her. Imposture hides through hiding, and masquerade hides through showing.
>
> (p. 8)

One can immediately sense from McGowan's gloss why the feminine position is "closer to subjectivity in its pure state." Masculine-identified subjects believe they possess the phallus; they do not question their existence as men. Their anxiety stops at castration anxiety, the fear that phallic power has limits. Masquerading feminine subjects, however, are prone to existential dread, the more terrifying sense that subjectivity recedes into nothingness, that there is a point where symbolic support slips away and that this is the "general state of things" (Zupančič, 2017, p. 56).

In Lacan's scheme of sexual difference, masculinity is a simulacrum of substantial subjectivity, and as such it cannot be recruited to sinthomatic writing. A person committed to imposture, to repressing castration and stashing the phallus, could not, as the masquerading Vinnie does, transform an optical illusion, a mask and the emptiness beneath it, into know-how, a new way of moving through the world with others that affirms the potentiality of the image while undermining "it as the be-all and end-all" (MacCannell, 2016, p. 83). Where masculinity fails, where it crinkles, fractures, and reveals itself, new images form and accrue, *nachträglich*.

~

Through deferred action, my birthplace figured its own *not-quite-here* political collapse. All that waiting—waiting in queue, waiting for utopia, waiting to emigrate—produced temporal detours, loci of queer potentiality. Failures of masculinity and its ideals presented especially fertile ground for late socialist animators, who invented its popular characters at the intervals between speech and listening: Goluboi shchenok, Cheburashka, Karlson, and the Soviet Winnie-the-Pooh, another Vinnie—Vinni-Pukh. Vinni's queerness, like those of the other characters, is accentuated by the very art of animation, which detaches voices from their human sources and places them in plastic, temporally lax, nonnormative bodies and unexpected or impossible situations.

Queer temporality is constituted by the object-voice, a silence made visible. And what theater scholar Peggy Phelan has asserted about the body in performance can also be said about the voice embodied by animation: It is a metonym that alludes not to the subjectivity of the performer but to another element of the performance—a character, a gesture, or a musical phrase (Phelan, 1993/1996, pp. 150–152). Like the acousmatic voice of Someone addressing the Hedgehog in the Fog, the gurgling baritone of actor Evgenii Leonov's Vinni-Pukh plays precisely this part: the former speaking "without sound" and thereby dissolving into enigmatic lack to be traversed by the fantasy of the viewer, and the latter evoking other Leonov roles, his mediated personalities and associations to the Soviet everyday life. Such vocal drag engenders intimacy and queers desire by prompting spectators to assume multiple identifications concurrently and therefore to question the self in linear time, even identity as such.

~

A. A. Milne's *Winnie-the-Pooh* originated in England and was inspired by stories the author created with his son, Christopher Robin, about Christopher's favorite teddy bear and other toy characters. "Winnie" was the name of a bear relocated from Winnipeg that Christopher visited at the London Zoo, and "Pooh" supposedly the name of a swan the boy saw once on holiday. While in *Winnie-the-Pooh* Milne appears as the author-narrator and Christopher the reader-protagonist, the text seems to have been forged collaboratively. Milne both observed Christopher's play with a toy bear and participated in it. He then transformed this narrated play into a book, one in which Milne is also occasionally a character conversing with Pooh and Christopher Robin. Perhaps because Milne's *Pooh* is a children's story told humorously from an adult's point of view by a nurturing narrator, it attracts an avid adult readership and has even generated so-called Poohology, a body of texts that mobilized the books, movies, and material culture of *Pooh* for didactic and satirical ends (Kidd, 2011, pp. 35–63).

Vinni-Pukh, translated faithfully by Boris Zakhoder in the early 1960s and then made into a three-part animated series by Fedor Khitruk for Soiuzmul'tfil'm between 1969 and 1972, also enjoyed immense popularity with a dual audience of children and adults, proving especially appealing to intelligentsia readers and spectators. Literature scholar Nataliia Smoliarova, waxing autobiographical in an academic article on the film series, tells of the warm welcome she received when in 1972 she started her first position as translator in one of the Moscow institutes. Her senior colleague boasted of the friendly atmosphere in the department: "We have here many couples, travel novels, shared children, and a copy of *Vinni-pukh*." Smoliarova considered herself lucky since both good colleagues and Zakhoder's translation were in short supply and high demand. There were long queues for the book in libraries and friendship circles; copies changed hands many times, and the less fortunate searched for it without success in stores and among fellow enthusiasts (Smoliarova, 2008, p. 287).

The most obvious change made by Khitruk in his film adaptation is the removal of Christopher Robin and his father-narrator from the story. Christopher's lines are given to Piatachok (Piglet) and in places to Rabbit, and Milne's to a less intrusive voice-over narration, with the effect that the distance between viewers and characters is narrowed and the self-reflective storytelling duties are transferred to the former. The potential for recognition and reflexivity on the part of the viewer is enriched, too, by occasional ruptures in the diegetic frame (Pukh pauses during his contemplative walks to stare directly into the camera) and the intertextuality occasioned by the voice of Leonov. The celebrated character actor not only brought to Khitruk's films his trademark natural acting style, slurred speech, warm facial expressions, and clumsiness; he also famously served as Vinni-Pukh's physical model.

The opening chapters of Milne's *Winnie-the-Pooh*, illustrated by *Punch* cartoonist Ernest H. Shepard, revolve around Pooh's insatiable appetite for honey. In the inaugural "We Are Introduced to Winnie-the-Pooh and Some Bees and the Stories Begin," Pooh fails to obtain honey from the top of a tree inhabited by bees. In the following "Pooh Goes Visiting and Gets Into a Tight Place," our hero climbs through a narrow hole into his friend Rabbit's home and eats so much honey that he gets stuck on his way out. Self-reflective narration is used liberally in these early chapters. Milne initially focuses on Pooh's relationship with Christopher Robin and introduces the good-mannered Rabbit in the second chapter, previewing other characters only briefly. The reader never forgets that Pooh is Christopher Robin's beloved toy, one might say his transitional object, and that Christopher is the narrator's 6-year-old son who asks his father "sweetly" to tell Pooh stories about himself "because he's *that* sort of bear" (Milne, 1926/2023, p. 4). Parenthetical italicized conversations that readers are led to assume took place between real father-author Milne and his son Christopher appear throughout. These layered metanarratives have been of great importance to the understanding of the Pooh stories and one of the principal reasons for their broad appropriation. Children's literature specialist Kenneth B. Kidd even suggests that the structure of Milne's book echoed the development of collaborative play in child psychoanalysis (2011, pp. 35–52).

Khitruk's first two films, *Vinni-Pukh* (1969) and *Vinni-Pukh idet v gosti* (*Vinni-Pukh Goes Visiting*; 1971), about 10 minutes each in length, in many respects are consistent with the original plot, reproducing much of the dialogue verbatim. But Khitruk's narrator, unlike Milne's, has no relationship to Vinni-Pukh or anyone else and only serves unobtrusively to introduce the story, offer sparse commentary, and utter a few valedictory lines at the end. In eliminating the framing devices that Milne uses to evoke the childlike make-believe world of the Hundred Acre Wood— a world of hybrid social groupings where forest animals, stuffed toys, and a boy congregate and have adventures—Khitruk obviates the need for Christopher Robin and human life more generally. He thereby intensifies and widens the fantasy space, creating a universe where Vinni-Pukh and his friends are very much alive: They are no longer talking animals or stuffed toys but, rather, anthropomorphic, "real" characters that feel more authentic when not placed in scenes with naturalistically drawn humans. The written word does not stand between them and the viewer, and the film induces identification and reflective engagement, implicitly summoning the audience to assume the position of Vinni-Pukh or the place evacuated of author-narrator Milne. Most obviously, Khitruk's version removes the father–son relationship and shifts its primary focus to the strikingly queer (non-oedipal?) alliance between Pukh and Piatachok.

The immediacy and queerness of Khitruk's world are also transmitted through naive animation. The scenes resemble children's colored-pencil drawings: flat, laconic, with saturated reds, yellows, and lush greens. Technical difficulties necessitated some of the simplicity in the art, limiting the movements of Pukh and Piatachok (for example, Pukh's front and back paws always moved in the same direction) but at the same time enhancing the characters' awkward charm (Leving, 2008, pp. 328–329, 336–343).

Khituk and Zakhoder further enliven Pukh by modifying and expanding the role of Piatachok. In substituting the piglet for Christopher Robin, they give Pukh a companion who, unlike the human Christopher, is not blatantly superior in intelligence or maturity. Piatachok, in fact, is quite admiring of Pukh and spends much of the films taking orders and breathlessly trying to keep up with the bear's swift pace. Voiced by the film actress Iia Savvina and sped up to a piercing treble, Piatachok reads as an infant or toddler, eliciting sympathy and enlarging the personality of his dear "Vinni."

Piatachok's part in the elaboration of Pukh's character is especially apparent in *Vinni-Pukh Goes Visiting*, based on Milne's second chapter. The honey-eating scene in Rabbit's abode is expanded in the Soviet version to demonstrate Pukh's servitude to the oral drive. The bear's superficial grasp of rules of comportment is utilized solely for the purpose of crude manipulation and the ultimate goal of procuring snacks. His perfunctory awareness of etiquette is unaccompanied by a true capacity for empathy, with the result that he overstays his welcome and eats everything Rabbit has in his cupboard. And yet Khitruk deepens, one might say *subjectivizes*, Vinni-Pukh through nuanced gestures and interactions with Piatachok. The bear gently bosses around his mate without appearing tyrannical. Like a parent might do to a small child, Pukh washes his little buddy's face before the meal. He then ties a napkin over Piatachok's mouth (but without force or malice) so that the piglet is unable to eat or say anything during the whole visit and disrupt his plans. Toward the end of the scene, Pukh reaches for Piatachok's hand several times before finally grabbing it and running off with him.

Khitruk's Vinni-Pukh is surlier and fatter than the British Pooh. The tiny and squeaking Piatachok serves to accentuate his friend's stoutness. Pukh's body is huge. It spills over, chagrins itself, announces its enormity. Pukh cannot help being overweight: He is all hunger and mouth, unable to stop ingesting. He invites our hunger and cannibalistic urges with his driven, out-of-control orality. His is an infantile mouth, a preoedipal body. Neither Pukh nor Piatachok perceives bodies as carriers of shame or markers of sexual difference. Pukh is innocent of the reality principle, and he will never grow up. Khitruk said as much in a letter to Zakhoder, explaining that he perceived Vinni-Pukh as a character who is

> always bursting with grandiose plans, too complex and unwieldy for the trivialities to which he wants to apply them. This is why the plans fall apart as soon as they come into contact with reality. He is constantly getting into trouble, not because of stupidity, but because his world does not accord with reality.
>
> (as cited in Leving, 2008, p. 328)

The Soviet Pukh is not a teddy bear or a naturalistic bear but a raspy-voiced man who remains a boy or failed adult. As in the Karlson and Cheburashka films, the stain of failure is immediately conveyed via Leonov's scratchy, cigarette-marred voice, housed in a naively drawn, clumsily rotund body. It is elaborated further through the bear's not-quite parental, self-serving friendship with Piatachok, as well as his id-driven motivation. Khitruk suggests that the relationship between Pukh and Piatachok is vaguely familial due to the loyalty and esteem of the soprano-voiced piglet for the much larger bear. But the films make equally explicit that the infantile Pukh is completely incapable of parenting anyone and might be even less informed about life than his junior mate, who protests, "no one goes visiting in the mornings" (Khitruk, 1971, 1:14).

In the second film, Khitruk and Zakhoder take the most liberties with Milne's text, mainly in the service of conveying late socialist cultural paradigms. While Shepard's Rabbit is drawn in a naturalistic style, Khitruk's is anthropomorphized, an unmistakable member of the Soviet intelligentsia. With large spectacles, nose in the air, finger raised, and lisped self-righteousness, he lectures and prevaricates more than Milne's meek figure (Leving, 2008, p. 328). Vinni-Pukh's voracious appetite and poor self-restraint in Rabbit's home acquire special relevance in a deficit economy. Rabbit is compelled to surrender the entire contents of his kitchen. He shudders at having to serve the honey and condensed milk but is too spineless and docile to refuse Pukh. Although Rabbit is cynical and insincere, initially lying to Pukh about not being home, he immediately yields to his visitor's demand just as he might satisfy the demands of the state.

Pukh's willfulness and drive for pleasure are thrown into sharp relief by the inertia and cheerless aridity of Rabbit. If Rabbit's intelligentsia masculinity is more fully achieved than Pukh's—civilized, moral, and castrated—it is also devoid of desire: bookish, overly polite, long-winded, and without virility. Indeed, Pukh's immature and queerly embodied masculinity is rendered endearing and triumphant in a world where being "mature" means living like the passive Rabbit.

~

The idea of Leonov-Pukh as a creative remedy for the libidinally drained Soviet intelligentsia reverberates with a scene bearing structural resemblance to *Vinni-Pukh Goes Visiting* in a different sort of film, a very popular romantic comedy made 8 years later. In Georgii Daneliia's *Autumn Marathon* (1979), Leonov makes a brief but memorable appearance as a Pukh-like character and helps stage similar themes and cultural logics among Brezhnev-era intellectuals.

Autumn Marathon is principally about a crisis of desire. It is a wry but not unsympathetic rendering of a likable 40-something university professor struggling with thorny midlife dilemmas. Incapable of refusing anyone's requests, thoroughly overcommitted, Andrei Buzykin (Oleg Basilashvili) can no longer manage the multiplying exigencies in his professional and private lives. Though well-intentioned, Andrei's efforts at placating his wife, mistress, needy friends, and clamoring colleagues ultimately disappoint and exasperate the very people he is desperate to please. Everyone seems to want something from Andrei, but what does Andrei want? As film scholar Lilya Kaganovsky (2009) points out, "Andrei takes no pleasure in either his wife or his mistress, and sex is implicitly replaced with eating" (eating without enjoyment, I would add). In an early scene that conveys Andrei's alienation, he sits with his back to his mistress, mechanically chewing his dinner while she talks about wanting to have his children (p. 186). Kaganovsky remarks, with Lacan in mind, that

> this is not simply another example of the prudishness of Soviet cinema, or the well-known pronouncement, "We have no sex." At stake here is a lack not merely of sex but of the "sexual relation." ... Relationships (between the sexes) presented in Soviet films deny the possibility of desire as an operative force, converting sexuality into its related, component parts: nurturing, family, marriage and children,

converting it, in other words, into demand:

> The "demand" coming from the state requires that subjects not only work and attend Party meetings, but also that they marry and reproduce. A subject out of bounds ... has to be contained [in a reproductive marriage, in the workplace]—his "desire" made identical to the "demand" of the state.
>
> (Kaganovsky, 2009, p. 186)

Andrei, however, is trapped in a rut of his own creation. "His attractive qualities—intelligence, sensitivity, kindness of soul"—are virtually eclipsed by his passivity. "He does not act but ... simply reacts to people and events as best he can, without any protest and a resigned smile" (Lawton, 2004, pp. 22–23). In Lacanian terms, Andrei is stuck at a point just short of desire: at the level of the Other's demand. He prefers addressing concrete demands and performing tasks (meeting his lover, helping a friend with translations, drinking with his neighbor, attending meetings) to dealing with desirousness: his mistress's fantasy of having children, his wife's cravings for intimacy. For Andrei and perhaps many of us, the encounter with the Other's desire, diffuse and enigmatic, is too anxiety producing. Yet desire enables and organizes subjectivity. The subject, like desire itself, requires lack in order to spring to life, to strive, and move ahead. In contrast to demand, desire has not one object but many; it wants to keep desiring (Fink, 1997, pp. 50–71).

If desire in this, psychoanalytic, sense "is a search for an object that promises a future," then, as Kaganovsky (2009) suggests, *Autumn Marathon*

> skips over "desire" and leaves us with something closer to "drive"—the circular movement around an objectless void. In the film, the repeated act of jogging that structures the narrative speaks to this objectless circulation. Every morning Andrei's foreign colleague, a Danish professor and fitness devotee, Bill, rings his doorbell and collects him to go jogging.
>
> (p. 186)

While one might quibble over Kaganovsky's comment that the drive's movement is "objectless" (since the void *is* the object of the drive), the circular structure of

Autumn Marathon is indisputable. The film begins and ends with a jogging session in the dark autumnal Leningrad hours. The two friends' "formulaic greeting accentuates the ritual and repetitive nature of this event: 'Morning!' says Bill in English. 'Morning!' repeats Andrei in English; 'Vy gotov?' ('Ready?'), asks Bill, 'gotov,' Andrei always answers" (Kaganovsky, 2009, p. 186).

For a moment in the film, forward movement seems possible. After a series of misunderstandings and arguments, Andrei's wife and mistress abandon him in dramatic fashion. Left alone, Andrei is delirious with relief, believing that he has found a way out of the impasse. But his celebration ends in a flash: mistress and wife in quick succession return, and the usual routine is resumed. The last scene confirms that all the characters, despite much frantic activity, have remained in the same place. When Bill shows up—in the evening this time—for their daily jog, Andrei agrees, and the film concludes with Bill in a tracksuit and Andrei still in the workday's dress shirt and tie, "jogging in the fading light, a row of streetlamps stretching before them into infinity. Andrei finally realizes that he is 'bezvol'nyi'— that he has no will" (Kaganovsky, 2009, pp. 186–187).

Unlike his neighbor Andrei, Vasilii Kharitonov, played by Leonov, has not succumbed to the tyranny of jogging and health discourses. Portly, working-class, and alcoholic, Kharitonov has a passion for vodka and mushrooms and little consideration for the academic's tendency to work at home. He drops in one Thursday (his day off), vodka in hand, and finds Andrei and Bill busy with a translation. Paying no mind to Andrei's mild protests, Kharitonov makes his way to the kitchen, swiftly pours the vodka, and insists that the three drink together. Andrei continues to resist feebly, but due to the professors' chronic passivity and politeness, they agree to have a shot, and then another, and a third—all without enthusiasm. A bit later, at the insistence of Kharitonov, the trio goes mushroom picking in a forest without mushrooms. Andrei finally becomes exasperated and walks off, leaving Bill with Kharitonov. Under the influence of a much more experienced drinker, the Danish professor ends up in a vodka-binging oblivion. After riding a bicycle into the wee hours all over the city looking for more alcohol, Bill is picked up by the police and taken to a detoxification clinic.

Much like the bespectacled Rabbit and the diminutive Piatachok, Andrei and Bill cannot seem to say "no" to Leonov's character. The ambivalent and analytical intelligentsia men are completely disarmed by Kharitonov-Pukh's insistent proposals, the monomaniacal force of his hunger and simplicity of his pleasure. Perhaps what Leonov's characters display is closer to drive than desire, but if it is drive, it is free of the obsessional defenses exhibited by Andrei and Bill.

~

In mourning the Soviet Union, I turned to the queer failure of Leonov-Pukh, his sudden appearance and popularization in the stagnation era. Was he the herald of utopia's collapse? Stagnation was not merely an effect of economy or discourse but also a central point of Brezhnev-era ideology. As the Soviet Constitution of October 1977 declared, socialism was now "developed." The Soviet Union interrupted itself on the road to communism, failing to reach its ultimate destination. The radiant tomorrow would never arrive. Kaganovsky (2009) elaborates:

> When the Stalinist system ... [had grown] exhausted, when self-sacrifice to the violence of the state finally resulted in the "graveyard" of socialism, we were left with "stagnation": that is to say, the production of subjects without desire. ... There was ... a "cultural logic of late socialism" that had ramifications in the sphere of popular culture. Literature and cinema responded to the economics of "stagnation" with a metaphorization of desire, by repeatedly staging its absence.
> (pp. 186–187)

I would qualify that rather than merely staging the absence of desire, *Autumn Marathon* poses desire and its redialectization as a problem. It presents a desire crisis generated by the deadlock in the stagnation-era subject with respect to the Other's demand. The drinking scene in Andrei's kitchen, though not especially long, made a tremendous impression on Soviet audiences and won Leonov recognition for a relatively minor role (Pesmen, 2000, pp. 182–183; Rollberg, 2009, p. 404). The resonance of that scenario may have rested partly in its similarity to the earlier Vinni-Pukh film, in which Leonov also was an interminable guest attempting to stretch time, to extend his visit and manipulate his host while remaining naively amused and sating himself. Perhaps Leonov resonated, too, because in both roles he offered at least a partial resolution of the desire problem. The repetitions enacted by both Vinni-Pukh and Kharitonov are playful and pleasure-seeking; they hark back not to a time before desire was eradicated but before it was born, an innocent earlier period. Their repetitive actions are not, like Andrei's, a circling around a traumatic void, the symptomatic compulsion to repeat. The void is not there because it has not been generated yet. The pleasure in fullness and in repetitive actions is not the psychotic's but the young child's.

~

In the third Khitruk film, *Vinni-Pukh i den' zabot* (*Vinni-Pukh and a Busy Day*; 1972), Pukh meets Donkey Ia (Eeyore in the Milne version), who is gloomy and self-pitying for somewhat vague but weighty reasons. When Pukh asks him, "What is the matter?" Ia answers, "Nothing, Pukh, nothing. We can't all and some of us don't. That's all there is to it." "Can't all what?" demands Pukh. "Have fun, sing, dance" (Khitruk, 1972, 2:28). The donkey, in other words, cannot enjoy. And he has an even bigger problem. Pukh soon observes that Ia is missing his tail. Not having noticed its absence previously, the tailless melancholic wonders whether it had been lost or stolen and laments its disappearance on his birthday, of all days! To cheer him up, Pukh resolves to get his friend a birthday present and perhaps even help him locate his tail.

Back home, Pukh searches for a suitable gift and settles on—what else?—a jar of honey. But, on the way to Ia, he predictably gets hungry and consumes the contents of the jar. Pukh then decides to give his friend the jar containing nothing, as well as the nothing in the jar: now Donkey could fill it with anything he wants! "How useful an empty jar will be," Pukh keeps exclaiming. It is not difficult to see the possible metaphors here. Ia is depressed, but he has the potential to desire because he has suffered an impossible loss; in other words, he is castrated. Pukh finds and returns the tail to its owner, affixing it with a bow—a sign of symbolic intervention—a memorial to the wound and a marker of its new, denatured status. Pukh also gives Ia an empty jar, the outline of something, a potential space, an emptiness that can be filled with many different objects. This is desire par excellence. Having given up the bodily object through symbolic castration—through alienation in language—the subject, in Freudian fashion, refinds the object in the world (Freud, 1925/1961d).

How can Vinni-Pukh, a mere child who does not know lack, who has not yet ceded anything, help the jaded Donkey? Pukh, after all, only understands primary process, pleasure. To the extent that he acknowledges others, it is via what Sigmund Freud (1915/1955b) deemed "the purified pleasure ego," an infantile, narcissistic mode of perception according to which the other, although separate, is just like him, wanting the same things he wants and in the same ways (p. 136). Was the stagnation-era audience supposed to see its salvation in this not-quite adult? Or, worse, a failed man, an eternal boy like Kharitonov?

The figure of Vinni-Pukh—which encompassed and utilized both Leonov's physical body and body of work—was an unlikely *sinthome* of late socialism, an effort to confront and revitalize its arrested libidinal and symbolic economies. Desire as lack—the search for an elusive object, the *not-hoped-for-yet*—while often missing in Brezhnev-era authoritative discourse, was evoked repeatedly in its animated films. Characters like Vinni-Pukh and Kharitonov, with their id-driven motivation, big bellies, and hearty appetites for food, drink, and homosocial relations, might have enacted a primitive and immature desire, but among their sanctimonious, enervated, and cerebral peers—the standard-bearers of late Soviet cultivated masculinity—they, at least, were able to enjoy.

One might wonder if in embracing Leonov's affable characters and their trusting acolytes, Brezhnev-era audiences were disavowing state violence—Stalinist purge campaigns that turned child against parent and neighbors against neighbor—or else reveling in childishness for its own sake, perhaps retreating to a "kitchen temporality" of escapism (D. McDonald, personal communication, October 13, 2014). I do not believe this was the case, especially in relation to the Vinni-Pukh films. In excising the fatherly Milne and his conversations with Christopher Robin, Khitruk positions the viewer in the paternal role, allowing him or her to act as a Third (or analyst) who intervenes in the self-contained and solipsistic world of Pukh and Piatachok by posing questions and causing desire. The viewer, in other words, eschews the need for an on-screen patriarch and assumes responsibility for interpreting the oracular speech and enigmatic behavior of the characters, converting drive into desire within the story and, by extension, within him- or herself.

~

I first heard the name Vinnie Myers in Dr. Forceps's waiting room. For an eternal 45 minutes I had been sitting next to a professionally dressed, handsome woman, probably in her late 30s. Peering at an open laptop balanced on her knees, she seemed entirely unperturbed by the doctor's abandonment. A nurse finally surfaced from a corridor leading to the examination rooms: An emergency had delayed Dr. Forceps, but not to worry, he was on his way, due to arrive in approximately half an hour.

"Golf game, you think?" My anemic attempt to engage the laptop votary.

She raised her eyes from the computer screen and grinned.

"I'm used to this. He runs very late sometimes. I have been coming for years to have my implant checked, but it's been a while since I was here last—I've been *bad*. I had cancer 7 years ago, unilateral mastectomy. It's hard to get motivated to have these checkups. It would be awful if the implant tore, if they had to cut me open again … and the areola tattoo probably would have to be redone."

Encouraged by Ms. Laptop's candor, I inquired further about her cancer history and reconstruction.

"My tumor was about the size of a dime, invasive ductal carcinoma, estrogen and progesterone positive. I was so young … I went for the most radical treatment. The reconstruction is fine, for what it is … although, you know, certain angles … in some poses it doesn't look hot. Overall, they do a good job here, and the implant holds up. But, whatever you do, *do not* get the tattoo here. The surgeons at FCH are not tattoo artists—they don't really know what they're doing. For the nipple and areola tattoos everyone goes to a guy in Maryland, Vinnie Myers."

"Wow, interesting … Is there nobody in New York City who can do this?"

"I know it must sound strange, but believe me, if you want it done right, if you want *the best*, you must go to Vinnie! He's an artist. I could show you his work—do you want to see?"

Inexplicably ebullient, she began unbuttoning her blouse in the crowded waiting room.

"*No … please!* I mean, erm … that's not necessary …"

"Oh, nobody here cares, it's fake anyway! You're sure you don't want to have a look?"

I waved off the idea. "It's okay, really, I don't have to see it right now. I will check out his work online—when I get home."

Later, in the exam room, I asked a nurse about the Maryland tattoo artist. She confirmed that Vinnie Myers was in high demand, a veritable legend. I'd have to make an appointment well in advance, some report an 8-month queue. It would be expensive, and health insurance probably would not cover it since Vinnie is not a doctor. If I had the tattooing done at Famous Cancer Hospital, my insurance would be obligated to pay. Also, if I wanted an areola tattoo, or any tattoo for that matter, I would have to wait at least 3 months after surgery.

When Vinnie was only a signifier, a mere gleam in my mind's eye, I'd just had mastopexy and nipple reconstruction. The new nipple, built from surrounding skin, soon became a disappointment. It shrank and flattened over time to a size substantially smaller than its authentic counterpart on the left. Obviously, it was too late for the trompe l'oeil version, but I figured that an areola tattoo and chiaroscuro effects on the fake nipple would create an illusion of greater projection.

The contralateral breast, too, was now an artifact of reconstruction and had acquired an inauthentic appearance. It no longer possessed a real areola because the nipple had been carved out and lifted with a concentric incision and another, vertical incision down the center of the lower part of the breast. The Houdini-like cutting and raising had left a thin white circular scar, a border around my nipple roughly where the areola used to be. The skin inside the circle was quite fair, almost the same hue as the rest of the breast, and would be difficult to match on the implanted right side.

I wasn't sure how my chest would look and feel eventually, and whether complementarity could be achieved. Maybe I should embrace the falseness and asymmetry, quit trying to make my breasts look "natural"! Isn't artifice the essence of creativity, the sublime—humanity itself—as Charles Baudelaire proclaimed? I pondered getting a decorative tattoo instead of the areola. I perused hundreds of online images of women with "mastectomy tattoos," young and old, saying *fuck cancer*, defiant, iridescent, making art of disease, vitality from mortal danger. I saw flat chests, scarred chests with and without implants smothered in filigree, roses, butterflies, cherry blossoms, hummingbirds, words, sentences, dissertations. So many options, so much beauty. I could not decide on an image. And what if the implant ruptured and another surgery was required? The prosthesis was not permanent.

Magazine articles highlight and extol the cosmetic advantages of decorative mastectomy tattoos. Regardless of whether they've had reconstruction, tattooed women prioritize covering up their scars and "taking back control" (Rauf, 2022). I relate to the aim of regaining agency and cloaking oneself in glamor, but the focus on scars seems odd, *as if scars are the biggest problem for people with missing body parts!* Another point of emphasis in media accounts: tattoos as symbols of "the end of one's cancer journey." Many of the Vinnie Myers videos show celebrating, tearful women, testifying to areola tattooing being the crowning moment, "the final piece" enabling them "to move on" (Today, 2015, 3:12). I was certain that I would not feel that sort of relief or optimism. I would not bring champagne in tumblers, my family and friends would not cheer, I would not cry, I would not stick a pushpin in Vinnie's giant map on the way out. Yet increasingly I experienced my mirror image as a violence. I decided to make the prosthesis look more like a breast and only then consider sheathing it in flowers and unicorns.

~

Exactly 3 months after my final lipofilling surgery, I contacted the "Vinnie Myers Team" about a consultation. I was asked to send three pictures, "right breast, left breast, and both sides," to determine the handling of my case. I heard back promptly via email from Vinnie Myers's daughter, Anna, who explained that Vinnie would proceed only if I agreed to have the natural side tattooed as well. During a follow-up phone call, I asked why I couldn't just have a unilateral procedure. Again, a forced choice. Complementarity was enforced: Satisfaction was guaranteed, and I would not be satisfied with unilateral results. It would be impossible to reproduce the pale tone of the left breast with the pigments they had available. The area around the left nipple would have to be darkened to match the tattooed areola on the right. The original had to be made to look like the copy.

Contrary to the instructions provided on the tattoo parlor's website, I was told to obtain a topical anesthetic from my doctor to bring to the appointment. I assumed it was for the left side since the right was already numb. My trepidation mainly concerned the pain of tattooing the natural breast. On the reconstructed side I expected to feel nothing as the needle perforated the skin, maybe a painless pressure. A month and a half later, on the drive down to Finksburg, I was nervous, eager for the ordeal to be over. I didn't realize I was en route to finding my *sinthome*.

~

Stepping into Vinnie's tattoo shop was like entering a museum. Galleries and catalogues of framed artistic tattoo reproductions covered the walls, but they seemed ghostly, pieces of a preserved and slowly decaying past. The life of the place clearly resided in the steady stream of cancer survivors expecting nipple and areola tattoos. Not that I was greeted with balloons and streamers. The environment was not festive or ceremonial, as the publicity videos promised. I had to bring my own party.

After a brief wait in one of the private rooms, Vinnie arrived, dapper and dark-witted. I handed him the anesthetic ointment, and he put it away without hesitation, substituting it with another tube. "We will use this one—it's stronger," he said under his breath. I was tempted to object but quickly surmised that the transaction was of questionable legality and to my advantage. In about 45 minutes I was getting a tattoo. He worked on the natural breast first; it wasn't pleasant, but I wouldn't call it painful. The anesthetic did its job. Vinnie talked the whole time, regaling me with stories of his wild adventures in Moscow. I happily gobbled up the friendly chatter. Suddenly it was time to tattoo the mastectomy side, to which anesthetic had not been applied. Vinnie grew serious, more focused. The needle touched skin, and then it happened. Pain. It hurt, a lot, and exquisitely. I felt it: *because it was mine, a part of my body*. I imagined the needle puncturing the epidermis and reaching the implant simultaneously, prosthetic and flesh, flesh and prosthetic, both extensions of *me*, mine to experience, a dead mass transforming into *I*, ego ideal into ideal ego.

I didn't want it to end, and then it was over. I sat up and inspected Vinnie's work in a full-length mirror. For the first time since the mastectomy, the mound on my chest resembled a breast; not the loved, amputated breast but nonetheless a breast. The pain I had experienced during the tattooing was in the service of an image that would hold me together. I was once again able to recognize and identify with my specular form. The tattoo is *realistic*; it is not *real*. It is a two-dimensional outcome of the suturing of a wound that brought its own violence: the inscription of the Real of my body with a sign. Now I could look in the mirror and say, *that is a breast— that is me*.

~

Prosthetic encounters, the interstitial experiences entailed in corporeal loss, necessitate the creative work of mourning, the identification with and release of the (missing) object, the *sinthome*. Mastectomy unveils the hole in reality: It shatters the body ego and floods the specular with the uncanny. Restoring the *I* after cancer, after amputation, is not merely a matter of patching the hole or bringing it to speech or generating testimony in the form of a book. To write the *sinthome* is to write via the imaginary, to represent the hole, to expose it by covering it up. The trompe l'oeil tattoo writes that hole. *I feel whole again* because I can function after cancer and mastectomy. This functioning, this regaining of knowledge about how to inhabit my body does not require denial of my lack. The hole remains. I know that one's chest area is whatever one wants it to be. Yet the writing of the image on flesh initiated a retroactive fastening to the symbolic: It had to look like a "breast" before it could look like "me."

References

Bracken, K., & Jensen, T. (2014, June 2). The Nipple Artist [Video]. *New York Times.* Retrieved August 28, 2024, from https://www.nytimes.com/video/health/100000002915699/the-nipple-artist.html

Daneliia, G. (Director). (1979). *Osennii marafon* [Autumn marathon] [Film]. Mosfil'm.

Fink, B. (1997). *A clinical introduction to Lacanian psychoanalysis: Theory and technique.* Harvard University Press.

Freud, S. (1955b). Instincts and their vicissitudes. In J. Strachey et al. (Eds. & Trans.), *The standard edition of the complete psychological works of Sigmund Freud* (Vol. 14, pp. 109–140). Hogarth Press. (Original work published 1915)

Freud, S. (1961d). Negation. In J. Strachey et al. (Eds. & Trans.), *The standard edition of the complete psychological works of Sigmund Freud* (Vol. 19, pp. 233–240). Hogarth Press. (Original work published 1925)

Kaganovsky, L. (2009). The cultural logic of late socialism. *Studies in Russian and Soviet Cinema, 3*(2), 185–199.

Khitruk, F. (Director). (1969). *Vinni-Pukh* [Animated short]. Soiuzmul'tfil'm.

Khitruk, F. (Director). (1971). *Vinni-Pukh idet v gosti* [Winnie-the-Pooh goes visiting] [Animated short]. Soiuzmul'tfil'm. Retrieved August 21, 2024, from https://www.dailymotion.com/video/x8i2gx7

Khitruk, F. (Director). (1972). *Vinni-Pukh i den' zabot* [Winnie-the-Pooh and a busy day] [Animated short]. Soiuzmul'tfil'm. YouTube. Retrieved August 21, 2024, from https://www.youtube.com/watch?v=EiQ1buBRYr0

Kidd, K. B. (2011). *Freud in Oz: At the intersections of psychoanalysis and children's literature.* University of Minnesota Press.

Kreuz, G. (2013, November 15). *Nipple tattooing artist Vinnie Myers helps breast cancer survivors* [Video and written text]. ABC 7 News (updated 2015, July 10). Retrieved August 28, 2024, from https://wjla.com/news/health/nipple-tattooing-artist-vinnie-myers-helps-breast-cancer-survivors-96904

Lacan, J. (2006c). The signification of the phallus. In *Écrits: The first complete edition in English* (B. Fink, Trans.; pp. 575–584). W. W. Norton & Company. (Original paper presented 1958)

Lacan, J. (2016). *The seminar of Jacques Lacan: Book XXIII. The sinthome* (J.-A. Miller, Ed.; A. R. Price, Trans.). Polity. (Original lectures presented 1975–1976)

Lawton, A. (2004). *Before the fall: Soviet cinema in the Gorbachev years.* New Academic Publishing, LLC.

Leving, I. (2008). "Kto-to tam vse-taki est'…": Vinni-pukh i novaia animatsionnaia este-tika ["There's someone really in there": Winnie-the-Pooh and the new wave of anima-tion aesthetics]. In I. Kukulin, M. Lipovetskii, & M. Maiofis (Eds.), *Veselye chelovechki: Kul'turnye geroi sovetskogo detstva* [Merry little fellows: Cultural heroes of Soviet child-hood] (pp. 315–353). Novoe literaturnoe obozrenie.

MacCannell, J. F. (2016). Lacan's imaginary: A practical guide. In S. Tomšič & A. Zevnik (Eds.), *Jacques Lacan: Between psychoanalysis and politics* (pp. 72–85). Routledge.

McGowan, T. (2018). The signification of the phallus. In S. Vanheule, D. Hook, & C. Neill (Eds.), *Reading Lacan's Écrits: From "Signification of the phallus" to "Metaphor of the subject"* (pp. 1–20). Routledge.

Milne, A. A. (1960). *Vinni-Pukh i vse ostal'nye* [Winnie-the-Pooh and everyone else] (B. Zakhoder, Trans.). Detskii mir.

Milne, A. A. (2023). *The original Winnie-the-Pooh book: The complete classic edition with original illustrations*. Independently published. (Originally published 1926)

Pesmen, D. (2000). *Russia and soul: An exploration*. Cornell University Press.

Phelan, P. (1996). *Unmarked: The politics of performance*. Routledge. (Originally published 1993)

Rauf, S. (2022, October 9). *Healing with ink: Breast cancer survivors take back control*. CBC News. Retrieved August 28, 2024, from https://www.cbc.ca/news/canada/montreal/breast-cancer-survivor-tattoo-mastectomy-1.6610708

Riviere, J. (1929). Womanliness as a masquerade. *International Journal of Psychoanalysis, 10*, 303–313.

Rollberg, P. (2009). *Historical dictionary of Russian and Soviet cinema*. Scarecrow Press Inc.

Smoliarova, N. (2008). Detskii "nedetski" Vinni-pukh [Winnie-the-Pooh: For children-not for children]. In I. Kukulin, M. Lipovetskii, & M. Maiofis (Eds.), *Veselye chelovechki: Kul'turnye geroi sovetskogo detstva* [Merry little fellows: Cultural heroes of Soviet child-hood] (pp. 287–314). Novoe literaturnoe obozrenie.

Today. (2015, October 16). *The healing tattoos of Vinnie Myers* [Video]. YouTube. Retrieved August 28, 2024, from https://www.youtube.com/watch?v=JoZsmckHoko

Today Show. (2015, October 16). *Meet tattoo artist Vinnie Myers' team: The mission and motivation* [Video]. Retrieved August 28, 2024, from https://www.today.com/video/meet-tattoo-artist-vinnie-myers-team-the-mission-and-motivation-545633859631

Zupančič, A. (2017). *What is sex?* MIT Press.

Epilogue, Rem(a)inder

While writing this book, after COVID-19, another implausible event: a 21st-century ground war in Europe, in my birthplace. On February 24, 2022, the Russian Armed Forces returned to Chernobyl and occupied it for 5 weeks. With their sights set on unreachable Kyiv, just 75 miles away, soldiers found 99 obdurate babushkas and incalculable amounts of radioactive waste. Russians were at it again: bringing tanks, digging trenches, building bunkers, setting fires, driving up radiation levels to Geiger-busting heights. The Russian army captured the Exclusion Zone in hopes of eventually taking the capital, but did its activities and attitudes exceed strategy, aim, and reason? Was Vladimir Putin's return to Chernobyl repetition compulsion, an unconscious attempt to reclaim the disaster, to restore and realize Soviet colonial and technological dreams?

In early March 2022, Russian forces seized the nuclear plant in Zaporizhzhya and continue to threaten the globe with shelling and mines. Many sites of Russian attack, indeed the entire war, hark back to the failures and heady visions of the unmourned Soviet past. A former KGB apparatchik assassinating opponents, waging genocidal conflict, attempting to reconstitute imperial geography and familiar psychic coordinates, territories charted long ago, retracing Soviet steps in efforts to reclaim what was never his.

~

Voice types—like bodies, sounds, and technologies—are bearers of historicity. Certain voices are popular in certain eras. Evgenii Leonov's broken-down, muffled baritone, an enunciation of failed masculinity, was the typical male voice of the Brezhnev-era screen. Masculinity, almost by definition, denies castration, its own limitations. When its imposture is exposed, so too is the *not-all*, the fact that the human is, at core, unfinished and that psychosomatic discomfort cannot be dissolved. Imposture itself, moreover, may be generated and used, *put on*. It may, in other words, transform into masquerade. The prosthetic is feminine.

In this vein, film scholar Oksana Bulgakowa (2014) asks why the desultory, soft, and breathy voices of Marlon Brando and Soviet actor Innokenty Smoktunovsky achieved canonical status in the 1950s, when ringing timbres were mandatory on stage and film just a decade before. Her answers visit territories beyond cinema history, connecting prevailing sonic expectations to technological

DOI: 10.4324/9781003498582-15

inventions, gendered embodiment, and sensory experience. Bulgakowa asserts that critical acclaim of Smoktunovsky's slurring inarticulateness was made possible by improvements in sound-on-film technology. Better microphones and the advent of magnetic tape recording permitted a wider range of frequencies. She also links the popular acceptance of Smoktunovsky's vocal style to changes in images and notions of Soviet masculinity, increasingly ambivalent, sensual, gentle, and open to intimacy (Bulgakowa, 2014, pp. 145–161).

In Soviet opera, two lyric tenors dominated the postwar period, reaching household-name status: Ivan Kozlovsky and Sergei Lemeshev. Both were stars of the Bol'shoi Theater, and both sang the role of the doomed poet Lensky in the most widely known Russian opera, Petr Tchaikovsky's *Eugene Onegin* (1878). Leme-shev's voice was immortalized in Aleksandr Ivanovskii and Gerbert Rappoport's *Muzykal'naia istoriia* (*A Musical Story*; 1940), a film that musicologist Anna Nis-nevich argues marks a radical shift in Soviet aesthetic and affective terrains. Whereas 1930s musical comedies like Grigorii Aleksandrov's *Volga-Volga* (1938) told the par-able of acoustic and social integration through use of simple numbers, *Muzykal'naia istoriia* contributed to the socialist discourse of *kul'turnost'* (cultivation), stressing inimitable talent, artistic expertise, and emotionally invested listening. According to Nisnevich (2014), *Muzykal'naia istoriia* and comparable films revived the late imperial Russian operatic canon to elevate audiences and show them novel forms of engagement, not merely with music but also with subjectivity (pp. 193–211). The Ukrainian-born Kozlovsky was championed by Joseph Stalin and eventually cel-ebrated for bringing the operatic repertoire to the masses. Kozlovsky frequently jux-taposed opera and popular art forms. He was particularly fond of alternating Russian arias and Ukrainian folk melodies in concert and on recordings.

It is no coincidence that the voices of Kozlovsky and Lemeshev were the cho-sen objects of exalted sensibility and transformative listening in this historical period, for the tenors had more in common than roles and *fach*. Both liberally employed a legato that was strikingly old-fashioned and feminine, more reminis-cent of 19th-century bel canto than the heroic phrasing commonly heard in the West in their day. Their plaintiveness and delicate pianissimi played with bounda-ries of gender and sense as they spirited away meaning into quiet upper regis-ters. One might well ask, recalling Bulgakowa: What does the popularity of tenors like Kozlovsky and Lemeshev tell us about postwar notions of masculinity? And might their mannered styles and lachrymose timbres—the very materiality of their voices—be registering brittleness in key facets of "developed socialism," includ-ing fatherhood, domestic life, romantic love, the gender system, the Great Russian cultural logics governing Soviet everyday life?

~

In Tchaikovsky's *Eugene Onegin*, Lensky courts fair and frivolous Olga Larina while visiting her provincial family estate with his world-weary Petersburg friend Onegin. In scene 1 of act 2, jaundiced Onegin takes revenge on Lensky for bringing him to a dull backwater by flirting with Olga at her sister Tatyana's name-day cel-ebration. Lensky is wildly jealous, humiliated, and impulsively challenges Onegin to a duel before the mortified eyes of the local beau monde. The social-whirly, melodramatic Larin Ball scene is followed by some of the most lyrical moments in the opera: Lensky's aria, "Where have you gone," a quiet interlude between erstwhile friends, and a deadly duel. The second scene of act 2 begins with the fore-shadowing of implacable tragedy. A cello-dominated prelude disclosing the full range of Lensky's thoughts yields to somber trombones and a pounding march. At this point, the curtain usually parts to reveal a winter landscape. The atmosphere is thick with foreboding.

In Alexander Pushkin's "novel in verse" (1825–1832), the serial from which the opera was adapted, Lensky's aria is an elegy the poet composes the night before the duel. Pushkin's textual version is mainly about Olga and clichéd Romanticism, but gay Tchaikovsky's libretto bears more ambiguity. After several rounds of "Ah, Olga, I did love you!" set to themes recalling Lensky's first-act arioso, a harmonic modulation and shift in rhythm signal a different addressee and a new idea:

> My beloved friend, my desired friend, come, come!
> My desired one, come, I am your betrothed …
> I wait for you, my desired one …
> Come, come, I am your betrothed!
> Where have you gone … golden days of my youth?
> (Tchaikovsky & Shilovsky, 1878/1999)

Who is the unnamed "desired one," the subject of Lensky's anguish? Is it his muse, Olga, or is it Onegin, his great, impossible love?

Legendary Soviet theater director Constantin Stanislavski instructed tenors sing-ing Lensky in the 1920s:

> Above all be manly. There is nothing more repulsive on the stage than a droopy, saccharine, effeminate tenor. Can there really be any room for sentimental self-pity in the spirit of the hot-headed, impulsive, proud young poet Lenski? … I want to plant in you an aversion to this kind of sentimentality, to the toying with the public affected by so many tenors nowadays.
> (Stanislavski & Rumyantsev, 1975/1998, p. 128)

Decades later, Kozlovsky and Lemeshev ignore Stanislavski's admonishment. The rival Bol'shoi tenors approach the role from an outwardly feminine position, in a manner and voice that contradict manliness and give the lie to sexual complemen-tarity. Kozlovsky's sentimental sugariness and Lemeshev's plaintive, "soggy" lilt (Stanislavski & Rumyantsev, 1975/1998, p. 128) reveal at once that Lensky will not find in Olga a passionate equal, that her preoccupation with shallow convention can-not meet his vulnerability. Their unsteadiness of tone also betrays the futility of Len-sky's love for Onegin and, more fundamentally, the failure of fantasy and its object. There exist, these plangent voices seem to suggest, those who live and die by the cut of excruciating lyricism, the experience and knowledge of the sexual nonrelation.

Lensky concludes his aria, Onegin arrives late, and they agree to begin, "why not?" A long pause, and then a barely audible pizzicato accompanying tenor and baritone. The entire duet is sung rhythmically, canonically, in hushed pianissimo. The adversaries stand apart, move closer, and gradually pace toward opposite sides of the stage. They sing together, but Onegin is consistently behind, echoing Lensky:

> Enemies! / The thirst for blood / drives us apart. / Not long ago we shared every- thing, / our meals, our thoughts, our leisure. / Now viciously, / like ancient foes, / we silently, cold-bloodedly / prepare to kill each other.

And then, in exalted crescendo, Onegin catches up, and they sing in unison, "Why can't we pause and laugh it off / before our hands are stained with blood ... / Can we not part as friends?" The answer, whispered four times: "No! No! No! No!" (Tchaikovsky & Shilovsky, 1878/1999).

Onegin fires first and Lensky is shot dead.

~

"Opera makes appalling demands on everyone: singers, musicians, directors, fund raisers, and designers (who more often than not fail)," opines playwright Tony Kush- ner in his introduction to the second edition of *The Queen's Throat*. "Opera is appall- ingly expensive, expansive, dilatory even, cost- and time-ineffective, and our ... social darwinist, profit-maximizing, budget-balancing world ought not to have made any place for it. Why has it done so? Opera subscriptions and audiences are growing!" (Kushner, 2001, pp. 4–5).

Psychoanalysis, too, is supremely inconvenient, time-consuming, extravagant. Astoundingly, it often succeeds by failing. "Who has the courage for psychoanaly- sis anymore?" rhetorically asks analyst Jamieson Webster.

> Who has the time and the energy in a world where 'being busy' is one's raison d'être? Forty-five minutes, three or four or even five times a week—with the terror that this arrangement will last a decade, maybe longer, two.
>
> (Webster, 2019, p. 1)

Yet many people continue to come for analysis. Our practices are growing.

Opera in this book is a means of conveying the impossibility of fully justify- ing or accounting for art, including the art of self-inscription, sublimation as *sinthome*. Psychoanalysis, like opera, is more art than science. But that doesn't mean opera and psychoanalysis are devoid of method, empty of ethics. On the contrary, both call for an ethics of the body and of desire, a deliberate confronta- tion with social norms and physical discomforts. Opera insists on the unmedi- ated voice, bare, without amplification. Psychoanalysis adjures the analysand to say whatever comes to mind, without censorship. In their unique ways, opera and psychoanalysis are committed to the marriage of music and words, and to the uncanny emergence of the object-voice: vertiginous heights where words become unintelligible, where meaning dissolves into its silent residue. And just as parapraxes betray unconscious thoughts and the subject's history, operatic voices carry personal and national pasts.

~

I cannot shake completely the extimate, object *a*, self-alienation, but I can accept it and hold myself together in the face of it. I can maintain the fantasy of wholeness while acknowledging a void—revealing it and then hiding it—with a sleight of hand. Each of us must find a way of dealing with a body marked by the signifier. The body is strange, it malfunctions, it doesn't always fit, but we make do, we acknowledge and, also, bind the strangeness so that we can be in our bodies, have sex, make art. The *sinthome* is this binding process. At the end of analysis, I identify with the sinthomatic act, I accept its work and its hole, the part of the work that cannot be completed and that sparks and references all my mad acts, fears, and aspirations. In identifying with the *sinthome*, I don't become it, I don't transform into object *a* and fall away: I sublimate; I maintain self-distance; I remain a subject.

References

Bulgakowa, O. (2014). Vocal changes: Marlon Brando, Innokenty Smoktunovsky, and the sound of the 1950s. In L. Kaganovsky & M. Salazkina (Eds.), *Sound, speech, music in Soviet and post-Soviet cinema* (pp. 145–161). Indiana University Press.

Kushner, T. (2001). Introduction. In W. Koestenbaum, *The queen's throat: Opera, homosexuality, and the mystery of desire* (pp. 1–8). Da Capo Press.

Nisnevich, A. (2014). Listening to *Muzykal'naia istoriia* (1940). In L. Kaganovsky & M. Salazkina (Eds.), *Sound, speech, music in Soviet and post-Soviet cinema* (pp. 193–211). Indiana University Press.

Stanislavski, C., & Rumyantsev, P. I. (1998). *Stanislavski on opera* (E. R. Hapgood, Ed. & Trans.). Routledge. (Originally published 1975)

Tchaikovsky, P., & Shilovsky, K. (1999). *Eugene Onegin* [Album recorded 1955 with the Bol'shoi Theater Orchestra and Chorus, Boris Khaikin, conductor]. Opera D'Oro. (Original work published 1878)

Webster, J. (2019). *Conversion disorder: Listening to the body in psychoanalysis*. Columbia University Press.

References

Abraham, N., & Torok, M. (1994). Mourning or melancholia: Introjection versus incorporation (N. T. Rand, Trans.). In N. Abraham, M. Torok, & N. T. Rand, *The shell and the kernel: Renewals of psychoanalysis* (Vol. 1, pp. 125–138). University of Chicago Press. (Original work published 1972)

Adorno, T. W. (1990). The curves of the needle (T. Y. Levin, Trans.). *October, 55,* 49–55. (Original work published 1928)

Aisenstein, M., & Gibeault, A. (1991). The work of hypochondria: A contribution to the study of the specificity of hypochondria, in particular in relation to hysterical conversion and organic disease. *International Journal of Psycho-Analysis, 72*(4), 669–681.

Alexievich, S. (2005). *Voices from Chernobyl: The oral history of a nuclear disaster* (K. Gessen, Trans.). Dalkey Archive Press. (Original work published 1997)

Audre Lorde in Berlin. (2018, March 21). *Audre Lorde—The complete last reading in Berlin* [Video]. YouTube. Retrieved August 12, 2024, from https://www.youtube.com/watch?v=Uo7TcxauHqw

Auslander, L. (1996). The gendering of consumer practices in nineteenth-century France. In V. De Grazia & E. Furlough (Eds.), *The sex of things: Gender and consumption in historical perspective* (pp. 79–112). University of California Press.

Azazello (Anatolyi Kalabin) Collection, 2015.075 (1972–1993). Wende Museum.

Badiou, A. (2009). Thinking the event [in dialogue with S. Žižek]. In P. A. Engelmann (Ed.), *Philosophy in the present* (English ed., pp. 1–48). Polity. (Original work published 2005 in German)

Baranskaya, N. (1990). A week like any other (P. Monks, Trans.). In *A week like any other: Novellas and stories* (pp. 1–62). Seal Press. (Original work published 1969)

Barber, S. M., & Clark, D. L. (2002). Introduction. Queer moments: The performative temporalities of Eve Kosofsky Sedgwick. In S. M. Barber & D. L. Clark (Eds.), *Regarding Sedgwick: Essays on queer culture and critical theory* (pp. 1–53). Routledge.

Barthes, R. (2001). *A lover's discourse: Fragments* (R. Howard, Trans.). Hill and Wang. (Original work published 1977)

Bendarjevskiy, A., & Maczelka, M. (Directors). (2011). *Chernobyl's heritage: The zone* [Film]. Urania Cinema. YouTube. Retrieved June 14, 2019, from https://www.youtube.com/watch?v=l-nvfu9QA8k

Benjamin, W. (1968). The work of art in the age of mechanical reproduction (H. Zohn, Trans.). In H. Arendt (Ed.), *Illuminations* (pp. 217–251). Harcourt Brace Jovanovich. (Original work published 1935)

Benvenuto, S. (2020). *Conversations with Lacan: Seven lectures for understanding Lacan*. Routledge.

Beumers, B. (2008). Comforting creatures in children's cartoons. In M. Balina & L. Rudova (Eds.), *Russian children's literature and culture* (pp. 153–171). Routledge.

Bezmozgis, D. (2011). *The free world* (1st ed.). Farrar, Straus and Giroux.

Birksted-Breen, D. (2016). *The work of psychoanalysis: Sexuality, time and the psychoanalytic mind*. Routledge.

Blackwell, A. (2012). *Visit sunny Chernobyl, and other adventures in the world's most polluted places*. Rodale, Inc.

Bogart, A., & Morris, H. (Directors). (2015). *The Babushkas of Chernobyl* [Film]. Chicken & Egg Pictures; Fork Films; PowderKeg Studios. YouTube. Retrieved August 18, 2024, from https://www.youtube.com/watch?v=q-WWiOUQeSY

Boym, S. (1994). *Common places: Mythologies of everyday life in Russia*. Harvard University Press.

Boym, S. (2001). *The future of nostalgia*. Basic Books.

Bracken, K., & Jensen, T. (2014, June 2). The Nipple Artist [Video]. *New York Times*. Retrieved August 28, 2024, from https://www.nytimes.com/video/health/100000002915699/the-nipple-artist.html

Brassier, R. (2007). *Nihil unbound: Enlightenment and extinction*. Palgrave Macmillan.

Brenner, L. (2017, September 5). Hypochondria. Retrieved August 28, 2024, from https://leonbrenner.com/2017/09/05/hypochondria/

Bulgakowa, O. (2014). Vocal changes: Marlon Brando, Innokenty Smoktunovsky, and the sound of the 1950s. In L. Kaganovsky & M. Salazkina (Eds.), *Sound, speech, music in Soviet and post-Soviet cinema* (pp. 145–161). Indiana University Press.

Carroll, L. (1978). *Prikliucheniia Alisy v strane chudes; Skvoz' zerkalo i chto tam uvidela Alisa, ili Alisa v zazerkal'e* [Alice adventures in Wonderland; What Alice saw on the other side of the looking glass, or Through the looking glass] (N. M. Demurova, Trans.). Nauka. (Original translation published 1967)

Carroll, L. (2010). *Alice in Wonderland*. Tribeca Books. (Original work published 1865)

Clément, C. (1988). *Opera, The undoing of women*. University of Minnesota Press.

Cleto, F. (1999). Introduction: Queering the camp. In F. Cleto (Ed.), *Camp: Queer aesthetics and the performing subject. A reader* (pp. 1–42). University of Michigan Press.

Coats, K. (2004). *Looking glasses and Neverlands: Lacan, desire, and subjectivity in children's literature*. University of Iowa Press.

Copjec, J. (2002). *Imagine there's no woman: Ethics and sublimation*. MIT Press.

Copjec, J. (2006). The object-gaze: Shame, hejab, cinema. *Filozofski vestnik, 27*(2), 11–29.

Daneliia, G. (Director). (1979). *Osennii marafon* [Autumn marathon] [Film]. Mosfil'm.

Derrida, J. (1995). Archive fever: A Freudian impression (E. Prenowitz, Trans.). *Diacritics, 25*(2), 9–63.

Derrida, J., & Dufourmantelle, A. (2000). *Of hospitality* (R. Bowlby, Trans.). Stanford University Press. (Original work published 1997)

De Veaux, A. (2004). *Warrior poet: A biography of Audre Lorde* (1st ed.). W. W. Norton & Company.

Dolar, M. (1991). "I shall be with you on your wedding-night": Lacan and the uncanny. *October, 58*, 5–23.

Dolar, M. (2006). *A voice and nothing more*. MIT Press.

Dollimore, J. (1991). *Sexual dissidence: Augustine to Wilde, Freud to Foucault*. Oxford University Press.

Dufourmantelle, A. (2019). *In praise of risk* (S. Miller, Trans.). Fordham University Press. (Original work published 2011)

Dulsster, D., & Vanheule, S. (2019). On Lacan and supervision: A matter of super-audition. *British Journal of Psychotherapy, 35*(1), 54–70.

Edelman, L. (2004). *No future: Queer theory and the death drive*. Duke University Press.

Eisenberg, E. (2005). *The recording angel: Music, records and culture from Aristotle to Zappa* (2nd ed.). Yale University Press. (Original work published 1987)

Entin, Y., & Gladkov, G. (1976). *Goluboi shchenok: Muzykal'naia skazka* [Blue puppy: A musical tale] [Audio recording]. Melodiia.

Esti. (Director). (2005a). *Natalie Dessay, la voix* [Natalie Dessay, the voice] [TV documentary, part 1]. France. YouTube. Retrieved August 19, 2024, from https://www.youtube.com/watch?v=JOCcaveUSzI&list=PL2m6FD0rcM3Evg6A93yktYdwT2ZbAoBAX&index=1

Esti. (Director). (2005b). *Natalie Dessay, la voix* [Natalie Dessay, the voice] [TV documentary, part 2]. France. YouTube. Retrieved August 19, 2024, from https://www.youtube.com/watch?v=V8QdaR90MPg

Esti. (Director). (2005c). *Natalie Dessay, la voix* [Natalie Dessay, the voice] [TV documentary, part 5]. France. YouTube. Retrieved August 19, 2024, from https://www.youtube.com/watch?v=HTFjxTGNn5c

Etkind, A. (2013). *Warped mourning: Stories of the undead in the land of the unburied*. Stanford University Press.

Feigelson, C. (1993). Personality death, object loss, and the uncanny. *International Journal of Psychoanalysis, 74*, 331–345.

Feldstein, R. (1995). The phallic gaze of Wonderland. In R. Feldstein, M. Jaanus, & B. Fink (Eds.), *Reading seminar XI: Lacan's four fundamental concepts of psychoanalysis; The Paris seminars in English* (pp. 149–174). State University of New York Press.

Fiennes, S. (Director). (2006). *The pervert's guide to cinema* [Film]. Mischief Films; Amoeba Film. Vimeo. Retrieved August 19, 2024.

Fink, B. (1995). *The Lacanian subject: Between language and jouissance*. Princeton University Press.

Fink, B. (1997). *A clinical introduction to Lacanian psychoanalysis: Theory and technique*. Harvard University Press.

Freeman, E. (2010). *Time binds: Queer temporalities, queer histories*. Duke University Press.

Freud, S. (1953a). Fragment of an analysis of a case of hysteria. In J. Strachey et al. (Eds. & Trans.), *The standard edition of the complete psychological works of Sigmund Freud* (Vol. 7, pp. 1–122). Hogarth Press. (Original work published 1905)

Freud, S. (1953b). The interpretation of dreams. In J. Strachey et al. (Eds. & Trans.), *The standard edition of the complete psychological works of Sigmund Freud* (Vols. 4–5, pp. 1–625). Hogarth Press. (Original work published 1900)

Freud, S. (1953c). The neuro-psychoses of defence. In J. Strachey et al. (Eds. & Trans.), *The standard edition of the complete psychological works of Sigmund Freud* (Vol. 3, pp. 41–61). Hogarth Press. (Original work published 1894)

Freud, S. (1953d). Project for a scientific psychology. In J. Strachey et al. (Eds. & Trans.), *The standard edition of the complete psychological works of Sigmund Freud* (Vol. 1, pp. 281–391). Hogarth Press. (Original work published 1895)

Freud, S. (1953e). Sexuality in the aetiology of the neuroses. In J. Strachey et al. (Eds. & Trans.), *The standard edition of the complete psychological works of Sigmund Freud* (Vol. 3, pp. 259–285). Hogarth Press. (Original work published 1898)

Freud, S. (1953f). Three essays on the theory of sexuality. In J. Strachey et al. (Eds. & Trans.), *The standard edition of the complete psychological works of Sigmund Freud* (Vol. 7, pp. 123–246). Hogarth Press. (Original work published 1905)

Freud, S. (1953g). Totem and taboo. In J. Strachey et al. (Eds. & Trans.), *The standard edition of the complete psychological works of Sigmund Freud* (Vol. 13, pp. 1–255). Hogarth Press. (Original work published 1912)

Freud, S. (1955a). Beyond the pleasure principle. In J. Strachey et al. (Eds. & Trans.), *The standard edition of the complete psychological works of Sigmund Freud* (Vol. 18, pp. 1–64). Hogarth Press. (Original work published 1920)

Freud, S. (1955b). Instincts and their vicissitudes. In J. Strachey et al. (Eds. & Trans.), *The standard edition of the complete psychological works of Sigmund Freud* (Vol. 14, pp. 109–140). Hogarth Press. (Original work published 1915)

Freud, S. (1955c). A metapsychological supplement to the theory of dreams. In J. Strachey et al. (Eds. & Trans.), *The standard edition of the complete psychological works of Sigmund Freud* (Vol. 14, pp. 217–235). Hogarth Press. (Original work published 1917)

Freud, S. (1955d). On narcissism: An introduction. In J. Strachey et al. (Eds. & Trans.), *The standard edition of the complete psychological works of Sigmund Freud* (Vol. 14, pp. 67–102). Hogarth Press. (Original work published 1914)

Freud, S. (1955e). The psychogenesis of a case of homosexuality in a woman. In J. Strachey et al. (Eds. & Trans.), *The standard edition of the complete psychological works of Sigmund Freud* (Vol. 18, pp. 145–172). Hogarth Press. (Original work published 1920)

Freud, S. (1955f). The "uncanny." In J. Strachey et al. (Eds. & Trans.), *The standard edition of the complete psychological works of Sigmund Freud* (Vol. 17, pp. 217–256). Hogarth Press. (Original work published 1919)

Freud, S. (1961a). Civilization and its discontents. In J. Strachey et al. (Eds. & Trans.), *The standard edition of the complete psychological works of Sigmund Freud* (Vol. 21, pp. 57–146). Hogarth Press. (Original work published 1930)

Freud, S. (1961b). The ego and the id. In J. Strachey et al. (Eds. & Trans.), *The standard edition of the complete psychological works of Sigmund Freud* (Vol. 19, pp. 1–66). Hogarth Press. (Original work published 1923)

Freud, S. (1961c). Inhibitions, symptoms and anxiety. In J. Strachey et al. (Eds. & Trans.), *The standard edition of the complete psychological works of Sigmund Freud* (Vol. 20, pp. 75–176). Hogarth Press. (Original work published 1926)

Freud, S. (1961d). Negation. In J. Strachey et al. (Eds. & Trans.), *The standard edition of the complete psychological works of Sigmund Freud* (Vol. 19, pp. 233–240). Hogarth Press. (Original work published 1925)

Freud, S. (1964). Constructions in analysis. In J. Strachey et al. (Eds. & Trans.), *The standard edition of the complete psychological works of Sigmund Freud* (Vol. 23, pp. 255–270). Hogarth Press. (Original work published 1937)

Fürst, J. (2012, March 31). *"When you come to Moscow, make sure that you have flowers in your hair (and a bottle of portwine in your pocket)": The life and world of the Soviet hippies under Brezhnev* [Conference presentation]. Reconsidering Stagnation International Workshop. Amsterdam, Netherlands.

Fürst, J. (2014). Love, peace and rock 'n' roll on Gorky Street: The "emotional style" of the Soviet hippie community. *Contemporary European History*, *23*(4), 565–587.

Fürst, J. (2016). If you're going to Moscow, be sure to have some flowers in your hair (and bring a bottle of port wine in your pocket). In D. Fainberg & A. Kalinovsky (Eds.), *Reconsidering stagnation in the Brezhnev era: Ideology and exchange* (pp. 123–146). Lexington Books.

Fürst, J. (2018). Liberating madness, punishing insanity. *Journal of Contemporary History*, *53*(4), 832–860.

Fürst, J. (2021). *Flowers through concrete: Explorations in Soviet hippieland*. Oxford University Press.

Fürst, J., & McLellan, J. (Eds.). (2017). *Dropping out of socialism: The creation of alternative spheres in the Soviet bloc*. Lexington Books.

Gaisberg, F. (1946). *Music on the record*. Robert Hale Ltd.

Gamburg, Y. (Director). (1976). *Goluboi shchenok* [Blue puppy] [Animated short]. Soiuzmul'tfil'm. Retrieved August 21, 2024, from https://www.youtube.com/watch?v=q KqtwkpCPTY

Gordeeva, I. (2017). Tolstoyism in the late-socialist cultural underground: Soviet youth in search of religion, individual autonomy and nonviolence in the 1970s–1980s. *Open Theology*, *3*(1), 494–515.

Grimm, J., Grimm, W., & Zipes, J. (2003). *The complete fairy tales of the brothers Grimm: All-new third edition* (J. Zipes, Trans.). Bantam Books. (Original work published 1987)

Grushin, O. (2010). *The line*. G. P. Putnam's Sons.

Guntrip, H. (1994). Confronting the critics on the reality of psychodynamic experience. In J. Hazell (Ed.), *Personal relations therapy: The collected papers of H. J. S. Guntrip* (pp. 371–398). Jason Aronson, Inc. (Original work published 1977)

Halberstam, J. (2005). *In a queer time and place: Transgender bodies, subcultural lives*. New York University Press.

Halberstam, J. (2011). *The queer art of failure*. Duke University Press.

Haughton, H. (2006). Alice's identity. In H. Bloom (Ed.), *Lewis Carroll's Alice's adventures in Wonderland* (pp. 193–203). Chelsea House Publishers.

Hollingsworth, C. (2009). Improvising spaces: Victorian photography, Carrollian narrative, and modern collage. In C. Hollingsworth (Ed.), *Alice beyond Wonderland: Essays for the twenty-first century* (pp. 85–100). University of Iowa Press.

Holquist, M. (1992). What is a Boojum? Nonsense and modernism. In D. J. Gray (Ed.), *Alice in Wonderland* (pp. 388–398). W. W. Norton & Company.

Humphrey, C. (2002). *The unmaking of Soviet life: Everyday economies after socialism*. Cornell University Press.

Idsøe, V. (Director). (2002). *Karlsson på taket* [Karlsson on the roof] [Film]. AB Svensk Filmindustrie.

Israel, K. (2000). Asking Alice: Victorian and other Alices in contemporary culture. In J. Kucich & D. F. Sadoff (Eds.), *Victorian afterlife: Postmodern culture rewrites the nineteenth century* (pp. 252–287). University of Minnesota Press.

Jayasekera, J., Zhao, A., Schechter, C., et al. (2023). Reassessing the benefits and harms of risk-reducing medication considering the persistent risk of breast cancer mortality in estrogen receptor–positive breast cancer. *Journal of Clinical Oncology*, *41*(4), 859–870. https://doi.org/10.1200/JCO.22.01342

Kachanov, R. (Director). (1969). *Krokodil Gena* [Crocodile Gena] [Animated short]. Soiuzmul'tfil'm. Retrieved August 21, 2024, from https://www.dailymotion.com/video/ xkb9ys

Kachanov, R. (Director). (1971). *Cheburashka* [Animated short]. Soiuzmul'tfil'm. Retrieved August 21, 2024, from https://www.dailymotion.com/video/x3ayizu

Kachanov, R. (Director). (1974). *Shapokliak* [Animated short]. Soiuzmul'tfil'm. YouTube. Retrieved August 21, 2024, from https://www.youtube.com/watch?v=ZPoFhdDeJqo

Kachanov, R. (Director). (1983). *Cheburashka idet v shkolu* [Cheburashka goes to school] [Animated short]. Soiuzmul'tfil'm. YouTube. Retrieved October 5, 2024, from https://www.youtube.com/watch?v=Fk3rvl6VfV0

Kaganovsky, L. (2009). The cultural logic of late socialism. *Studies in Russian and Soviet cinema, 3*(2), 185–199.

Katz, M. B. (2016). *Drawing the iron curtain: Jews and the golden age of Soviet animation.* Rutgers University Press.

Khitruk, F. (Director). (1969). *Vinni-Pukh* [Animated short]. Soiuzmul'tfil'm.

Khitruk, F. (Director). (1971). *Vinni-Pukh idet v gosti* [Winnie-the-Pooh goes visiting] [Animated short]. Soiuzmul'tfil'm. Retrieved August 21, 2024, from https://www.dailymotion.com/video/x8i2gx7

Khitruk, F. (Director). (1972). *Vinni-Pukh i den' zabot* [Winnie-the-Pooh and a busy day] [Animated short]. Soiuzmul'tfil'm. YouTube. Retrieved August 21, 2024, from https://www.youtube.com/watch?v=EiQ1buBRYr0

Kidd, K. B. (2011). *Freud in Oz: At the intersections of psychoanalysis and children's literature.* University of Minnesota Press.

Kirshner, L. (2018). The presence of the analyst. English version retrieved August 20, 2024, from https://www.academia.edu/38092225/The_Presence_of_the_Analyst_docx. (Original work published 2018 in German)

Klein, M. (1984). A contribution to the psychogenesis of manic-depressive states. In R. Money-Kyrle (Ed.), *Love, guilt and reparation and other works, 1921–1945* (pp. 262–289). Free Press. (Original work published 1935)

Kliuchkin, K. (2008). Zavetnyi mul'tfil'm: Prichiny populiarnosti "Cheburashki" [A cherished cartoon: Reasons for the popularity of "Cheburashka"]. In I. Kukulin, M. Lipovetskii, & M. Maiofis (Eds.), *Veselye chelovechki: Kul'turnye geroi sovetskogo detstva* [Merry little fellows: Cultural heroes of Soviet childhood] (pp. 360–377). Novoe literaturnoe obozrenie.

Kobrin, K. (2007). Chelovek brezhnevskoi epokhi na Beiker Street: K postanovke problemy "pozdnesovetskogo viktorianstva" [Brezhnev-era man on Baker Street: Toward the question of "post-Soviet Victorianism"]. *Neprikosnovennyi zapas, 53*(3), 147–160.

Koestenbaum, W. (1993). *The queen's throat: Opera, homosexuality, and the mystery of desire* (1st ed.). Vintage Books.

Koestenbaum, W. (with Kushner, T.). (2001). *The queen's throat: Opera, homosexuality, and the mystery of desire.* Da Capo Press. (Original work published 1993)

Kornhaber, D. (2020). *Silent film: A very short introduction.* Oxford University Press.

Kovalevskaia, I. (Director). (1969). *Bremenskie muzykanty* [Bremen town musicians] [Animated short]. Soiuzmul'tfil'm. YouTube. Retrieved August 21, 2024, from https://www.youtube.com/watch?v=d7NpFhucGbg

Kreuz, G. (2013, November 15). *Nipple tattooing artist Vinnie Myers helps breast cancer survivors* [Video and written text]. ABC 7 News (updated 2015, July 10). Retrieved August 28, 2024, from https://wjla.com/news/health/nipple-tattooing-artist-vinnie-myers-helps-breast-cancer-survivors-96904

Kushner, T. (2001). Introduction. In W. Koestenbaum, *The queen's throat: Opera, homosexuality, and the mystery of desire* (pp. 1–8). Da Capo Press.

Lacan, J. (1938). Family complexes in the formation of the individual (C. Gallagher, Trans.). Unpublished manuscript. Retrieved August 28, 2024, from http://www.lacaninireland.com/web/wp-content/uploads/2010/06/FAMILY-COMPLEXES-IN-THE-FORMATION-OF-THE-INDIVIDUAL2.pdf

Lacan, J. (1966–1967). *The seminar of Jacques Lacan: Book XIV* (C. Gallagher, Trans.). Unpublished manuscript. Retrieved October 5, 2024, from http://www.lacaninireland. com/web/wp-content/uploads/2010/06/14-Logic-of-Phantasy-Complete.pdf

Lacan, J. (1967–1968). *The seminar of Jacques Lacan: Book XV* (C. Gallagher, Trans.). Unpublished manuscript. Retrieved October 5, 2024, from http://www.lacaninireland. com/web/wp-content/uploads/2010/06/Book-15-The-Psychoanalytical-Act.pdf

Lacan, J. (1991). *The seminar of Jacques Lacan: Book II. The ego in Freud's theory and in the technique of psychoanalysis, 1954–1955* (J.-A. Miller, Ed.; S. Tomaselli, Trans.). W. W. Norton & Company. (Original lectures presented 1954–1955)

Lacan, J. (1992). *The seminar of Jacques Lacan: Book VII. The ethics of psychoanalysis, 1959–1960* (J.-A. Miller, Ed.; D. Porter, Trans.). W. W. Norton & Company. (Original lectures presented 1959–1960)

Lacan, J. (1998a). *The seminar of Jacques Lacan: Book XI. The four fundamental concepts of psychoanalysis* (J.-A. Miller, Ed.; A. Sheridan, Trans.). W. W. Norton & Company. (Original lectures presented 1964)

Lacan, J. (1998b). *The seminar of Jacques Lacan: Book XX. On feminine sexuality: The limits of love and knowledge, 1972–1973* (J.-A. Miller, Ed.; B. Fink, Trans.). W. W. Norton & Company. (Original lectures presented 1972–1973)

Lacan, J. (2006a). The mirror stage as formative of the *I* function as revealed in psychoanalytic experience (B. Fink, Trans.). In *Écrits: The first complete edition in English* (B. Fink, Trans.; pp. 75–82). W. W. Norton & Company. (Original work published 1949)

Lacan, J. (2006b). Presentation on transference. In *Écrits: The first complete edition in English* (B. Fink, Trans.; pp. 176–185). W. W. Norton & Company. (Original work published 1952)

Lacan, J. (2006c). The signification of the phallus. In *Écrits: The first complete edition in English* (B. Fink, Trans.; pp. 575–584). W. W. Norton & Company. (Original paper presented 1958)

Lacan, J. (2007). *The seminar of Jacques Lacan: Book XVII. The other side of psychoanalysis* (J.-A. Miller, Ed.; R. Grigg, Trans.). W. W. Norton & Company. (Original lectures presented 1969–1970)

Lacan, J. (2014). *The seminar of Jacques Lacan: Book XX. Anxiety* (J.-A. Miller, Ed.; A. R. Price, Trans.). Polity. (Original lectures presented 1962–1963)

Lacan, J. (2015). *The seminar of Jacques Lacan: Book VIII. Transference* (J.-A. Miller, Ed.; B. Fink, Trans.). Polity. (Original lectures presented 1960–1961)

Lacan, J. (2016). *The seminar of Jacques Lacan: Book XXIII. The sinthome* (J.-A. Miller, Ed.; A. R. Price, Trans.). Polity. (Original lectures presented 1975–1976)

Lacan, J. (2017). *The seminar of Jacques Lacan: Book V. Formations of the unconscious* (J.-A. Miller, Ed.; R. Grigg, Trans.). Polity. (Original lectures presented 1957–1958)

Lacan, J. (2020). *The seminar of Jacques Lacan: Book IV. The object relation* (J.-A. Miller, Ed.; A. R. Price, Trans.). Polity. (Original lectures presented 1956–1957)

Laplanche, J. (1998). *Essays on otherness* (J. Fletcher, Ed.; L. Thurston, Trans.). Routledge.

Laurent, E. (1992). Quatre remarques sur le souci scientifique de Jacques Lacan [Four remarks on Jacques Lacan's scientific concerns]. In M.-P. de Cossé Brissac, F. Giroud, R. Dumas, et al. (Eds.), *Connaissez-vous Lacan?* [Do you know Lacan?] (pp. 41–43). Seuil.

Lawton, A. (2004). *Before the fall: Soviet cinema in the Gorbachev years*. New Academic Publishing, LLC.

Lelio, S. (Director). (2017). *A fantastic woman* [Film]. Fabula; Komplizen Film.

Leving, I. (2008). "Kto-to tam vse-taki est'…": Vinni-pukh i novaia animatsionnaia estetika ["There's someone really in there": Winnie-the-Pooh and the new wave of animation aesthetics]. In I. Kukulin, M. Lipovetskii, & M. Maiofis (Eds.), *Veselye chelovechki: Kul'turnye geroi sovetskogo detstva* [Merry little fellows: Cultural heroes of Soviet childhood] (pp. 315–353). Novoe literaturnoe obozrenie.

Lin, L. (2017). *Freud's jaw and other lost objects: Fractured subjectivity in the face of cancer*. Fordham University Press.

Livanov, V. (Director). (1973). *Po sledam bremenskikh muzykantov* [On the trail of the Bremen town musicians] [Animated short]. Soiuzmul'tfil'm. YouTube. Retrieved August 26, 2024, from https://www.youtube.com/watch?v=X3xNJSpOgWk

Lorde, A. (1997). *The cancer journals* (Special ed.). Aunt Lute Books. (Original work published 1980)

Lorde, A. (2007). *Sister outsider: Essays and speeches*. Crossing Press. (Original work published 1984)

Losev, L. (1984). *On the beneficence of censorship: Aesopian language in modern Russian literature*. O. Sagner in Kommission.

MacCannell, J. F. (2016). Lacan's imaginary: A practical guide. In S. Tomšič & A. Zevnik (Eds.), *Jacques Lacan: Between psychoanalysis and politics* (pp. 72–85). Routledge.

MacFadyen, D. (2005). *Yellow crocodiles and blue oranges: Russian animated film since World War II*. McGill–Queen's University Press.

Maiofis, M. (2008). Milyi, milyi trikster: Karlson i sovetskaia utopiia o "nastoiashchem detstve" [Sweet, sweet trickster: Karlson and the Soviet utopia of "real childhood"]. In I. Kukulin, M. Lipovetskii, & M. Maiofis (Eds.), *Veselye chelovechki: Kul'turnye geroi sovetskogo detstva* [Merry little fellows: Cultural heroes of Soviet childhood] (pp. 241–286). Novoe literaturnoe obozrenie.

Matviyenko, S., & Roof, J. (2018). Introduction. In S. Matviyenko & J. Roof (Eds.), *Lacan and the posthuman* (pp. 9–21). Palgrave Macmillan.

McGowan, T. (2018). The signification of the phallus. In S. Vanheule, D. Hook, & C. Neill (Eds.), *Reading Lacan's Écrits: From "Signification of the phallus" to "Metaphor of the subject"* (pp. 1–20). Routledge.

Meltzer, D. (2018). *The Kleinian development part 2: Richard week-by-week*. The Harris Meltzer Trust. (Original work published 1978)

Milne, A. A. (1960). *Vinni-Pukh i vse ostal'nye* [Winnie-the-Pooh and everyone else] (B. Zakhoder, Trans.). Detskii mir.

Milne, A. A. (2023). *The original Winnie-the-Pooh book: The complete classic edition with original illustrations*. Independently published. (Originally published 1926)

Milner, M. (1952). Aspects of symbolism in comprehension of the not-self. *International Journal of Psycho-Analysis, 33*(2), 181–195.

Muñoz, J. E. (2019). *Cruising utopia: The then and there of queer futurity* (10th anniversary ed.). New York University Press. (Original work published 2009)

Mussorgsky, M. (1992). *Khovanshchina* [Album recorded with the Kirov Opera and Orchestra, St. Petersburg, Valery Gergiev, conductor]. Philips. (Original work published 1881)

Nancy, J.-L. (2008). *Corpus* (R. A. Rand, Trans.). Fordham University Press.

Nietzsche, F. W. (1961). *Thus spoke Zarathustra* (R. J. Hollingdale, Trans.). Penguin Publishing Group. (Original work published 1884)

Nietzsche, F. W. (1962). *Philosophy in the age of the Greeks* (M. Cowan, Trans.). Regnery Publishing. (Original work published 1873)

Nikolaieva, M. (1996). The "serendipity" of censorship. *Para*doxa, 2*(3–4), 379–386.

Nisnevich, A. (2014). Listening to *Muzykal'naia istoriia* (1940). In L. Kaganovsky & M. Salazkina (Eds.), *Sound, speech, music in Soviet and post-Soviet cinema* (pp. 193–211). Indiana University Press.

Norshtein, Y. (Director). (1975). *Ezhik v tumane* [Hedgehog in the fog] [Animated short]. Soiuzmul'tfil'm. YouTube. Retrieved August 25, 2024, from https://www.youtube.com/watch?v=ThmaGMgWRlY

Ohayon, M. (Director). (2016). *Cristina* [Film]. Kavana Entertainment.

Parsons, M. (1999). The logic of play in psychoanalysis. *International Journal of Psychoanalysis, 80*(5), 871–884.

Perelberg, R. J. (2021). The empty couch: Love and mourning in times of confinement. *International Journal of Psychoanalysis, 102*(1), 16–30.

Pesmen, D. (2000). *Russia and soul: An exploration.* Cornell University Press.

Phelan, P. (1996). *Unmarked: The politics of performance.* Routledge. (Originally published 1993)

Plokhy, S. (2018). *Chernobyl: The history of a nuclear catastrophe.* Basic Books.

Pontieri, L. (2012). *Soviet animation and the Thaw of the 1960s: Not only for children.* John Libbey Publishing.

Rackin, D. (Ed.). (1991). *Alice's adventures in Wonderland and through the looking glass: Nonsense, sense, and meaning* (1st ed.). Twayne Publishers.

Raleigh, D. J. (2012). *Soviet baby boomers: An oral history of Russia's Cold War generation* (1st ed.). Oxford University Press.

Rauf, S. (2022, October 9). *Healing with ink: Breast cancer survivors take back control.* CBC News. Retrieved August 28, 2024, from https://www.cbc.ca/news/canada/montreal/breast-cancer-survivor-tattoo-mastectomy-1.6610708

Riviere, J. (1929). Womanliness as a masquerade. *International Journal of Psychoanalysis, 10*, 303–313.

Robinson, P. A. (2002). *Opera, sex, and other vital matters.* University of Chicago Press.

Rollberg, P. (2009). *Historical dictionary of Russian and Soviet cinema.* Scarecrow Press Inc.

Rousselle, D. (2020). *The truth about coronavirus.* Ebrary. Retrieved August 28, 2024, from https://ebrary.net/141868/psychology/truth_coronavirus

Russell, J. (2017). *Nietzsche and the clinic: Psychoanalysis, philosophy, metaphysics.* Karnac.

Russell, J. (2019). *Psychoanalysis and deconstruction: Freud's psychic apparatus.* Routledge.

Santanelli di Pompeo, F., Paolini, G., Firmani, G., & Sorotos, M. (2022). History of breast implants: Back to the future. *JPRAS Open: An International Open Access Journal of Surgical Reconstruction, 32*, 166–177. https://doi.org/10.1016/j.jpra.2022.02.004

Sbriglia, R., & Žižek, S. (2020). *Subject lessons: Hegel, Lacan, and the future of materialism.* Northwestern University Press.

Sedgwick, E. K. (1993a). How to bring your kids up gay: The war against effeminate boys. In E. K. Sedgwick (Ed.), *Tendencies* (pp. 154–164). Duke University Press. (Original work published 1991)

Sedgwick, E. K. (1993b). Privilege of unknowing: Diderot's *The nun.* In E. K. Sedgwick (Ed.), *Tendencies* (pp. 23–51). Duke University Press. (Original work published 1988)

Sedgwick, E. K. (1993c). Tales of the avunculate: Queer tutelage in *The importance of being earnest.* In E. K. Sedgwick (Ed.), *Tendencies* (pp. 52–72). Duke University Press.

Sedgwick, E. K. (2003). Shame, theatricality, and queer performance: Henry James's *The art of the novel.* In E. K. Sedgwick (Ed.), *Touching feeling: Affect, pedagogy, performativity* (pp. 35–66). Duke University Press.

Siefert, M. (1995). Aesthetics, technology, and the capitalization of culture: How the talking machine became a musical instrument. *Science in Context, 8*(2), 417–449.

Siegelbaum, L. H. (2008). *Cars for comrades: The life of the Soviet automobile.* Cornell University Press.

Smith, M., & Morra, J. (2007). Introduction. In M. Smith & J. Morra (Eds.), *The prosthetic impulse: From a posthuman present to a biocultural future* (pp. 1–14). MIT Press.

Smoliarova, N. (2008). Detskii "nedetski" Vinni-pukh [Winnie-the-Pooh: For children-not for children]. In I. Kukulin, M. Lipovetskii, & M. Maiofis (Eds.), *Veselye chelovechki: Kul'turnye geroi sovetskogo detstva* [Merry little fellows: Cultural heroes of Soviet childhood] (pp. 287–314). Novoe literaturnoe obozrenie.

Smolkin-Rothrock, V. (2011). Cosmic enlightenment: Scientific atheism and the conquest of space. In J. T. Andrews & A. A. Siddiqi (Eds.), *Into the cosmos: Space exploration and Soviet culture* (pp.159–194). University of Pittsburgh Press.

Sontag, S. (1999). Notes on camp. In F. Cleto (Ed.), *Camp: Queer aesthetics and the performing subject; A reader* (pp. 51–65). University of Michigan Press. (Original work published 1964)

Sorokin, V. (2008). *The queue* (S. Laird, Trans.). New York Review Books Classics. (Original work published 1983)

Stanislavski, C., & Rumyantsev, P. I. (1998). *Stanislavski on opera* (E. R. Hapgood, Ed. & Trans.). Routledge. (Originally published 1975)

Stathopoulos, G. (2017). Hypochondria: A review of its place in psychoanalytic theory. *Psychoanalytic Quarterly*, *86*(2), 359–381.

Stepantsev, B. (Director). (1968). *Malysh i Karlson* [The Kid and Karlson] [Animated short]. Soiuzmul'tfil'm. Retrieved August 21, 2024, from https://www.dailymotion.com/video/x41pyqe

Stepantsev, B. (Director). (1970). *Karlson vernulsia* [Karlson returns] [Animated short]. Soiuzmul'tfil'm. Retrieved August 21, 2024, from https://www.dailymotion.com/video/x41pyqe

Sterne, J. (2003). *The audible past: Cultural origins of sound reproduction*. Duke University Press.

Stiegler, B. (1998a). *Technics and time: Vol. 1. The fault of Epimetheus* (R. Beardsworth & G. Collins, Trans.). Stanford University Press. (Original work published 1994)

Stiegler, B. (1998b). *Technics and time: Vol. 2. Disorientation* (S. Barker, Trans.). Stanford University Press. (Original work published 1996)

Stockton, K. B. (2009). *The queer child, or growing sideways in the twentieth century*. Duke University Press.

Susan G. Komen. (n.d.). *Breast cancer risk factors: BRCA1 and BRCA2 inherited gene mutations in women*. Retrieved August 12, 2024, from https://www.komen.org/breast cancer/risk-factor/gene-mutations-genetic-testing/brca-genes/

Symes, C. (2004). *Setting the record straight: A material history of classical recording*. Wesleyan University Press.

Tarkovsky, A. (Director). (1979). *Stalker* [Film]. Mosfil'm.

Taylor, A. (Director). (2005). *Žižek!* [Film]. Zeitgeist Films. YouTube. Retrieved August 13, 2024, from https://www.youtube.com/watch?v=7FItgC3H9xw

Tchaikovsky, P., & Shilovsky, K. (1999). *Eugene Onegin* [Album recorded 1955 with the Bol'shoi Theater Orchestra and Chorus, Boris Khaikin, conductor]. Opera D'Oro. (Original work published 1878)

Tchaikovsky, P., & Tchaikovsky, M. (1993). *Pique dame* [Album recorded with the Kirov Opera and Orchestra, St. Petersburg, Valery Gergiev, conductor]. Philips. (Original work published 1890)

Today. (2015, October 16). *The healing tattoos of Vinnie Myers* [Video]. YouTube. Retrieved August 28, 2024, from https://www.youtube.com/watch?v=JoZsmckHoko

Today Show. (2015, October 16). *Meet tattoo artist Vinnie Myers' team: The mission and motivation* [Video]. Retrieved August 28, 2024, from https://www.today.com/video/meet-tattoo-artist-vinnie-myers-team-the-mission-and-motivation-545633859631

Van Haute, P., & Geyskens, T. (2012). *A non-oedipal psychoanalysis? A clinical anthropology of hysteria in the works of Freud and Lacan.* Leuven University Press.

Vanier, A. (2012). Winnicott and Lacan: A missed encounter? (K. Valendinova, Trans.). *Psychoanalytic Quarterly, 81*(2), 279–303.

Verdery, K. (1996). The "etatization" of time in Ceauşescu's Romania. In K. Verdery (Ed.), *What was socialism, and what comes next?* (pp. 39–58). Princeton University Press. (Original work published 1992)

Verdi, G., & Piave, F. M. (1997). *Rigoletto* [Album recorded with the Orchestra and Chorus of Teatro alla Scala, Tullio Serafin conductor]. EMI. (Originally recorded in 1955, original work published 1851)

Verhaeghe, P. (2015). Today's madness does not make sense. In P. Gherovici & M. Steinkoler (Eds.), *Lacan on madness: Madness yes you can't* (pp. 68–80). Routledge.

Verhaeghe, P., & Declercq, F. (2002). Lacan's analytical goal: *Le sinthome* or the feminine way. In L. Thurston (Ed.), *Re-inventing the symptom: Essays on the final Lacan* (pp. 59–83). The Other Press.

Vysotsky, V. (1977). *Alisa v strane chudes* [Alice in Wonderland] [Audio recording]. Melodiia.

Wang, J., Li, B., Luo, M., Huang, J., Zhang, K., Zheng, S., Zhang, S., & Zhou, J. (2024). Progression from ductal carcinoma in situ to invasive breast cancer: Molecular features and clinical significance. *Signal Transduction Targeted Therapy, 9*, Article 83. https://doi.org/10.1038/s41392-024-01779-3

Webster, J. (2019). *Conversion disorder: Listening to the body in psychoanalysis.* Columbia University Press.

Wills, D. (2007). Technology or the discourse of speed. In M. Smith & J. Morra (Eds.), *The prosthetic impulse: From a posthuman present to a biocultural future* (pp. 237–264). MIT Press.

Wills, D. (2021). *Prosthesis.* Stanford University Press. (Original work published 1995)

Winnicott, D. W. (1974). Fear of breakdown. *International Review of Psycho-Analysis, 1*(1–2), 103–107.

Winnicott, D. W. (2005). *Playing and reality.* Routledge Classics. (Original work published 1971)

Yurchak, A. (2006). *Everything was forever, until it was no more: The last Soviet generation.* Princeton University Press.

Zhuk, S. I. (2010). *Rock and roll in the Rocket City: The West, identity, and ideology in Soviet Dniepropetrovsk, 1960–1985.* Johns Hopkins University Press.

Žižek, S. (1993). *Tarrying with the negative: Kant, Hegel, and the critique of ideology.* Duke University Press.

Zupančič, A. (2017). *What is sex?* MIT Press.

Index

Note: Page numbers followed by "n" refer to end notes.

For Product Safety Concerns and Information please contact our EU
representative GPSR@taylorandfrancis.com
Taylor & Francis Verlag GmbH, Kaufingerstraße 24, 80331 München, Germany

www.ingramcontent.com/pod-product-compliance
Lightning Source LLC
Chambersburg PA
CBHW052003270326
41929CB00015B/2777